Case Studies in Gerontological Nursing for the Advanced Practice Nurse

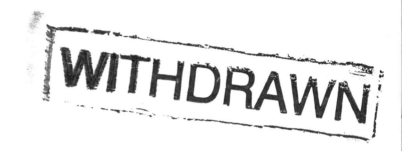

Case Studies in Gerontological Nursing for the Advanced Practice Nurse

Editors

Meredith Wallace Kazer, PhD, APRN, A/GNP-BC, FAAN
Leslie Neal-Boylan, PhD, RN, CRRN, APRN, FNP-BC

Ⓦ**WILEY-BLACKWELL**

A John Wiley & Sons, Inc., Publication

Registered office: John Wiley & Sons Ltd, The Atrium, Southern Gate, Chichester, West Sussex, PO19 8SQ, UK

Editorial offices: 2121 State Avenue, Ames, Iowa 50014-8300, USA
The Atrium, Southern Gate, Chichester, West Sussex, PO19 8SQ, UK
9600 Garsington Road, Oxford, OX4 2DQ, UK

For details of our global editorial offices, for customer services and for information about how to apply for permission to reuse the copyright material in this book, please see our website at www.wiley.com/wiley-blackwell.

Library of Congress Cataloging-in-Publication Data

Case studies in gerontological nursing for the advanced practice nurse / editors, Meredith Wallace Kazer, Leslie Neal-Boylan.
    p.   ;   cm.
  Includes bibliographical references and index.
  ISBN-13: 978-0-8138-2378-2 (pbk.: alk. paper)
  ISBN-10: 0-8138-2378-1 (pbk.: alk. paper)
  1. Geriatric nursing–Case studies.   I. Kazer, Meredith Wallace, PhD, RN.
II. Neal-Boylan, Leslie.
  [DNLM: 1. Nursing Care–Case Reports.   2. Aged. WY 152]
RC954.c42   2012
618.97'0231–dc23

                          2011017809

A catalogue record for this book is available from the British Library.

Set in 10/12pt Palatino by Toppan Best-set Premedia Limited
Printed and bound in Singapore by Fabulous Printers Pte Ltd

1   2012

Contents

Contributors

EDITORS

Meredith Wallace Kazer, PhD, APRN, A/GNP-BC, FAAN
Associate Professor and Graduate Program Director
School of Nursing
Fairfield University
Fairfield, CT

Leslie Neal-Boylan, PhD, RN, CRRN, APRN, FNP-BC
Professor and Graduate Program Coordinator
Nursing Department
Southern Connecticut State University
New Haven, CT

CONTRIBUTORS

Ivy M. Alexander, PhD, APRN, ANP-BC, FAAN
Professor
Director—Adult, Family, Gerontological and Women's Health Primary
    Care Specialty
Yale University School of Nursing
New Haven, CT

Marie Boltz, PhD, APRN, BC
Associate Director for Practice, Hartford Institute for Geriatric Nursing
Assistant Professor, New York University College of Nursing
New York, NY

Kimberlee-Ann Bridges, MSN, RN-BC, CNL
Surgical Unit Clinical Nurse Leader
Danbury Hospital
Danbury, CT

Frieda R. Butler, PhD, MPH, FAAN, FGSA
Gerontological Consultant and Professor Emerita
College of Health and Human Services
Department of Global and Community Health
George Mason University
Fairfax, VA

Dympna Casey, RGN, BA, MA, PhD
Aras Moyola
School of Nursing and Midwifery
National University of Ireland
Galway, Ireland

Donna Packo Diaz, MS, RN
Coordinator
APDA Parkinson Center
Hospital of Saint Raphael
New Haven, CT

Karen Dick, PhD, GNP-BC, FAANP
Graduate Program Director and Clinical Associate Professor
College of Nursing and Health Sciences
University of Massachusetts Boston
Boston, MA

Ashley Domingue, MSN, RN, ANP-BC, GNP-C
Foundation Medical Partners
Nashua, NH

Annemarie Dowling-Castronovo, PhD(c), RN
Assistant Professor and Jonas Scholar
Evelyn L. Spiro School of Nursing
Wagner College
Staten Island, NY

Everol M. Ennis, Jr., MSN, APRN, A/GNP-BC
Nurse Practitioner
Community Health Services, Inc.
Hartford, CT

Bonnie Cashin Farmer, PhD, RN
Associate Professor
School of Nursing
University of Southern Maine
Portland, Maine

Susan C. Frazier, MS, NP-C, GNP-BC
Steward Skilled Care Team
Fall River, MA

Patricia C. Gantert, MSN, RN-BC
Medical Educator/Diabetes Resource Nurse
St. Vincent's Medical Center
Bridgeport, CT

Christine M. Goldstein, LCSW-R, OSW-C
Good Samaritan Home Health Agency
Bay Shore, NY

Susan A. Goncalves, DNP(c), MS, RN-BC
Nurse Manager Med/Surg Unit
St. Vincent's Medical Center
Bridgeport, CT

Philip A. Greiner, DNSc, RN
Associate Dean for Faculty Development in Scholarship and Teaching
    and Professor
College of Health Professions
Pace University
Pleasantville, NY

Kendra M. Grimes, MSN, APRN, GNP-BC
Yale University School of Nursing
New Haven, CT

Shelley Yerger Hawkins, DSN, APRN, FNP, GNP, FAANP
Associate Professor of Nursing
Coordinator, Nurse Practitioner Programs
University of Arkansas Medical Sciences
Little Rock, AR

Rebecca Herter, MSN, RN
A/GNP Candidate
Yale University School of Nursing
New Haven, CT

Melanie J. Holland, BSN, MS
Adjunct Professor
Quinnipiac University
Hamden, CT
Outreach Nurse
St. Vincent's Medical Center
Bridgeport, CT

Cynthia S. Jacelon, PhD, RN, CRRN, FAAN
Associate Professor
School of Nursing
University of Massachusetts
Amherst, MA

Jaclyn R. Jones, MSN, APRN, NP-C
Yale School of Nursing
Yale University
New Haven, CT

Evanne Juratovac, PhD, RN (GCNS-BC)
Assistant Professor, Frances Payne Bolton School of Nursing
Faculty Associate, University Center on Aging and Health
Case Western Reserve University
Cleveland, OH

Jina Ko, MSN, RN, ANP-C
Nurse Practitioner
White Memorial Medical Center
Los Angeles, CA

Barbara L. Kramer, MSN, RN, CHPN
Palliative Care Coordinator
Good Samaritan Home Health Agency and Catholic Home Care
Bay Shore, NY

Alison Kris, PhD, RN
Assistant Professor
Fairfield University
School of Nursing
Fairfield, CT

Devon Kwassman, MSN, RN
A/GNP Candidate
Yale University School of Nursing
New Haven, CT

Kimberly O. Lacey, DNSc, MSN, CNS
Assistant Professor
Department of Nursing
Southern Connecticut State University
New Haven, CT

Amanda LaManna, MSN, RN, NP-C
Adult Nurse Practitioner
Miami University Student Health Services
Oxford, Ohio

Antoinette Larkin, RGN, H. Dip. Gerontology
Clinical Nurse Specialist in Elderly Care
Portiuncula Hospital
Ballinalsoe
Galway, Ireland

Julie M. L. Lautner, MSW, MSN, RN
A/GNP Candidate
Yale University School of Nursing
New Haven, CT

Kathleen Lovanio, MSN, APRN, F/ANP-BC
Assistant Professor, VANA
Fairfield University School of Nursing
Fairfield, CT

Geraldine Marrocco, EdD, APRN, CNS, ANP-BC
Assistant Professor
Yale University School of Nursing
New Haven, CT

Bernard McCarthy, MSc
Lecturer
School of Nursing and Midwifery
National University of Ireland
Galway, Ireland

Elizabeth McGann, DNSc, RN, GCNS-BC
Professor of Nursing
Department of Nursing
Quinnipiac University
Hamden, CT

Anne Moore, DNP, RN
Director of Spine and Surgical Business Planning
Hospital of Saint Raphael
New Haven, CT

Kathy Murphy, RN, BA, DipN, RNT, MSc, PhD
Professor of Nursing
School of Nursing and Midwifery
National University of Ireland
Galway, Ireland

Nicholas R. Nicholson, Jr., PhD, MPH, RN, PHCNS-BC
Postdoctoral Fellow
Geriatric Clinical Epidemiology and Aging Related Research
School of Medicine
Yale University
New Haven, CT

Kenneth S. O'Rourke, MD
Associate Professor
Section on Rheumatology and Immunology
Wake Forest University School of Medicine
Winston-Salem, NC

Maureen E. O'Rourke, RN, PhD
Adjunct Assistant Professor of Internal Medicine-Hematology/
    Oncology
Wake Forest University School of Medicine
Winston-Salem, NC

Kelly Smith Papa, MSN, RN
Director of Education
Alzheimer's Resource Center of Connecticut
Plantsville, CT

Lynn Price, JD, MSN, MPH, FNP-BC
Associate Professor
Department of Nursing
Quinnipiac University
Hamden, CT

Valerie C. Sauda, RN-BC, MS
Geriatric Nurse Service Instructor
Nursing Department
Eastern Maine Community College
Bangor, ME

Mary Shelkey, PhD, ARNP
Assistant Professor
College of Nursing
Seattle University
Seattle, WA

Eileen O'Connor Smith, BSN, RN-C
Director of Nursing
Alzheimer's Resource Center of Connecticut
Plantsville, CT

Cathi A. Thomas, MS, RN, CNRN
Assistant Clinical Professor, Neurology
Parkinson Disease and Movement Disorder Center
Boston University Medical Campus
Boston, MA

Christine Tocchi, PhD(C), MSN, APRN, GNP-BC
Pre-Doctoral Scholar
Yale University School of Nursing
Yale University
New Haven, CT

Claire Welford, RGN, DipNS, BNS–Hons., MSc, PGC–TLHE
School of Nursing and Midwifery
National University of Ireland
Galway, Ireland

Cora D. Zembrzuski, PhD, APRN
Gero-psychiatric Consultant
MedOptions, Inc.
Behavioral Health Consultants
Old Saybrook, CT

Introduction

By Meredith Wallace Kazer and Leslie Neal-Boylan

Older adults are the fastest growing population cohort worldwide. In the U.S., the Administration on Aging (2009) reports that there were over 38.9 million older adults in the country, which reflects a 13.0% increase over the last decade for a total of 12.8% of the total population. One in every eighth person in the U.S. is an older adult. If individuals survive to the age of 65, they will likely live an average of 18.6 more years for an average life span of approximately 84 years. It is predicted that the older adult population will increase from 40 million in 2010 to 55 million in 2020, which represents a 36% increase for this decade. The fastest growing population of older adults is the 85+ population, which is expected to increase from 5.7 million in 2010 to 6.6 million in 2020.

The rapid growth of older adults in the U.S. positions this population in almost every care setting in which clinicians practice. Except for those clinicians who choose to work solely with maternal clients, most clinicians will care for older adults in an array of care environments. Even pediatric clinicians will encounter older adult parents as grandparents raising grandchildren, and these situations will require knowledgeable and experienced clinicians to assist in negotiating the many challenges of older adulthood. However, geriatric education or education that focuses on the care of this population has not kept pace with the increased prevalence of older adults in health care settings. In the latest available survey, Gilje, Lacey, and Moore (2007) revealed that just over 50% of baccalaureate nursing programs surveyed offered a standalone geriatric course. In order to provide cost-effective and evidence-based care to meet the great needs of the rising population of older adults, geriatric education is needed in all educational institutions that prepare clinicians to care for older adults. Most importantly, resources with which to facilitate geriatric education are greatly needed.

This book was developed as a resource for geriatric clinical education. Using real cases, this book provides thoughtful clinical scenarios through which clinicians can enhance clinical reasoning and gain geriatric nursing knowledge. The cases in this book were chosen to illustrate both typical and atypical situations that occur in geriatric practice. Readers are encouraged to go beyond simply trying to find the answers regarding the diagnoses and treatment plans for the patients involved in these cases toward the development of new ideas and knowledge. The usefulness of each case is enhanced if readers consider various scenarios for the patient in light of how the patient's conditions or circumstances might affect the family within the care setting. Remembering that the patient is part of an environment will help enhance readers' understanding of the condition from multiple perspectives.

This book is organized around 6 sections that focus on conditions and environments that impact older adults. The first section provides an overview of issues that impact the geriatric population. Contained within this section is a case study that discusses the elements of successful aging. The section proceeds with an issue that is becoming more prevalent within health care education—the need for cultural competence. The Administration on Aging (2009) reports that in 2008, 19.6% of older adults were minorities: 8.3% were African American, 6.8% were persons of Hispanic origin (who may be of any race), approximately 3.4% were Asian or Pacific Islander, and less than 1% were American Indian or Native Alaskan. By the year 2010, these minority populations are projected to increase from 5.7 million in 2000 (16.3% of the older adult population) to 8.0 million in (20.1% of older adults) and then to 12.9 million in 2020 (23.6% of older adults). This drastic increase in the cultural diversity of older adults requires that clinicians analyze their views and values regarding other cultures, learn essential elements of these cultures that impact health care choices, and facilitate the delivery of culturally competent health care interventions across care settings.

Section 1 proceeds to focus on two other major issues that impact older adults. Ageism, which is defined as a negative attitude or bias toward older adults that results in the belief that older people cannot or should not participate in societal activities or be given equal opportunities afforded to others (Holohan-Bell & Brummel-Smith, 1999), affects health care of older adults and impacts access to services. Ageism has the power to deprive older adults of their dignity and respect and may facilitate the disengagement of older adults from society. Ageism also has the potential to influence policies and care decisions for older adults. The rising costs of health care, limited reimbursement options for older adults, and low income among older adults also impact health care greatly. The median income of older adults in 2008 was only $25,503 for males and $14,559 for females, and approximately 3.7

million older adults (9.7%) were below the poverty level in 2008. Section 1 includes cases that address both of these issues.

Section 2 focuses on common health conditions that affect older adults. In developing a framework for cases in this section, a review-of-systems approach was used. Thus, the cases reflect health care conditions that impact all systems from head to toe. Because cardiac conditions are major challenges as patients age, this section begins with a case study that focuses on this system. Common skin conditions, bowel and bladder issues, and musculoskeletal concerns are represented within the early cases in this section. Other commonly occurring conditions such as stroke, sexually transmitted diseases, chronic obstructive pulmonary disease, Parkinson disease, and osteoporosis are also featured within this section.

There is a common misconception prevalent in health care that health promotion activities are not useful for older adults in their later years. Many clinicians incorrectly believe that after 60, 70, or 80 years of poor health behaviors such as drinking, smoking, or poor nutrition, older adults cannot benefit from programs focused on improving health practices acquired early in life and continued into older adulthood. The reality is that older adults are certainly not "too old" to stop smoking and drinking excessive amounts of alcohol, improve food choices, start exercising, develop sleep hygiene habits, and enhance their overall health and safety. Older adults may benefit from health promotion activities, even in their seventh, eighth, ninth, and tenth decades of life. Section 3 provides case studies in which older adults find themselves in need of health promotion activities and successfully engage in them. Contained within this section are cases discussing older adults challenged with primary prevention interventions, such as immunizations, smoking cessation, and good sleep hygiene development. This section also discusses secondary prevention strategies such as screening for prostate cancer.

While the majority of older adults live in their own homes, the Administration on Aging (2009) reports that approximately 31% (11.2 million) of noninstitutionalized older adults live alone (8.3 million women; 2.9 million men). As individuals age, living alone presents a number of challenges to living a quality life. For many older adults, institutional living and assisted living are often alternatives to living alone; but these alternatives also involve challenges. Section 4 presents case studies on the challenges of living alone and in institutions. The transition between environments, homeless older adults, and lack of fit in care environments are also among the cases presented in this section.

Many older adults approach their later years cognitively intact. However, a syndrome commonly known as the three Ds (delirium, depression, and dementia) occurs frequently in the older adult population. Section 5 presents cases that illustrate the similarities and difference in the presentation of the three Ds and provides information to help clinicians to effectively detect these conditions and to implement early treatment. In so doing, the consequences of these cognitive and psychological conditions may be prevented.

Finally, the last section of this book presents cases on special issues among older adults that may impact levels of independence. Polypharmacy and its impact on one older adult is the focus of the first case study in this section. The section continues to explore the challenge of driving, as well as the challenge of continued sexual health among older adults, amidst declining function and overall health. Pain management and end-of-life decision making cases are also present in this section to help clinicians anticipate and manage these special issues among the older adult population.

As readers progress through this book, they will be interested in and impressed with the depth and breadth of the case studies in gerontological nursing. Each section focuses on a different area of concern for older adults and contains cases that illustrate the issue in a manner that enhances the readers' understanding. Using this pedagogical method of learning, readers will enhance their knowledge and understanding regarding the vast array of issues of interest to clinicians who provide advanced care to older adults. Consequently, improved health care may be provided, resulting in improvement of the quality of life of the fastest growing U.S. population.

REFERENCES

Administration on Aging (2009). Profile of Older Americans. Washington, D.C: *Journal of Professional Nursing, 23,* 21–29.

Gilje, F., Lacey, L., & Moore, C. (2007). Gerontology and geriatric issues and trends in U.S. Nursing programs: A national survey.

Holohan-Bell, J., & Brummel-Smith, K. (1999). Impaired mobility and deconditioning. In J. Stone, J. Wyman, & S. Salisbury (Eds.), *Clinical gerontological nursing. A guide to advanced practice* (pp. 267–287). Philadelphia, PA: W.B. Saunders.

Abbreviations and Acronyms

AAA	Area Agency on Aging
ABG	arterial blood gas
ABMT	autologous bone marrow transplantation
ACE	angiotensin-converting enzyme
ACOG	American College of Obstetricians and Gynecologists
ACS	American Cancer Society
AD	Alzheimer disease
ADH	antidiuretic hormone
ADL	activities of daily living
ADR	adverse drug reactions
A-fib	atrial fibrillation
AHI	apnea-hypopnea index
AHRQ	Agency for Healthcare Research and Quality
AIMS	Abnormal Involuntary Movement Scale
AL	assisted living
AM/CL	amoxicillin/clavulanate
AMI	acute myocardial infarction
ANA	antinuclear antibody
AP	anteroposterior
APDA	American Parkinson Disease Association, Inc.
ARN	American Rehabilitation Nurse
ART	antiretroviral therapy
ASA	American Society of Anesthesiologists
ASO titre	antistreptolysin O titre
ATC	around the clock
ATS	American Thoracic Society
BKA	below-the-knee amputation
BM	bowel movement
BMI	body mass index
BPH	benign prostatic hypertrophy
BUN	blood urea nitrogen
C&S	culture and sensitivity
CAD	coronary artery disease

CAM	confusion assessment method
CAP	community-acquired pneumonia
CA-UTI	catheter-associated urinary tract infection
CBC	complete blood count
CBT	cognitive behavioral therapy
CCRC	continuing care retirement community
CDC	Centers for Disease Control
CDT	Clock Drawing Test
CES-D	Center for Epidemiologic Studies Depression Scale
CFO	chief financial officer
CHF	congestive heart failure
CMC	carpometacarpal
CMP	comprehensive metabolic panel
CMS	Centers for Medicare and Medicaid Studies
CN	cranial nerve
COPD	chronic obstructive pulmonary disease
COX-2	cyclooxygenase-2
CP	chest pain
CPAP	continuous positive airway pressure
CPR	cardiopulmonary resuscitation
CrCl	creatinine clearance
CSDD	Cornell scale for depression in dementia
CT	computer tomography
CTA	clear to auscultation
CVA	cerebrovascular accident
DAT	dementia of Alzheimer's type
D/C	discharge
DCCT	Diabetes Control and Complications Trial
DDX	differential diagnosis
DIP	distal interphalangeal
DJD	degenerative joint disease
DNR	do not resuscitate
DOE	dyspnea on exertion
DRE	digital rectal examination
DSM-IV	Diagnostic and Statistical Manual of Mental Disorders
DVT	deep vein thrombosis
DXA	dual-energy x-ray absorptiometry
EAI	elder assessment instrument
ECT	electroconvulsive therapy
ED	emergency department
EDS	excessive daytime sleepiness
EEG	electroencephalography
EKG	electrocardiogram
ELISA	enzyme-linked immunosorbent assay
EMG	electromyogram
EMS	emergency medical system

EOAD	early onset Alzheimer disease
EOG	electrooculography
EOM	extraocular movement
ER	emergency room
ESR	erythrocyte sedimentation rate
ESS	Epworth Sleepiness Scale
FAST	functional assessment staging tool
FBS	fasting blood sugar
FEV1	forced expiratory volume in 1 second
FVC	forced vital capacity
GD	global depression
GDR	gradual dose reduction
GDS	Geriatric Depression Scale
GERD	gastroesophageal reflux disease
GFR	glomerular filtration rate
GFRS	Geriatric Functional Rating Scale
HAD	HIV-associated dementia
HART	highly active antiretroviral therapy
HbA1c	hemoglobin A1c
HCAP	health care associated pneumonia
HCP	health care provider
HCTZ	hydrochlorothiazide
HDL	high-density lipoprotein
HIV	human immunodeficiency virus
HOH	hard of hearing
HPA	hypothalamic-pituitary-adrenal
HRQOL	health related quality of life
HRSA	Health Resources and Services Administration
HT	hormone therapy
HTN	hypertension
HZ	herpes zoster
IA	intraarticular
IADL	instrumental activities of daily living
IBS	irritable bowel syndrome
ICS	intercostal space
IDSA	Infectious Diseases Society of America
IM	intramuscular
INR	international normalized ratio
I/O	intake and output
IT	intensive therapy
IV	intravenous
LDL	low-density lipoprotein
LI	limited information
LLN	lower limit of normal
LR	likelihood ratio
LSO	lumbarsacral orthosis

MCL	midclavicular line
MCP	metacarpophalangeal
MDR	multidrug resistant
MI	myocardial infarction
MMSE	Mini-Mental State Examination
MRI	magnetic resonance imaging
MRSA	methicillin-resistant *staphylococcus aureus*
NASS	National Association of Spine Surgeons
NC	nasal cannula
NCSDR	National Center on Sleep Disorders Research
NG	nasogastric
NHLBI	National Heart Lung and Blood Institute
NIDDM	Non-insulin dependent diabetes mellitus
NIH	National Institutes of Health
NKA	no known allergies
NKDA	no known drug allergies
NKF	National Kidney Foundation
NKFA	no known food allergies
NNRTI	nonnucleoside reverse transcriptase inhibitor
NP	nurse practitioner
NRT	nicotine replacement therapies
NSAID	nonsteroidal antiinflammatory drug
NSF	National Sleep Foundation
NTG	nitroglycerin
OA	osteoarthritis
OFI	oral fluid intake
OP	osteoporosis
ORIF	open reduction internal fixation
OTC	over the counter
PainAD	pain assessment for advanced dementia
PC	palliative care
PCA	patient controlled analgesia
PCR	polymerase chain reaction
PERRLA	pupils are equal, round, and reactive to light and accommodation
PHN	postherpetic neuralgia
PI	protease inhibitor
PIP	proximal interphalangeal
PO	by mouth
PPD	pack per day; purified protein derivative
PPI	proton-pump inhibitor
PR	pulmonary rehabilitation
PSA	prostate specific antigen
PSG	polysomnography
PSI	pneumonia severity index
PSQI	Pittsburgh Sleep Quality Index

PTSD	posttraumatic stress disorder
PVD	peripheral vascular disease
PVR	post void residual
RA	rheumatoid arthritis or risk disease
RCVA	right cerebrovascular accident
REM	rapid eye movement
RF	rheumatoid factor
ROM	range of motion
SBGM	self–blood glucose monitoring
SIADH	syndrome of inappropriate diuretic hormone hypersecretion
SOB	shortness of breath
SPT	suprapubic tube
SS	specific suggestion
SSRI	selective serotonin reuptake inhibitor
START	Screening Tool to Alert doctors to Right Treatment
STI	sexually transmitted infection
STOPP	Screening Tool of Older Person's Potentially inappropriate prescriptions
T2DM	Type 2 diabetes mellitus
TAH BSO	total abdominal hysterectomy and bilateral salpingo-oopherectomy
TB	tuberculosis
TBW	total body water
TC	tai chi
TCM	transitional care model
TENS	trancutaneous electrical nerve stimulation
TIA	transient ischemic attack
TIBC	total iron binding capacity
TM	tympanic membrane
TMS	trimethoprim-sulfamethoxazole
TPN	total parenteral nutrition
TRUS	transrectal ultrasound
TSH	thyroid stimulating hormone
TZD	thiazolidinedione
UA	urinalysis
UI	urinary incontinence
USPSTF	U.S. Preventative Services Task Force
UTI	urinary tract infection
VA	Veteran's Administration
VCF	vertebral compression fracture
VS or V/S	vital sign
VZV	varicella-zoster virus; varicella-zoster vaccine
WBC	white blood cell
WOCN	wound ostomy continence nurse

Section 1

The Aging Population

Case 1.1 Recipe for Successful Aging

By Christine Tocchi, PhD(C), MSN, APRN, GNP-BC

Mrs. R presents to the primary-care practice for an annual examination. She is new to the practice and has several health questions she would like to discuss regarding aging as she is now a "senior" and needs to stay healthy to care for her 88-year-old mother with early stage Alzheimer disease. Mrs. R is 65 years old and describes her overall health as good. She was diagnosed with hypertension and hypercholesterolemia approximately 15 years ago and has been seeing her former primary physician every 6 months for checkups. Mrs. R also has osteoarthritis of the right knee with occasional pain and stiffness. She is concerned that she may need to have knee replacement surgery in the future. Mrs. R recently relocated to a new apartment to accommodate being the primary caregiver for her mother. Mrs. R is not sure how to manage her mother's routine health care.

Mrs. R has a past medical history of hypertension, hypercholesterolemia, and osteoarthritis of the right knee. Her past surgical history includes a tonsillectomy at age 7 and cholecystectomy at age 41. Her medications are: HCTZ, 12.5 mg daily; atorvastatin, 20 mg daily; and Tylenol Arthritis, 2 tablets as needed for knee pain with an average of once a day administration and twice a day "on bad days". She has a mammogram annually. Her last Pap smear was 2 years ago. She had a colonoscopy at age 55. Both tests revealed no abnormal findings. TB: unknown. She has no known allergies (NKA). Her functional status reveals that she is independent in all activities of daily living and instrumental activities of daily living. She drives her own automobile. Her father died at age 63 of myocardial infarction (MI). Her mother is

Case Studies in Gerontological Nursing for the Advanced Practice Nurse, First Edition.
Edited by Meredith Wallace Kazer, Leslie Neal-Boylan.
© 2012 John Wiley & Sons, Inc. Published 2012 by John Wiley & Sons, Inc.

alive, age 88, with a history of mild stage Alzheimer disease, hypercholesterolemia, and osteoarthritis of both knees. Mrs. R is not sure of her paternal and maternal grandparents' health history. Mrs. R has 2 brothers ages 69 and 67 living in Puerto Rico with unknown health history. She has 2 younger brothers living in the United States. Her 60-year-old brother has a health history of MI at age 48, hypertension, and diabetes mellitus. Her 57-year-old brother has hypercholesterolemia. Mrs. R also has 2 sisters living in the United States. One sister, age 62, has diabetes mellitus, hypertension, and a history of breast cancer. Her 55-year-old sister is alive and in good health. Mrs. R also has 3 children: 2 sons, ages 42 and 40, are both in good health; and her daughter, age 37, is also in good health. She has 8 grandchildren.

Mrs. R is a recently retired home health aide. She has a high school diploma and has received certification as a home health aide. She is divorced and currently residing in a 2-bedroom apartment of a 2-family house with her 88-year-old mother. Mrs. R is the primary caregiver for her mother. One sister lives locally and works full-time. This sister lives with her family on the first floor of the 2-family house. The sister sporadically assists with primary caregiving of mother when she is not working. Mrs. R's other siblings live within 20 miles but only visit during the holidays. Mrs. R's children all live locally, work full-time, and have children. Mrs. R provides child care for her daughter's 7- and 10-year-olds after school 3 days per week. Her son's family comes to dinner every Sunday. Mrs. R has a boyfriend whom she sees approximately 3 times per week. The couple dines at a local restaurant weekly without her mother.

Mrs. R states that her finances are adequate and include Social Security and a "small" amount of savings. She also does alterations occasionally for a local tailor for extra income. Mrs. R has a 20 pack year history of smoking. She has not smoked for 25 years. Mrs. R denies a history of alcohol abuse or use of recreational drugs. She has approximately 1 glass of wine per day with dinner. Mrs. R is sexually active. She denies dyspareunia or sexual problems with herself or her partner. She has no history of sexually transmitted diseases.

Hobbies: Mrs. R enjoys cooking and has a weekly card game with her girlfriends. Most of her day is spent shopping, doing housework, babysitting, and overseeing the care of her mother.

Mrs. R currently denies any pain, discomfort, or constitutional symptoms. She does state that she has intermittent right knee pain associated with arthritis. The pain and stiffness occur on cold or rainy days and with extended walking or sitting. The pain is described as a "bad ache," 7 on a scale of 1–10; and its duration is 30 minutes to 1 hour. Stretching, heat, and Tylenol Arthritis are all effective. She averages 2 Tylenol Arthritis tablets per day and twice a day on "bad days". She denies headache. Mrs. R states that she has noticed some difficulty with blurred vision at night when driving and requires reading glasses for any "close work". She denies any hearing loss or tinnitus. She denies nasal congestion, drainage, epistaxis, sore throat, or a cough. On a rare occasion, she has experienced dyspnea on exertion without chest pain or palpitations, which is relieved with rest. Mrs. R also denies any abdominal pain, nausea, vomiting, constipation, or diarrhea. On occasion, she has experienced indigestion after a large meal, which is relieved with Tums. She complains of rare stress incontinence with laughing or sneezing, but no urge incontinence, dysuria, hematuria, or retention difficulties. She wakes to void once per night. Mrs. R denies any vaginal drainage. She denies any joint pain except knee pain. She denies muscle weakness, paresthesia, edema, or difficulty with balance or gait. Mrs. R denies episodes of lightheadedness, vertigo, syncope, tremors, or falls in the past 6 months. She describes her mood as good, without depressive symptoms, anxiety, or mood swings. She also describes her memory as good with rare "forgetfulness" of names or misplacing things but "it always comes to me in a couple of minutes".

OBJECTIVE

Mrs. R is a 65-year-old female in no acute distress. Her BP is 126/78; her pulse is 78; and her respirations are 12. She is 64 inches tall and weighs 125 lb. Her head is normocephalic. PERRLA. External ear canals are without drainage, erythema, or swelling. Her TMs are intact. Her neck is supple. There is no evidence of lymphadenopathy, thyroidomegaly, or carotid bruits. Her thorax is symmetrical, and her breath sounds are clear to auscultation. Cardiac examination reveals S1, S2 with no murmurs, gallops, or clicks. Her abdominal examination is benign. Her extremities have no evidence of cyanosis, clubbing, or edema. Her neurological examination is nonfocal, without evidence of rigidity, myoclonus, cogwheeling, or tremors. She has a positive get-up-and-go test, and her Romberg sign is negative.

CRITICAL THINKING

What are the current statistics on life-expectancy trends of the older adult population that will guide recommendations for care for Mrs. R?

How can Mrs. R successfully age without becoming dependent on others for physical support?

What are the current rates of disability in older adults and methods to prevent disability?

What are the most important areas to assess in Mrs. R. in order to help to promote health and prevent disease and complications associated with chronic illness?

What is the plan of treatment for Mrs. R based on her history and physical examination results?

RESOLUTION

What are the current statistics on life-expectancy trends of the older adult population that will guide recommendations for care for Mrs. R?

The growth in the number and proportion of older adults in the United States is increasing at an unprecedented rate. The older adult population is currently 12.8% of the U.S. population; 1 in 8 Americans are greater than 65 years of age. It is estimated that this population will increase to approximately 20% by the year 2030 (U.S. Department of Health and Human Services, 2008). The older adult population comprises a large heterogeneous group of age categories and ethnicity. Older adults like Mrs. R are frequently characterized as young old (65–75 years of age), old old (75–85 years of age), or oldest old (those 85 years of age and greater). The baby boomers (those born between 1946 and 1964) will start turning 65 in 2011, and the number of older people will increase dramatically during the 2010–2030 period. The oldest-old population is the fastest growing segment of the population and is projected to grow rapidly after 2030, when the baby boomers move into this age group. The U.S. Census Bureau projects that the population age 85 and over could grow from 5.3 million in 2006 to nearly 21 million by 2050 (Federal Interagency Forum on Aging-Related Statistics, 2006).

With the expected increase in the number of older adults, there is also an anticipated change in the racial/ethnic composition of this cohort. It is projected that by 2030, more than 1 in 3 older adults will be from 1 of 4 minority groups: African American, Asian/Pacific, Hispanic, and American Indian (Federal Interagency Forum on Aging-Related Statistics, 2010).

Because of the projected increase in the older-adult population, the health and the usage of health care services of this group will be of great concern to public policy. Population information will be needed in order to evaluate their impact on Medicare and Medicaid (Kramarow, Lubitz, Lentzner, & Gorina, 2007). Some states have higher concentrations of older adults and will need to analyze available resources to accommodate the projected rise of this population. Presently, the majority of older adults reside in 10 states: Florida, Pennsylvania, West Virginia, Iowa, North Dakota, Rhode Island, Maine, South Dakota, Arkansas, and Connecticut (Administration on Aging, 2009). Health care resources, transportation options, availability of caregivers, and health policy will all be affected by the increase in the number of older adults.

Life expectancy: The decline in adult mortality over the past half century has contributed to the steady increase in life expectancy. In 2004, the average life expectancy at birth in the United States was 75.2 and 80.4 for men and women. At age 65, the average male was expected to live another 17.1 years and females another 20 years (Centers for Disease Control and Prevention, 2006). The extended life span of humans is largely due to advances in medical science that have prevented or decreased the occurrence of acute illness. Chronic disease and degenerative illness have replaced acute illness as the leading causes of death for older adults.

How can Mrs. R successfully age without becoming dependent on others for physical support?
Successful aging allows older adults like Mrs. R to maintain autonomy and remain living independently in the community. However, there is a lack of a universal definition or measurement of successful aging. The World Health Organization, the White House Conference on Aging, and the National Institute of Aging have emphasized that successful aging goes beyond avoidance of disease and disability. Rowe and Kahn (1997), whose model was used in the MacArthur Research Network on Successful Aging, defined successful aging as including low probability of disease and disease-related disability, high cognitive and physical functional capacity, and active engagement in life. Other components in the literature identify life satisfaction, presence of illness, longevity, personality, environment, and self-rated health (McReynolds & Rossen, 2004).

Research suggests that good lifestyle choices have an essential role in successful aging. The literature indicates that adequate physical activity, even initiated in later years, contributes to high physical and cognitive functioning and overall health (Aranceta, Perez-Rodrigo, Gondra, & Orduna, 2001; Fillit et al., 2002; Houde & Melillo, 2002; Mattson, Chan, & Duan, 2002; Oguma, Sesso, Paffengarger, & Lee, 2002). Specifically, physical activity increases muscle tone, flexibility, cardiovascular health, positive mood, and cognition. It also prevents falling, which is a significant health issue for older adults.

Nutrition is a powerful and modifiable lifestyle factor that can delay or prevent chronic disease in later life and potentially may add extra years of health, productivity, and functioning (Shikany & White, 2000). The leading causes of death of older adults in the United States (which include coronary heart disease, cancer, and stroke) are associated with diet. However, older adults like Mrs. R are at risk of undernutrition due to physiological changes related to digestion, metabolism, and nutrients. Many older adults may have poor nutritional intake because of a decrease in sense of taste or an increase in chewing or swallowing difficulties.

Social support contributes to physical and cognitive function and engagement in life (Lange-Collette, 2002). Psychologists believe social support provides a stress buffering effect on health (Cohen, 2004). Stress is thought to activate physiological systems such as the sympathetic nervous system and the hypothalamic-pituitary-adrenal (HPA) cortical axis (Cohen, Kessler, & Gordon, 1995). Prolonged activation of these systems is thought to place an individual at risk for a variety of physical and psychological illnesses. Social support may interrupt the stress–physical decline cycle. Maintaining active social relationships and involvement may provide the necessary emotional support to deter the chronic activation of the sympathetic nervous system and HPA axis. Social support may also promote a sense of fulfilling important social roles, enhance feelings of self-control and competency, and facilitate healthful lifestyle behaviors that prevent chronic illness and disability, such as exercise and healthy nutrition (Krause, Herzog, & Baker, 1992; Mendes de Leon, Glass, & Berkman, 2003).

What are the current rates of disability in older adults and methods to prevent disability?
The World Health Organization (2010) defined disability as an umbrella term, covering impairments, activity limitations, and participation restrictions. Research indicates that older adults have significantly increased prevalence of disability, particularly non-Caucasians; and the suggested contributing factor is the current epidemic of obesity (Seeman, Merkin, Crimmins, & Karlamangia, 2010). Older obese adults are more likely than nonobese cohorts to have certain chronic conditions and report higher levels of disability (Kramarow et al., 2007). Prevention of disability is a significant factor for maintaining independence and successful aging. Maintaining a healthy lifestyle and managing chronic illness are important methods in prevention of disability.

Chronic disease: Chronic illness causes most death among older Americans (Kramarow et al., 2007). Results from the National Health Interview Survey indicated that nearly one-third of older adults in 2004–2005 reported having been diagnosed with some form of health disease, and approximately half reported having been diagnosed with arthritis. An individual's risk for having more than one chronic condition increases with age in 62% of Americans greater than 65 years of age; 1 in 5 Americans have multiple chronic conditions (Volgeli et al., 2007). The most prevalent conditions for the older adult population include arthritis (57%), hypertension (55%), pulmonary disease (38%), diabetes (17%), cancer (17%), and osteoporosis (16%) (Partnership for Solutions National Program Office, 2004).

To manage chronic illness, older adults like Mrs. R often have multiple health care providers. The average number of physicians seen by Medicare patients ranges from 4 (with 1 chronic condition) to 14 (with 5 or more conditions) (Volgeli et al., 2007). As the number of health care providers increases, it is increasingly more challenging for patients to comprehend, recall, and reconcile instructions (National Academy of Social Insurance, 2003). Also, patients with multiple conditions tend to take more medications and are more likely to suffer adverse drug events (Boyd, Darer, Boult, Fried, Boult, & Wu, 2005; Gandi et al., 2003; Gurwitz et al., 2003; Tinetti, Bogardus, & Agostini, 2004).

What are the most important areas to assess in Mrs. R. in order to help to promote health and prevent disease and complications associated with chronic illness?

Older adults often present with complex medical problems that have been managed by multiple providers and have lengthy medication lists, several health concerns, and misconceptions about normal aging and health management. The goal of the first primary care visit is to properly evaluate the older adult with attention to their special needs. Subsequent visits will focus on addressing any additional health concerns, health promotion, and prevention.

The purpose of the initial assessment is to complete a comprehensive history and a physical examination and to assess for common geriatric syndromes (Table 1.1.1) and iatrogenic illnesses. Iatrogenic illnesses are

TABLE 1.1.1. Common Geriatric Syndromes.

Iatrogenic Illness
Weight loss and malnutrition
Cognitive impairment
Depression
Urinary incontinence
Immobility & gait disorders
Falls
Visual and hearing impairments
Dizziness
Syncope
Sleep disorders
Pressure ulcers
Pain

TABLE 1.1.2. Health Maintenance.

Eye exam
Hearing exam
Colonoscopy
Mammogram
Pap smear
Bone density test
Dental exam
Foot exam
Functional ability test
Social support

TABLE 1.1.3. Immunizations.

Pneumonia
Influenza
Tetanus
Zoster

any illnesses that result from a diagnostic procedure or therapeutic intervention, that are not natural consequences of the patient's disease, and that are associated with medications, diagnostic and therapeutic interventions, nosocomial infections, and environmental hazards. Also essential to the care of older adults is complete health maintenance (Table 1.1.2) and immunization records (Table 1.1.3).

What is the plan of treatment for Mrs. R based on her history and physical examination results?

Hypertension. Order laboratory diagnostics to identify secondary causes and screen for target organ damage. Initial diagnostic evaluation may include assessment of kidney function (electrolytes), urine screening for protein or microalbumin, blood sugar levels, and an electrocardiogram. Continue hydrochlorothiazide.

Hypercholesteremia. Order lipid panel. Continue atorvastatin.

Osteoarthritis. Tylenol Arthritis, 1–2 tablets as needed but not to exceed 3 doses per day. Referral to orthopedic specialist for evaluation of osteoarthritis of the right knee.

Physical activity. Thirty minutes of physical activity per day is recommended for health promotion and prevention. This will be especially important in this case with Mrs. R's history of hypertension and risk for coronary heart disease and diabetes mellitus.

Nutrition. Low fat diet with emphasis on fruits, vegetables, complex carbohydrates, and protein.

Referrals. Gastroenterology for colonoscopy and gynecology for annual examination, Pap smear, mammography, and dexometry.

Recommendations. Ophthalmology for funduscopic examination. Mrs. R should have her mother assessed by a geriatrician to discuss pharmacological and nonpharmacological treatment options for Alzheimer disease.

Overall, this case underscores an opportunity for earlier identification of disease to improve treatment outcomes. Beyond the personal plan of care, the provider may pursue opportunities to offer staff education to accomplish this goal in the future.

REFERENCES

Administration on Aging (2009). *A profile of older Americans*. Washington, DC: Department of Health and Human Services.

Aranceta, J., Perez-Rodrigo, C., Gondra, J., & Orduna, J. (2001). Community-based program to promote physical activity among elderly: The Gerobilbo Study. *Journal of Nutrition, Health, & Aging, 5*, 238–242.

Boyd, C. M., Darer, J., Boult, C., Fried, L. P., Boult, L., & Wu, A. W. (2005). Clinical practice guidelines and quality of care for older patients with multiple comorbid diseases: Implications for pay for performance. *Journal of the American Medical Association, 294*, 716–724.

Centers for Disease Control and Prevention (2006). *Faststats: Life expectancy*. Retrieved from http://www.cdc.gov/nchs/fastats/lifexpec.htm table 11

Cohen, S. (2004). Social relationships and health. *The American Psychologist, 59*, 676–684.

Cohen, S., Kessler, R. C., & Gordon, L. U. (1995). Strategies for measuring stress in psychiatric and physical disorders. In S. Cohen, R. C. Kessler, & L. U. Gordon (Eds.), *Measuring stress* (pp. 3–28). New York: Oxford University Press.

Federal Interagency Forum on Aging-Related Statistics (2006). Older Americans 2006: Key indicators for well-being. Hyattsville, MD. Retrieved from http://www.agingstats.gov/Agingstasdotnet/Main_Site/Data/2006_Documents/OA_2006.pdf

Federal Interagency Forum on Aging-Related Statistics (2010). Older Americans 2010: Key indicators of well-being. Hyattsville, MD. Retrieved from http://www.agingstats.gov/agingstatsdotnet/Main_Site/Data

Fillit, H. M., Butler, R. N., O'Connell, A. W., Albert, M. S., Birren, J. E., Cotman, C. W., . . . Tully, T. (2002). Achieving and maintaining cognitive vitality and aging. *Mayo Clinic Proceedings, 77*, 681–696.

Gandi, T. K., Weingrt, S. N., Borus, J., Seger, A. C., Peterson, J., Burdick, E., . . . Bates, D. W. (2003). Adverse drug events in ambulatory care. *The New England Journal of Medicine, 348*, 1556–1564.

Gurwitz, J. H., Field, T. S., Harrold, L. R., Rothschild, J., Debellis, K., Seger, A. C., . . . Bates, D. W. (2003). Incidence and preventability of adverse drug events among older persons in the ambulatory setting. *Journal of the American Medical Association, 289,* 1107–1116.

Houde, S. C., & Melillo, K. D. (2002). Older adults: An integrative review of research methodology and results. *Journal of Advanced Nursing, 38,* 219–234.

Kramarow, E., Lubitz, J., Lentzner, H., & Gorina, Y. (2007). Trends in the health of older Americans, 1970–2005. *Health Affairs, 26,* 1417–1425.

Kraus, N., Herzog, A. R., & Baker, E. (1992). Providing support to others and well-being in later life. *Journal of Gerontology: Psychological Sciences, 47,* P300–P311.

Lange-Collette, J. (2002). Promoting health among perimenopausal women through diet and exercise. *Journal of the American Academy of Nurse Practitioners, 14,* 172–177.

Mattson, M. P., Chan, S. L., & Duan, W. (2002). Modification of brain aging and Neurodegenerative disorders by genes, diet, and behavior. *Physiological Reviews, 82,* 637–672.

McReynolds, J. L., & Rossen, E. K. (2004). Importance of physical activity, nutrition, and social support for optimal aging. *Clinical Nurse Specialist CNS, 18,* 200–206.

Mendes de Leon, C. F., Glass, T. A., & Berkman, L. F. (2003). Social engagement and disability in a community population of older adults: The New Haven EPESE. *American Journal of Epidemiology, 157,* 633–642.

National Academy of Social Insurance (2003). *Medicare in the 21ˢᵗ century: Building a better chronic care system.* Washington, DC: National Academy of Social Insurance.

Oguma, Y., Sesso, H. D., Paffengarger, R. S., & Lee, I. M. (2002). Physical activity and all cause mortality in women: A review of the evidence. *British Journal of Sports Medicine, 36,* 162–172.

Partnership for Solutions National Program Office (2004). Chronic conditions: Making the case for ongoing care. Partnerships for Solution: John Hopkins University.

Rowe, J. W., & Kahn, R. L. (1997). Successful aging. *The Gerontologist, 37,* 435–440.

Seeman, T. E., Merkin, S. S., Crimmins, E. M., & Karlamangia, A. S. (2010). Disability trends among older Americans: National health and nutrition examination surveys, 1988–1994 and 1999–2004. *American Journal of Public Health, 100,* 100–107.

Shikany, J. M., & White, G. L. (2000). Dietary guidelines for chronic disease prevention. *Southern Medical Journal, 93,* 1138–1151.

Tinetti, M. E., Bogardus, S. T., & Agostini, J. V. (2004). Potential pitfalls of disease-specific guidelines for patients with multiple conditions. *The New England Journal of Medicine, 351,* 2870–2874.

U.S. Department of Health and Human Services (2008). *Population of older adults.* Rockville, MD: U.S. Department of Health and Human Services, Office of the Surgeon General. Retrieved from http://aspe.hhs.gov/dalcp/reports/

Volgeli, C., Shields, A. E., Lee, T. A., Gibson, T. B., Marder, W. D., Weiss, K. D., & Blumental, D. (2007). Multiple chronic conditions: Prevalence, health consequences, and Implications for quality, care management, and costs. *Society of General Internal Medicine, 22,* 391–395.

World Health Organization (2010). Disabilities. Retrieved from http://www.who.int/topics/disabilities/en/

ADDITIONAL RESOURCES

Administration on Aging (2007). *A profile of older Americans*. Washington, DC: Department of Health and Human Services.

Population Reference Bureau (2003). Which states are the oldest? Retrieved from www.prb.org/articles/2003/whichstatearetheoldest.aspx

Case 1.2 Cultural Competence Is a Journey

By Jina Ko, MSN, RN, ANP-C,
and Julie M. L. Lautner, MSW, MSN, RN

Ms. L is an 82-year-old woman complaining of lower abdominal pain for 2 weeks. Her 16-year-old grandniece, Joan, is with her today and is translating on Ms. L's behalf. Ms. L recently arrived in the U.S. from Taiwan to be with her sister MengFei, age 74, and her sister's family. Ms. L speaks Taiwanese, Japanese, and some Mandarin. Her English is very limited. Ms. L is not married and does not have any children. Her health history is sparse with no reported medical or surgical history, allergies, or medications. Joan reports that Ms. L occasionally sees a traditional Chinese herbalist for "better health."

When the provider comes into the room, Ms. L has not changed into a gown as instructed and is sitting on a chair next to Joan. During the initial assessment, Ms. L seems reluctant to reveal any specific health history to the provider; but as Joan translates, Ms. L points to her lower abdomen-pelvis area and reports ongoing pain for "many years" that has recently gotten "much worse". Ms. L agrees and nods to subsequent questions or responds in short, abrupt, negative statements, as both Ms. L and Joan seem increasingly uncomfortable with the more focused line of questioning. The provider becomes impatient with Ms. L's vague answers and detached demeanor as the time allotted for the history and physical is quickly dwindling away. She instructs Ms. L to change into her gown and sit on the examining table while she steps out. Ms. L appears reluctant to change, and begins speaking rapidly with Joan. Joan tells the provider that Ms. L has never been undressed in front of a health care provider before. The provider tries to assure Ms. L that she needs her to change into the gown in order to perform

Case Studies in Gerontological Nursing for the Advanced Practice Nurse, First Edition.
Edited by Meredith Wallace Kazer, Leslie Neal-Boylan.
© 2012 John Wiley & Sons, Inc. Published 2012 by John Wiley & Sons, Inc.

the exam and steps out, assuming that Ms. L will understand once the exam begins. Upon returning to the room, Ms. L is gowned and sitting on the table, but remains silent and does not offer any eye contact. The provider begins the abdominal part of the physical examination without using Joan to translate the process since their allotted time is almost over. When asked to get into position for a pelvic exam, Ms. L becomes increasingly agitated. The provider asks Joan to explain that this is a normal part of the exam and that it is necessary to examine her for the source of her pain. Ms. L shakes her head and refuses. The provider begrudgingly relents and tells Joan that she will have to schedule Ms. L for abdominal and transvaginal ultrasounds instead. Ms. L does not return for her ultrasounds as scheduled, and subsequent calls to the household to reschedule are unsuccessful.

CRITICAL THINKING

What do you know about cultural diversity in the geriatric population? What is cultural competence and why does it matter to those in health care?

Would a lesson in cultural competence have aided the provider and improved her care for this individual, or would her interaction have remained the same?

Time constraints can be challenging in practice. Was the provider right to rush the exam? As it turns out, Ms. L has valid reasons for her discomfort with the exam process. Would a more comprehensive history have improved care? Why or why not?

What could the provider have done better in this first visit to establish a better foundation for care with Ms. L?

What are some guiding principles behind cultural competence that can further help practitioners to become more proficient?

RESOLUTION

What do you know about cultural diversity in the geriatric population? What is cultural competence and why does it matter to those in health care?

The U.S. is an increasingly diverse population, particularly among older adult groups. The Centers for Disease Control and Prevention indicate that while the non-Hispanic Caucasian population will decrease from 83% of all older adults in 2003 to only 72% in 2030, other racial and ethnic older adult group numbers will increase dramatically (2007). More specifically, the Hispanic/Latino older adult population will increase by nearly 50% during that same time frame, the African American older adult population will increase by 20%, and the Asian older adult population will increase nearly 60%—the largest older adult population group increase in the U.S. The evidence is clear that ethnic and cultural diversity is on the rise in the U.S., particularly among older adult populations; and clinicians must be able to work with and among a diverse population base in order to provide the best, most comprehensive care.

A clear, singular definition of cultural competence does not exist. In their work *Towards a Culturally Competent System of Care*, Cross and colleagues provide a pivotal foundation upon which current interpretations and extrapolations of cultural competence derive (Cross, Bazron, Dennis, Isaacs, 1989). They write, "Cultural competence is a set of congruent behaviors, attitudes, and policies that come together in a system, agency or among professionals and enable that system, agency or those professions to work effectively in cross-cultural situations" (Cross et al., 1989, p. iv). The authors cite the following key elements that contribute to becoming more culturally competent: 1) valuing diversity, 2) having the capacity for cultural self-assessment, 3) being conscious of the dynamics inherent when cultures interact, 4) having institutionalized culture knowledge, and 5) having developed adaptations to service delivery reflecting an understanding of cultural diversity (Cross et al., 1989).

The work of Cross and colleagues was significant in that it moved beyond previous ideas of cultural awareness, knowledge, or sensitivity, ideas which had failed to include the coalescing of behaviors, policies, and attitudes that allow agencies and organizations to work effectively in cross-cultural situations (Adams, 1995, as cited by the Center for Effective Collaboration and Practice, n.d.). Instead, cultural competence calls upon agencies, organizations, policies, and policy builders to recognize the need for **successful** communication and working relationships in order to participate in the breakdown of potentially biased and stereotyped care that frequently undermines and underserves large portions of the population. The need for **self-assessment** emphasizes that stereotyped, biased, or racist viewpoints are incompatible with and are opposed to successful cross-cultural work, particularly on the individual level.

Over the last 20 years, the literature on cultural competence in health care has expanded greatly. Most readers of this text have been exposed to the concept of cultural competence at some point, as health care professionals have been on the front lines of the cultural competence movement. Having been faced with the complexities of working with diverse populations, providers understand that failed interactions can have life-or-death consequences. Despite these lessons, few can say with confidence that they are truly culturally competent. All too often, cultural competence is interpreted as an end point without the need for ongoing critical followup and assessment; yet this is far from accurate.

Would a lesson in cultural competence have aided the provider and improved her care for this individual, or would her interaction have remained the same?

Most health care organizations and individual providers are well intentioned and care about their communities and patients. Yet, despite lessons in cultural competency and exposure to a diverse health care community, many remain a part of the larger culture that attempts, but fails, to provide the most comprehensive and supportive intercultural care. Cultural competence is not a concrete destination. Instead, cultural competence is an act of "becoming," with continuous followup, self-analysis, and education. Becoming culturally competent requires the attention and focus of the individual provider during each and every patient interaction, with peers in the workplace, and on professional and academic policies that may inadvertently discriminate against other groups.

Time constraints can be challenging in practice. Was the provider right to rush the exam? As it turns out, Ms. L has valid reasons for her discomfort with the exam process. Would a more comprehensive history have improved care? Why or why not?

Approximately 6 weeks after the initial visit, Ms. L returned to the office, this time with Ms. L's younger sister, MengFei. MengFei is a patient in the same office but under the care of another provider. MengFei asks if they can use a language translation line, the one she uses with her provider, since her English is not as good as Joan's. During the initial conversation, MengFei reveals that Ms. L has been reluctant to return to the office because she has only ever taken traditional Chinese medicine in the past, has never had to completely undress before a provider, and is frequently nervous and afraid of her new surroundings, since she only recently arrived in the U.S. MengFei also reveals that Ms. L was taken hostage during World War II and was repeatedly raped and brutalized by her captors, leaving her infertile, with severe urinary incontinence issues, and with chronic pelvic pain that no longer seems to be helped by traditional medicines. MengFei notes that Ms. L's symptoms have recently worsened. Because of her past, Ms. L never married and was isolated by her community for many years. MengFei reports that the family was only recently reunited and that she has sponsored Ms. L to come to the U.S. so that she can live out her remaining years in peace and good health. MengFei also reports that the younger children in the family do not know of Ms. L's past and that Ms. L would have been humiliated if Joan, her grandniece, were to know about her experiences.

In hindsight, this information is significant; it reveals much about Ms. L's past and explains much of her behavior during the visit. It should be noted, however, that the provider may not have needed these disclosures from the family had she been more patient and empathetic from the outset. Time constraints in the clinical setting are indeed challenging; however, sitting with a patient and listening to what is being said—and what is not being said—can be beneficial for both the patient and the provider. Discovering that an individual has a history of abuse, assault, or other history of trauma should not be the sole incentive behind decelerating our ever-accelerating clinical visits.

What could the provider have done better in this first visit to establish a better foundation for care with Ms. L?
Any interaction with a patient should begin where the patient is, rather than where the provider would like him or her to be. Health care providers have their own unique and important agendas in addressing the health needs of any individual patient; and taking the time to understand and accept where the patient stands at any given point in time can be a challenge. Nevertheless, it is extraordinarily important. Older adults come to a provider's practice with a lifetime of experiences, memories, challenges faced and overcome, and previous exposures to illness and health care systems. Despite every appearance of sameness, one can never assume a common understanding of language, culture, or experience. In this particular case, there are numerous ways that the clinician failed to see the differences between herself and the patient and, as a result, failed in the patient's overall care.

Research indicates that the use of trained health care interpreters is an effective and appropriate means of providing support to limited–English speaking patients (Jacobs, Lauderdale, Meltzer, Shorey, Levinson, & Thisted, 2001; Ngo-Metzger et al., 2007). Numerous federal and national agencies, including the U.S. Department of Health and Human Services Office of Minority Health, now have guidelines on the use of family interpreters (2010). The State of California currently requires that all commercial health and dental providers provide professional translators, "if not in person, then at least by telephone or video conferencing" (Sundaram, 2009). By using Joan as Ms. L's interpreter, the clinician failed to acknowledge any embarrassment or discomfort Ms. L might feel by having to answer personal questions in front of her teenage relative. Similarly, it was unlikely that Ms. L would have explained her discomfort with the lithotomy position through Joan, as Ms. L would likely feel ashamed of her past. While some family translators are useful and acceptable to the patient, the clinician can never generalize that this is the case. Instead, the clinician should give the patient the power to choose the most suitable translator and embrace the choice of the professional translator or family member as a step towards a more cooperative health care relationship.

Next, the clinician appears to interpret Ms. L's short, restricted responses as normal for her ethnic and cultural group. However, the clinician failed to see beyond the surface of Ms. L's presentation. Ms. L's underlying history of rape prevented her from feeling comfortable in the lithotomy position, yet the provider's response was one of frustration in not obtaining a full examination. Instead of accepting Ms. L's discomfort with compassion and empathy, the provider again failed to see the patient's unique story as one deserving of her time and energy.

Finally, the provider excluded Ms. L from the examination process by failing to explain her actions during the physical portion of the exam. This further alienated the patient and dismissed Ms. L, who was already limited by language and culture, as an active participant in her own health care. By talking throughout an examination and explaining each step along the way, the provider engages the patient in the process and reinforces open dialogue and supportive care.

What are some guiding principles behind cultural competence that can further help practitioners to become more proficient?
First, as mentioned briefly above, **start where the patient is**. Accept discomfort or mistrust in the health care setting as a challenge to be overcome with compassion and empathy. Determine language proficiency and ask about comfort with translators. Some patients will feel more comfortable with a family member, while others will not. Use professional health care translators as much as possible. Second, **don't generalize**. In an outcome-driven, time-limited health care environment, the biggest hazard of cultural competence is unnecessarily and inappropriately stereotyping individuals and groups (Gregg & Saha, 2006). Assuming to know or understand an entire ethnic or cultural group, without anticipating within-group differences, limits a provider's ability to assess and interpret individual distinctions and fails to acknowledge the unique experiences and characteristics of each patient. Education, acculturation level, place of birth, languages spoken, and past trauma or experiences in war, among other things, greatly influence an individual's identity and fluency within and among different cultures.

Think about and confront your own particular biases. Do you assume because a patient has limited–English speaking ability that he or she is not literate or educated? Are you surprised when an Asian patient maintains direct eye contact throughout a visit and is forthright in her answers? How do you react to a patient's accent? Do you make assumptions about patients based on their attire, be it western or traditional? Be cautious and cognizant of your own generalizations. Although they may seem on the surface to aid you in the practice, these generalizations may limit your ability to see patients for who they truly are. Finally, **don't be afraid to ask specifics about the patient's ethnic**

or cultural identity. Inquiring in a sensitive and curious, but honest, manner gives patients a safe place to openly share beliefs and values. This allows providers easy insight into the patient's thoughts and lifestyle, while connecting with the patient and establishing a trusting provider-patient relationship. Good rapport in health care partnerships is crucial in providing individualized and effective care, as well as empowering patients to take control of their own health. This is the essence of cultural competence.

There are a number of excellent outside resources that can aid individual providers and their agencies in developing more comprehensive and appropriate cultural competency skills. Health care providers are patient advocates and must stand up to fight racism, sexism, classism, and all forms of discrimination. Therefore, it is the provider's responsibility to continually seek ways to effectively care for patients of all ethnicities and ages, understanding that cultural competence is not a destination, but an ever evolving journey.

REFERENCES

Adams, D. (1995). *Health issues for women of color: A cultural diversity perspective.* Thousand Oaks, CA: SAGE. Publications as cited on the Center for Effective Collaboration and Practice Web site. Retrieved on July 17, 2010 from http://cecp.air.org/

Centers for Disease Control and Prevention and The Merck Company Foundation. (2007). *The state of aging and health in America 2007.* Whitehouse Station, NJ: The Merck Company Foundation; 2007.: Retrieved from www.cdc.gov/aging and www.merck.com/cr

Cross, T., Bazron, B., Dennis, K., & Isaacs, M. (1989). *Towards a culturally competent system of care, volume I: A monograph on effective services for minority children who are severely emotionally disturbed.* Washington, DC: Georgetown University Child Development Center, CASSP Technical Assistance Center.

Goode, T. D., & Dunne, C. (2004). *Cultural self-assessment. From the curricula enhancement module series.* Washington, DC: National Center for Cultural Competence, Georgetown University Center for Child and Human Development.

Gregg, J., & Saha, S. (2006). Losing culture on the way to competence: The use and misuse of culture in medical education. *Academic Medicine, 81*(6), 542–547. doi:10.1097/01.ACM.0000225218.15207.30

Jacobs, E., Lauderdale, D., Meltzer, D., Shorey, J., Levinson, W., & Thisted, R. (2001). Impact of interpreter services on delivery of health care to limited–English-proficient patients. *Journal of General Internal Medicine, 16*(7), 468–474. doi:10.1046/j.1525-1497.2001.016007468.x

Ngo-Metzger, Q., Sorkin, D., Phillips, R., Greenfield, S., Massagli, M., Clarridge, B., & Kaplan, S. (2007). Proficient patients: The importance of language concordance and interpreter use. *Journal of General Internal Medicine, 22*, 324–330. doi:10.1007/s11606-007-0340-z

Sundaram, V. (2009). *Immigrants gain rights to medical interpreters.* Retrieved July 20, 2010. Retrieved from http://news.newamericamedia.org/news/view_article.html?article_id=05234777cbb7c6e5f9caec245e3e9942

ADDITIONAL RESOURCES

Center for Effective Collaboration and Practice, part of the American Institutes for Research, is a great resource with information on specific issues and a Web site dedicated specifically to cultural competence. Web site: http://cecp.air.org/

Management Sciences Health—A Provider's Guide to Quality and Culture is a tremendous resource for addressing and improving intercultural health care delivery. Web site: www.msh.org

National Center for Cultural Competence through the Georgetown University Center for Child and Human Development has another excellent Web site with a plethora of information. Web site: http://www11.georgetown.edu/research/gucchd/nccc/

Tsend, W. S. and Streltzer, J. *Cultural Competence in Health Care* (2007) is a comprehensive text on intercultural communication, advocacy, and social justice in the health care environment. Available online through Springer U.S. online. doi: 10.1007/978-0-387-72171-2

Unequal treatment: *Confronting Racial and Ethnic Disparities in Health Care* (2003). Written by the Board on Health Sciences Policy and available through the National Academies Press online: http://books.nap.edu/openbook.php?isbn=030908265X&page=R1#pagetop

Case 1.3 The Ugly Face of Ageism

By Shelley Yerger Hawkins, DSN, APRN, FNP, GNP, FAANP

Mrs. U presents to the primary care practice for an initial visit. She has been a patient at another local practice; but due to changes in insurance with her recent retirement, she is required to change providers. Mrs. U is a 70-year-old woman who is generally healthy with Type 2 diabetes mellitus (T2DM) and osteoarthritis of the knees and hips. At the time that she was diagnosed with T2DM 5 years ago, Mrs. U met with a diabetes educator and subsequently developed an individualized management plan that she has tried to maintain.

However, she does not regularly exercise or perform self–blood glucose checks outside of having her glucose checked when having a follow-up visit for her T2DM. She claims that she had her glucose checked 3 months, ago and "It was fine." Mrs. U has no surgical history. Her last menstrual period was 16 years ago. She has never married and has no children. She has a high school education and spent most of her life working in retail sales which allowed her to live a modest lifestyle and build a small savings toward retirement. She enjoys going to church twice a week and has several longtime female friends. One of those friends never married; and they are especially close.

She has no history of smoking or alcohol use. She admits that caffeine consumption is "a bad habit" since she consumes 2–3 eight-ounce cups of coffee daily and has an equal number of Diet Cokes. She drinks 1–2 eight-ounce glasses of water daily from the tap since she avoids the expense of purchasing bottled water. She has two siblings, a 74-year-old brother and a 68-year-old sister, with families who are not geographically accessible without long-distance travel. Both

Case Studies in Gerontological Nursing for the Advanced Practice Nurse, First Edition.
Edited by Meredith Wallace Kazer, Leslie Neal-Boylan.
© 2012 John Wiley & Sons, Inc. Published 2012 by John Wiley & Sons, Inc.

siblings are reasonably healthy and have T2DM. Both parents are deceased, having died from heart disease and marginally managed late life T2DM. During her visit, review of systems is negative with the exception of frequent urination. She acknowledges that she noticed "some" urinary frequency and urgency during the past several months attributing it to the stress associated with retirement.

She experienced one episode of having an accident when she could not make it to the bathroom in time to urinate. This occurred during the daytime. She denies any nocturia, burning, pain, color changes, or odor associated with urination. She denies a history of vaginal infections or urinary tract infections. Denies fatigue or falls. Mrs. U states that her best friend has been wearing a sanitary napkin since she has constant problems with urinary leaking and that she does not want to get to that point in her life. She has daily bowel movements and has not experienced any changes with her defecation patterns.

Medications: Glucophage, 500 mg twice daily; Aleve, as needed

Allergies: NKDA

OBJECTIVE

Awake, alert, and oriented x4. Mild kyphosis. Dress is appropriate for setting and season. Responds to questions appropriately but often avoids eye contact. Follows commands and moves carefully when changing from a sitting-to-standing position. Neurological exam intact with 2+ deep-tendon reflexes bilaterally intact. Gross vision and hearing tests are normal.

PERRLA. Tympanic membranes intact without cerumen. Weight: 145 lb; height: 5 ft 5 inches; BP: 135/80; P: 80; RR: 16; T: 97.2. Skin dry and intact. Cardiac exam reveals normal S1 and S2 without adventitious sounds. Lungs clear to auscultation. Normoactive bowel sounds; umbilicus midline; and no scars or pulsations. No suprapubic distention or tenderness. No hepatosplenomegaly. Perineum without redness, discharge, or excoriation. Peripheral pulses intact with trace pedal edema.

Good upper extremity range of motion with no joint tenderness or erythema noted. Lower extremity range of motion slightly decreased in knees and hips. No joint tenderness or erythema noted over lower joint sites.

ASSESSMENT

Urinary Incontinence (UI): Mrs. U has urinary frequency and urgency during the past 3–4 weeks, coupled with urinary leakage that has resulted in uncontrolled urination prior to reaching a bathroom. It is important to note that older adults often develop UI, and both the patient and provider tend not to discuss it.

Urinary Tract Infection (UTI): Many older adults do not present with the classic signs and symptoms such as burning, dysuria, frequency, nocturia, urgency, strong odor, fever, or back pain. Atypical presentations such as new onset of UI or increase in incontinent episodes may be indicative of a UTI. Thus, a bladder infection may be the source of her symptoms.

Uncontrolled T2DM: Mrs. U has T2DM which can alter the neurological integrity of the bladder over time. Given that she has experienced increased urinary frequency and urgency, it may be that her glucose is elevated. There are no medical records to review; and, even though Mrs. U states that her last glucose was "fine," there are no documented readings.

DIAGNOSTICS

It is essential that health care providers perform a comprehensive health history and physical examination when an older patient experiences changes in physical or psychological health. Often, when older adults present with an atypical presentation, essential diagnostic testing that would help establish an accurate diagnosis is excluded.

Mrs. U is a new patient at the practice, and her medical records have not been transferred from her previous practice. Unfortunately in this case, ageism is affecting the health care provider's selection of diagnostic testing and subsequent plan of care. Ageism can affect differential treatment, since beliefs and attitudes about older adults can translate into discriminatory practices, especially in a cost-conscious climate. The health care provider elects to exclude a urinalysis since Mrs. U is experiencing "normal" urinary changes due to aging that are likely being exacerbated by stress due to her recent lifestyle changes. Since Mrs. U does have T2DM, an HbA1c and metabolic panel are ordered.

Test results: HbA1c: 7.1 mg/dL; metabolic panel within normal limits.

CRITICAL THINKING

What is the most likely differential diagnosis and why?

What is the plan of treatment?

What is the plan for follow-up care?

Does the patient's psychosocial history impact how the clinician might treat her?

How would diagnostic testing and subsequent treatment be different for this patient without the influence of ageism?

ADVANCED PRACTICE CRITICAL THINKING

How can the use of telemedicine with older adults discourage ageism?

What web-based resources can the clinician offer to older adult patients with UI?

RESOLUTION

What is the most likely differential diagnosis and why?
Urinary incontinence is an obvious differential diagnosis, given that Mrs. U is a 70-year-old female who presents with urinary frequency and urgency. Overall, she is feeling well but is bothered by these symptoms. UI is not a normal part of aging. It is a loss of urine control due to a combination of factors including genitourinary pathology, age-related changes, comorbid conditions, medications, and/or functional impairments (Reuben et al., 2010). It is well established in the literature that patients do not typically talk about details related to urinary habits and that many providers do not ask probing questions to establish that, indeed, a patient does have UI (Smith, 2006). Furthermore, the health care provider should explore the possibility that the urinary changes are associated with the patient's T2DM. UI has been associated with the neuropathic and microvascular changes that occur in the urinary system in patients with T2DM. Research demonstrates that men and women with DM are more likely to experience UI and experience more severe leakage than nondiabetic patients (Lifford, Curhan, Hu, Barbieri, & Grodstein, 2005). Unfortunately, in this case the provider's professional behaviors are affected by ageism; and Mrs. U's urinary signs and symptoms are interpreted as normal and with no possible physiological basis. Often, ageism results in either a misdiagnosis or a patient being destined to live with UI and its potential complications without assistance.

Another possible differential diagnosis is a urinary tract infection. Even though Mrs. U does not present with the classic signs and symptoms of a UTI, this diagnosis must be explored. Health care providers working with older adults must understand that what they "see" as an initial presentation of illness may not be the baseline status for the patient (Gray-Micelli, Aselage, & Mezey, 2010). According to Gray-Micelli (2008), a critical component of geriatric assessment is looking beyond the symptoms to determine if a reversible underlying cause exists. Mrs. U presents with new onset of UI or an increase in UI that is suggestive of a UTI; the classic signs and symptoms such as burning, dysuria, nocturia, strong odor, changes in urine appearance, fever, and low back or abdominal pain are absent (Mauk, 2010). However, since no urinalysis was ordered, there are no objective data to support a diagnosis of UTI.

Uncontrolled T2DM is another differential diagnosis since Mrs. U was diagnosed with T2DM 5 years ago and since the provider has no medical records to determine the extent of her control.

She tells the provider that she does not perform self–blood-glucose monitoring (SBGM) and that her last lab was 3 months ago. Even though complications of T2DM such as cardiovascular disease, balance and gait disturbances, and retinopathy are often presenting symptoms in an older adult, acute symptomatology such as polyuria and UI must be explored (Mauk, 2010). It is unlikely though that her T2DM is the source of her recent urinary changes since her HbA1c is 7.1 mg/dL. According to the American Diabetes Association 2010 guidelines, HbA1c should be <7.0 mg/dL.

What is the plan of treatment?
Based on the data collected by this health care provider, a diagnosis of UI is established, keeping in mind that ageism has played a significant role in the interaction of this health care provider with this older adult patient. Even though much detail was not obtained surrounding Mrs. U's urinary changes, the provider explained to Mrs. U that given her age she is highly susceptible to urinary changes and that this is a normal part of aging. She was advised to stop drinking carbonated beverages and caffeinated coffee since both may cause bladder irritation and spasms resulting in urinary frequency and urgency (Bradway & Cacchione, 2010). She was advised to eliminate these bladder irritants from her diet one at a time with evaluation of effectiveness in 7–10 days. She was advised to increase her water consumption to 6–8 eight-ounce glasses of water daily. Mrs. U agreed to sign a release for her medical records from her previous health care provider.

What is the plan for follow-up care?
Mrs. U was asked to schedule a follow-up appointment in 3–4 weeks. By that time, she should experience some improvement in her urinary frequency and urgency due to dietary changes. Hopefully, she will have adapted to her lifestyle change, too, since leaving the work force is also a normal part of aging. Once her medical records have been transferred, a more comprehensive review of her overall health can be made. It is probable that tighter control of her glucose will be a focus given her age, recent lifestyle change, and strong family history of

T2DM. The provider does not believe that Mrs. U will incorporate behavioral changes into her lifestyle; therefore, minimal time will be spent on dietary, exercise, and blood-glucose monitoring since she seems to maintain adequate control of her T2DM.

Does the patient's psychosocial history impact how the clinician might treat her?
Mrs. U has experienced a major developmental milestone with her retirement. However, since this is a normal part of aging, the provider will probably spend minimal or no time discussing it. Recognition of this life change should be addressed by acknowledging it and engaging in some conversation about her thoughts and feelings as well as her future plans. Furthermore, Mrs. U did mention that her friend uses sanitary napkins to manage her urinary frequency and that she did not want to "reach that point". A prudent provider who approaches all patients with the idea that everyone should receive comparable health care regardless of age would talk with Mrs. U about the use of absorbent products and that they should not be relied upon as the sole, or even as a primary, strategy for management of UI (Bradway & Cacchione, 2010). Urinary problems are embarrassing and can lead to social isolation and depression. Mrs. U is especially susceptible since she recently retired and will likely be spending much more time alone.

ADVANCED PRACTICE CRITICAL THINKING

How would diagnostic testing and subsequent treatment be different for this patient without the influence of ageism?
It is absolutely essential to diagnostically exclude all possible differential diagnoses regardless of the patient's age. In this situation, the influence of ageism caused the provider to have a narrow scope and prejudicial attitude with diagnosis and management. A urinalysis must be ordered in order to rule out bacteriuria. In this case, the patient experienced symptomatic bacteriuria since she had urinary frequency and urgency, as opposed to asymptomatic bacteriuria whereby the patient presents without signs or symptoms. Risk factors for UTI in Mrs. U include T2DM, female gender, and recent onset of urinary frequency and urgency. A reasonably prudent provider who was practicing without the influence of ageism would have ordered a urinalysis at the time of the patient's office visit. The urinalysis would have yielded >10^5 cfu/mL confirming pyuria. Bactrim DS, one tablet twice daily by mouth for 10 days, would have been prescribed. Mrs. U would have been scheduled to return for another urinalysis within 1 week of completing the antibiotic unless she developed new symptomatology (Reuben et al., 2010).

How can the use of telemedicine with older adults discourage ageism?
Ageism is systematic stereotyping of and discrimination against people
because of old age (Kane, Preister, & Neumann, 2007). Attitudinal and
behavioral components are typically present so that both prejudicial
beliefs and attitudes exist along with discrimination against or inappropriate negative treatment toward old age. Often, older adults have
availability and accessibility challenges to health care resources due to
factors such as limited or no transportation, lack of funds to support
travel to and from health care sites, and lack of health care providers
trained in geriatrics. As a result, resources and opportunities for health
care often are not provided or deemed appropriate since allocation of
resources favor younger patients. Even though there continues to be
ambivalence regarding use of telemedicine devices with older adults
due to sensory and cognitive changes resulting from aging, the amount
of ongoing research in this area continues to grow, since bringing health
care into the older adult patient's home can resolve many of these
issues. By offering remote monitoring of physiological indicators, educational interventions, and the mere interaction with a health care
provider in a home setting, health care resources are made available to
older adults. Various types of telemedicine devices can help to discourage the concept of ageism.

**What Web-based resources can the clinician offer to older adult
patients with UI?**
American Geriatrics Society at http://www.americangeriatrics.org
American Journal of Nursing, *How to Try This* at http://links.lww.
    com/A311
ConsultGeriRN.org at http://consultgerirn.org
National Association for Continence at http://www/nafc.org
National Institute of Aging at http://www.nia.nih.gov/
    Healthinformation/Publications/urinary.htm
Society of Urologic Nurses and Associates at http://www.suna.org
Wound, Ostomy, and Continence Nurses Society at http://www.wocn.
    org

REFERENCES

American Diabetes Association (2010). Retrieved on August 7, 2010, from
    http://www.diabetes.org/diabetes-statistics
Bradway, C., & Cacchione, P. (2010). Teaching strategies for assessing and
    managing urinary incontinence in older adults. *Journal of Gerontological
    Nursing, 36*(7), 18–26.
Gray-Micelli, D. (2008). *Modification of assessment and atypical presentation in older
    adults with complex illness.* Retrieved from the Hartford Institute for Geriatric
    Nursing Web site at http//hartfordign.org/uploads/File/gnec_state_of_
    science_papers/gnec_atypical_presentations.pdf

Gray-Micelli, D., Aselage, M., & Mezey, M. (2010). Teaching strategies for atypical presentation of illness in older adults. *Journal of Gerontological Nursing*, *36*(7), 38–43.

Kane, K., Preister, R., & Neumann, D. (2007). Does disparity in the way disabled older adults are treated imply ageism? *The Gerontologist*, *47*(3), 271–279.

Lifford, K., Curhan, G., Hu, F., Barbieri, R., & Grodstein, F. (2005). Type 2 diabetes mellitus and risk of developing urinary incontinence. *Journal of the American Geriatrics Society*, *53*(11), 1851–1857.

Mauk, K. (2010). *Gerontological nursing: Competencies for care* (2nd ed.). Boston, MA: Jones & Bartlett.

Reuben, D., Herr, K., Pacala, J., Pollock, B., Potter, J., & Semla, T. (2010). *Geriatrics at your fingertips* (12th ed.). New York: American Geriatrics Society.

Smith, D. (2006). Urinary incontinence and diabetes: A review. *Journal of Wound, Ostomy, and Continence Nursing*, *33*(6), 619–624.

ADDITIONAL RESOURCES

Kagan, S. (2008). Ageism in cancer care. *Seminars in Oncology Nursing*, *24*(4), 246–253.

Ory, M., Hoffman, M., Hawkins, M., Sanner, B., & Mockenhaupt, R. (2003). Challenging aging stereotypes: Strategies for creating a more active society. *American Journal of Preventive Medicine*, *25*(3), 164–171.

Palmore, E. (1999). *Ageism: Negative and positive*. New York: Springer.

Tannenbaum, C., Brouillette, J., Michaud, J., . . . Valiquette, L. (2009). Responsiveness and clinical utility of the Geriatric Self-Efficacy Index for Urinary Incontinence. *Journal of the American Geriatrics Society*, *57*(3), 470–475.

Case 1.4 If Only We Had National Health Insurance

By Philip A. Greiner, DNSc, RN

Mr. B arrives for his regularly scheduled appointment at a private, internal medicine practice near his home. After Mr. B waited briefly to be seen, the clinician who provides primary care to Mr. B knocks and enters the examination room. The clinician greets Mr. B and asks him how he is feeling today. Mr. B promptly raises his voice and replies, "How am I feeling? How would you feel if you got a bill like this?" He waives what appears to be a bill from Medicare in front of the clinician and speaks with anger about his recent Medicare bill. The clinician listens carefully to his content and tone. It seems that Mr. B had received a statement from his Medicare Advantage Plan provider indicating the amount of the last office visit expenses that Mr. B was responsible for paying. It is quite clear that Mr. B is unhappy with this bill.

By asking some further questions for clarification, the clinician engages Mr. B; and he becomes calmer and less confrontational. The clinician proceeds through the objective part of the exam; but she suggests that Mr. B should meet with her and the office billing manager after the visit to determine what elements of his care were not covered by Medicare and to revise his plan of health care accordingly. Mr. B agrees to this plan. He also expresses his gratitude for this suggestion and apologizes for his tone, but his frustration about the cost of health care and the confusing nature of the billing process is evident.

Upon further assessment Mr. B is found to have no health complaints. He has no surgical history. He is a widow with 3 adult children. He has a high school education and has spent most of his life working as a courier. He is involved in an intimate relationship with a

Case Studies in Gerontological Nursing for the Advanced Practice Nurse, First Edition.
Edited by Meredith Wallace Kazer, Leslie Neal-Boylan.
© 2012 John Wiley & Sons, Inc. Published 2012 by John Wiley & Sons, Inc.

"girlfriend". He states that they practice safe sex. He has no history of smoking. He drinks alcohol socially. He has 1 brother who is healthy; and both of his parents are deceased, having died from unknown causes when he was in his early thirties.

OBJECTIVE

Mr. B is a healthy older adult who is currently being well managed for hypertension with lisinopril 5 mg daily and for osteoarthritis, for which he takes acetaminophen as needed. During this visit, his blood pressure is elevated to 154/92; and his pulse is rapid at 92. He states, "I am very scared because I don't have the kind of money to pay this bill." Although he is anxious, he is awake, alert, and oriented. He has erect posture and is clean and well kept. His clothes are appropriate for the weather. He is 5 ft 7 inches and weighs 140 lb. His oxygen saturation is at 98%, and his lungs are clear. He has no pedal edema. He does not smoke; he drinks socially; and he walks daily for exercise. He states that he takes his medication every day without fail and needs only an occasional acetaminophen to control his arthritis pain.

After completing the history and physical examination, the clinician and Mr. B meet with the billing manager. Mr. B states that, since he is healthy, he opted several months ago to change traditional Medicare to a Medicare Advantage Plan (Medicare Part C) that emphasized health promotion and clinical prevention in keeping with the purpose of periodic primary provider visits. While the premium for this plan was lower than what he had been paying, office visits required a larger deductible and higher co-payments for services as compared to traditional Medicare. Mr. B thought he was selecting a less-expensive health plan than traditional Medicare without realizing that he would need to pay more out-of-pocket expenses for illness visits to the primary care provider. Given Mr. B's good health status, the nurse practitioner (NP) confirmed that the Medicare Advantage Plan was appropriate for Mr. B. The business manager also verified his income status, which was high enough to disqualify him for additional coverage through Medicaid.

The office manager asked Mr. B some basic questions about his Medicare coverage. Upon further questioning, it was determined that Mr. B was unclear of the choices he made during his selection of policy options when he opted for the Medicare Advantage Plan. This situation is common among older adults who were used to traditional Medicare coverage or are newly eligible for Medicare coverage. The advent of Medicare Part C, Medicare Advantage Plans, allowed insurance companies to market their various plans to older adults. While the Center for Medicare and Medicaid Studies (CMS) requires all Medicare

Advantage Plans to have certain services and to provide assistance to older adults to help them understand these plans, it is easy to become overwhelmed and confused in the process. The Medicare.gov Web site can be very helpful in determining the types of coverage available in the area and the costs associated with the various plans; but it means that the older adult must have computer access, be used to searching online, be comfortable navigating the Internet, or have assistance with the process.

ASSESSMENT

Hypertension: While Mr. B's blood pressure was elevated today, it was likely because of his anger and frustration related to the medical insurance coverage change and his lack of understanding of health insurance coverage options. The clinician rechecks Mr. B's blood pressure after his meeting with her and the billing manager and before making any changes in his medication. She also confirms that he is taking his prescribed medications as per his plan and that he is maintaining moderate physical activity most days a week, limiting alcohol, and eating a diet representative of the major food groups.

Osteoarthritis—stable: The clinician confirms that Mr. B's arthritis pain is well managed with over-the-counter medications as per his plan and that he is working to maintain physical activity.

CRITICAL THINKING

Are there various Medicare Part C plans available in the geographic or service area?

What would be the next steps in working with Mr. B?

What resources are available in the service area to assist Mr. B with Medicare questions?

Are assistance and education, such as those described above, billable services?

RESOLUTION

Are there various Medicare Part C plans available in the geographic or service area?

The answer to this question should be a resounding "Yes!" But all too often clinicians are removed from the billing process and are less knowledgeable about payment plans than they need to be. A quick source available to all clinicians is the regional Area Agency on Aging (AAA) (Department of Health & Human Services, 2010). These federally funded agencies are located in every region of the United States and provide information and assistance to older adult residents, their caregivers, and the general public within their area. Each of these agencies must provide an area plan for enhancing the services for older adults in their area, current information on the older adult population, and services to assist older adults and their caregivers in obtaining available services, including information on Medicare and related health plan options in the region.

What would be the next steps in working with Mr. B?
It is important that the clinician anticipate the broader care needs of patients, not just the presenting health problems. One of the challenges of working in most clinical settings is the emphasis placed on timely patient management by the clinician. The clinician can make the case for having others within the health care team prepared to lend assistance in working to meet patient needs and for having systems in place for capturing relevant data to assist in care delivery. In addition, The Joint Commission requires reporting on the environment of care. The environment of care includes the physical plant, utilities, and service contracts for needed services; but it can also include space and Internet access if deemed necessary for adequate delivery of care. This approach may also require all involved to think of expanding the idea of the care delivery team to include other people within the agency who may not be first line providers. Consider involving the most appropriate people within the organization to best meet the needs of the patient. Review how the patient care team in this case study resolved the patient care needs:

Together with the business manager, the clinician reviewed Mr. B's Medicare Advantage Plan in detail with him to identify ways that he could minimize out-of-pocket costs and maximize his health care benefit. One of the key features of his plan was preventive health visits. Mr. B agreed to schedule a preventive health visit. The business manager called the Medicare Advantage Plan administrator and arranged for a representative to visit Mr. B to go over current plan options and to prepare for the next open enrollment period if changes to Mr. B's plan were needed. Mr. B was also encouraged to ask for information and support when he felt confused by his health care, as the education of patients about their chronic disease and related health care coverage is a critical part of patient-centered care.

The clinician took Mr. B's BP after the discussion with the billing manager and found that it had returned to 128/80. Thus, the clinician made no changes in his medication. She encouraged him to continue taking his prescribed medication and to maintain his fitness and nutritional schedule. She also suggested that he might consider adding yoga or other means of stress management to his daily health routine. Finally, she suggested that he buy a home BP monitor to track his blood pressure. She provided him with a copy of normal BP guidelines and advised him to call the office if his blood pressure is above the range on 3 consecutive readings. She also advises Mr. B to call and make an appointment if his arthritis pain increases or he has any other change in his health status. In this way, Mr. B may be able to take better control over his health and may avoid unnecessary medical appointments that he cannot afford.

What resources are available in the service area to assist Mr. B with Medicare questions?

Clinicians are often asked to address issues that they feel are outside of their areas of expertise. Information on health care coverage may be an area with which many providers are unfamiliar. While it is not practical that clinicians be familiar with all aspects of every plan, they should have a general working knowledge of the health insurance options for their service population. More importantly, they should know where patients or family members can obtain information and guidance related to available health plans.

As mentioned above, the regional Area Agency on Aging is a primary resource for older adults to find information on available Medicare Advantage Plans in the state. Many states also provide information on state Internet sites and related links, such as those for the Department of Public Health, the Office of the Insurance Commissioner, or the Office of the Attorney General. Information on plan availability should also be available from the organization's business office or insurance contact.

Are assistance and education, such as those described above, billable services?

Patient education to manage chronic health problems is considered an integral part of the provision of care. It is the clinician's responsibility to explore areas where the patient is unable to adhere to the mutually defined plan of care, identify potential and real barriers to adherence, and modify the plan of care based on an assessment of the patient's needs. In this case study, the patient was unable to adhere to the plan of care due to his failure to understand his insurance coverage. Improper use of services and misunderstanding of coverage options are barriers to access to care and are concerns that the clinician should address. Health literacy, computer literacy, access to information, and the ability to incorporate information into health action are areas to which the clinicians should attend. This patient-centered approach to care makes it necessary for the clinicians to know a great deal about their patients and the service area.

The clinician should meet with the Chief Financial Officer (CFO) and/or billing officer to determine the most appropriate billing codes to use in such situations. In every case, the documentation of the services provided, the need for such services, and the outcome of the service provision are keys to the reimbursement for these services. Describe how the lack of information about health plans presented a barrier to care access, how the clinician assessed the need for intervention, how the patient responded to the plan components, and the outcome(s) of the intervention, especially any revisions in the plan of care. The ability to link the intervention to the issue of access to care for ongoing chronic disease management is important to obtaining reimbursement.

TOOLBOX

Questions that may be added to Annual Patient Information and Intake forms:

- **Do you use a computer, smart phone, or iPad on a regular basis?**
- **Are you able to use the Internet on your own or with some help?**
- **Do you or a close friend get information from Internet sources?**
- **If asked to find information on the Internet, do you feel confident that you could find the information on your own?**
- **Which icon (picture or word) on your computer screen would you click to get to the Internet?**

REFERENCES

Department of Health & Human Services (2010). *Home Page*. Retrieved July 30, 2010, from Administration on Aging Web site: www.hhs.gov/open/contacts/aoa.html

Medicare (2010). *Medicare Home Page*. Retrieved July 39, 2010, from the Medicare Web site: http://www.medicare.gov/

Section 2

Common Health Challenges of Aging

Case 2.1 The Heart of It All

By Jaclyn R. Jones, MSN, APRN, NP-C

Mrs. S, a 78-year-old female, presents to the clinic complaining of difficulty catching her breath and persistent indigestion. She is a well-established patient at the clinic. With the exception of today's visit, she describes her overall health as good. Her medical history includes hypertension, dyslipidemia (both well controlled with medications and lifestyle management), and osteoarthritis. Her surgical history consists of a Cesarean section 40 years ago and a total right knee replacement 5 years ago without complications. She is recently widowed and lives alone within a retirement community complex. She has 2 daughters and 5 grandchildren who live in different states. She is a nonsmoker and drinks 2–3 glasses of wine per month. Her physical activity is limited secondary to osteoarthritis of her knees and hips; but she participates in aquatic aerobics every Monday and Wednesday morning although, since her husband's death 6 months ago, she has not been going regularly. She is actively involved in the retirement community, where she serves as a board member and is one of the social chairs for the clubhouse. Her mother, a lifelong smoker, died at age 65 from lung cancer; her father had a history of hypertension and died at age 80 from pneumonia. Her sister is a breast cancer survivor. There is no other significant family history.

Upon review of systems, she reports fatigue, general weakness, and indigestion discomfort on and off for 2 weeks. Her indigestion typically lasts for 5–20 minutes. She has had bouts of heartburn that typically

Case Studies in Gerontological Nursing for the Advanced Practice Nurse, First Edition.
Edited by Meredith Wallace Kazer, Leslie Neal-Boylan.
© 2012 John Wiley & Sons, Inc. Published 2012 by John Wiley & Sons, Inc.

resolve with over-the-counter (OTC) antacids, but these have not helped lately. Within the past few days, she's noticed shortness of breath (SOB), activity intolerance related to dyspnea on exertion (DOE), nausea, a nonproductive cough, and an epigastric/reflux burning sensation. Her chief complaints today are shortness of breath (SOB) and indigestion pain that does not radiate. She denies palpitations, headache, fever, chills, vomiting, and diarrhea. Her medications include losartan, 50 mg daily; lovastatin, 10 mg daily; naproxen, 250 mg twice daily as needed for pain. She is allergic to penicillin.

OBJECTIVE

Mrs. S is ambulatory, awake, alert and oriented x4. She is noticeably short of breath and appears anxious. Weight: 150 lb; height: 5 ft 4 inches; BP: 80/60; P: 106; T: 98.6; RR: 24. Chest/lungs: Diminished at bases although difficult to assess related to patient's inability to take a deep breath due to discomfort. No chest tenderness on palpation. Cardiac: Rate irregular, tachycardic; S1, S2, and S4 sounds noted. Skin: Diaphoretic, cool.

ASSESSMENT

Myocardial infarction: Patient has many symptoms that indicate cardiovascular origin, including DOE, SOB, nausea, diaphoresis, and substernal burning discomfort. She has cardiac risk factors including hypertension, age, and dyslipidemia.

Pneumonia: Mrs. S complains of fatigue, weakness, new onset of cough, and difficulty breathing, all of which point to possible respiratory infection. Older adults often do not present with classic symptoms of pneumonia that include fever, cough, and dyspnea. Sometimes the only indication is a change in the level of cognition.

Gastroesophageal Reflux Disease (GERD): She is exhibiting substernal burning pain and cough, which are signs and symptoms reflective of reflux. Chest pain from GERD can often imitate pain of a cardiac origin.

Anxiety/depression: The patient recently lost her husband. Shortness of breath, fatigue, and weakness could be a panic attack with possible underlying depression.

DIAGNOSTICS

EKG reveals some ST depression in leads V1 and V2 suggestive of posterior heart ischemia. Cardiac enzymes and CXR should be deferred to emergency department.

CRITICAL THINKING

What is the most likely differential diagnosis and why?

What is the plan of treatment?

What is the plan for follow-up care?

Does the patient's psychosocial history impact how the clinician might treat this patient?

What if the patient also had kidney failure?

With the differentials listed, what are the best treatment options for this patient?

Are there any standardized guidelines that the clinician should use to assess or treat this patient?

RESOLUTION

What is the most likely differential diagnosis and why?
This patient is suffering from an acute myocardial infarction (AMI). Myocardial infarctions (MI) are some of the most common causes of death in the United States. The mortality for those over the age of 70 is double compared to younger adults (<65 years). MIs are more common in men than in premenopausal women, but this equalizes after menopause (Fauci et al., 2008). Chest pain is commonly regarded as the hallmark and necessary diagnostic symptom of patients with AMI; yet approximately one-third of MI patients, most of whom were over the age of 75, present without chest pain (Canto et al., 2000). Older adults often present with atypical symptoms that include dyspnea, epigastric distress, weakness, fatigue, syncope, and possibly altered mental status (Rosenthal, Williams, & Naughton, 2006). Mrs. S presents with epigastric discomfort, dyspnea, weakness, and fatigue. The office EKG shows evidence suggestive of an AMI. However, up to 25% of

patients with AMI have normal or misread EKGs; thus EKGs are not diagnostic (McCarthy, Beshansky, D'Agostino, & Selker, 1993).

What is the plan of treatment?
Mrs. S should be sent to the emergency department for a full cardiac workup to rule out myocardial infarction. While awaiting the arrival of the emergency medical system (EMS), oxygen via nasal cannula can be administered as well as a chewable aspirin. In cases of persistent chest/epigastric pain, sublingual nitroglycerin (NTG) may offer relief if it is available in the office; but since Mrs. S is hypotensive, a contraindication to NTG, it should not be administered to her. (Winters & Katzen, 2006).

What is the plan for follow-up care?
Regardless of the diagnosis, Mrs. S should have a follow-up appointment after being discharged from the hospital. With a confirmed MI, she should be referred to a cardiologist. Her primary care provider should continue to follow her for all other health care needs.

Does the patient's psychosocial history impact how the clinician might treat this patient?
Research shows that almost half of post–MI patients have either major or minor depression (Ziegelstein, 2001). Additionally, multiple studies have found that patients with depression have an increased risk of morbidity and mortality after an AMI (Rugulies, 2002; Frasure-Smith, Lesperance, Juneau, Talajic, & Bourassa, 1999; Frasure-Smith, Lesperance, & Talajic, 1995). This, coupled with Mrs. S's recent loss of her husband, warrants ongoing mental health assessment. She may benefit from mental health counseling, grief support groups, and possible pharmacological antidepressant therapy.

What if the patient also had kidney failure?
The complexity of concurrent coronary artery disease and kidney failure is best managed by a cardiologist, who has the training to treat such comorbidities, particularly since renal disease can potentiate another ischemic episode, as well as the possible renal toxic side effects of cardiovascular medications. As a primary care provider, it is crucial to evaluate any and all prescribed medications that may be contraindicated or cautionary with kidney failure.

With the differentials listed, what are the best treatment options for this patient?
1. **AMI**—The best treatment option is within an emergency room setting, where the patient will receive oxygen, 160–325 mg aspirin (if not already given), and IV medications that might include NTG, morphine, atropine, and thrombolytic therapy. Depending on the type of AMI, timing, and available resources, the patient may undergo cardiac catheterization with possible percutaneous coronary intervention (Rosenthal et al., 2006; Ryan et al., 1996).

2. **Pneumonia**—Following a **diagnosis** with chest X-ray, antibiotic therapy should be **initiated**. Sputum culture is not required for diagnosis and treatment, unless there is suspicion of drug-resistant bacteria. If the patient has multiple risk factors or comorbidities, hospitalization may be warranted (Rosenthal, et al., 2006).

3. **GERD**—There is no gold standard diagnostic tool for gastroesophageal reflux disease. Diagnosis **can** be made on history alone or by trial of proton-pump inhibitor (PPI).The patient should be given a trial of high dose proton pump inhibitors (PPIs) and educated on lifestyle modifications, including avoidance of large meals before bedtime, abstaining from lying down after eating, and decreasing or eliminating high-fat, high-carbohydrate, and acidic foods, as well as caffeine and alcohol (Goroll & Mulley, 2009).

Are there any standardized guidelines that the clinician should use to assess or treat this patient?

The American College of Cardiology and the American Heart Association have jointly published guidelines for general management of patients with AMI, management of patients with ST-elevation MI, and management of patients with unstable angina/non-ST-elevation MI (ACC/AHA, 2007; Anteman et al., 2004). The guidelines focus on treatment of MIs within emergency departments, and they also offer guiding principles for medical management post-MI after discharge from the hospital.

REFERENCES

ACC/AHA (2007). Guidelines for the management of patients with unstable angina/non-ST-elevation myocardial infarction: Executive summary: A report of the American College of Cardiology/American Heart Association task force on practice guidelines (writing committee to revise the 2002 guidelines for the management of patients with unstable Angina/ Non-ST-elevation myocardial infarction): Developed in collaboration with the American College of Emergency Physicians, the Society for Cardiovascular Angiography and Interventions, and the Society of Thoracic Surgeons: Endorsed by the American Association of Cardiovascular and Pulmonary Rehabilitation and the Society for Academic Emergency Medicine. (2007). *Circulation, 116*(7), 803–877. doi:10.1161/ CIRCULATIONAHA.107.185752.

Antman, E. M., Anbe, D. T., Armstrong, P. W., Bates, E. R., Green, L. A., Hand, M., . . . Jacobs, A. K. (2004). ACC/AHA guidelines for the management of patients with ST-elevation myocardial infarction. *Circulation, 110*(9), e82–293.

Canto, J. G., Shlipak, M. G., Rogers, W. J., Malmgren, J. A., Frederick, P. D., Lambrew, C. T., . . . Kiefe, C. I. (2000). Prevalence, clinical characteristics, and mortality among patients with myocardial infarction presenting without chest pain. *JAMA: The Journal of the American Medical Association, 283*(24), 3223–3229. doi:10.1001/jama.283.24.3223.

Fauci, A. S., Kasper, D. L., Longo, D. L., Braunwald, E., Hauser, S. L., Jameson, J. L., & Loscalzo, J. (Eds.). (2008). *Harrison's principles of internal medicine* (17th ed.). McGraw-Hill.

Frasure-Smith, N., Lesperance, F., Juneau, M., Talajic, M., & Bourassa, M. G. (1999). Gender, depression, and one-year prognosis after myocardial infarction. *Psychosomatic Medicine, 61*(1), 26–37.

Frasure-Smith, N., Lesperance, F., & Talajic, M. (1995). Depression and 18-month prognosis after myocardial infarction. *Circulation, 91*(4), 999–1005.

Goroll, A. H., & Mulley, A. G. (2009). *Primary care medicine: Office evaluation and management of the adult patient* (6th ed.). Philadelphia, PA: Wolters Kluwer Health/Lippincott Williams & Wilkins.

McCarthy, B. D., Beshansky, J. R., D'Agostino, R. B., & Selker, H. P. (1993). Missed diagnoses of acute myocardial infarction in the emergency department: Results from a multicenter study. *Annals of Emergency Medicine, 22*(3), 579–582. doi:10.1016/S0196-0644(05)81945-6.

Rosenthal, T. C., Williams, M. E., & Naughton, B. J. (Eds.). (2006). *Office care geriatrics* (1st ed.). Philadelphia, PA: Lippincott Williams & Wilkins. Retrieved from http://ovidsp.ovid.com/ovidweb.cgi?T=JS&NEWS=N&PAGE=fulltext&AN=01382628/1st_Edition/5&D=books

Rugulies, R. (2002). Depression as a predictor for coronary heart disease: A review and meta-analysis. *American Journal of Preventive Medicine, 23*(1), 51–61. doi:10.1016/S0749-3797(02)00439-7.

Ryan, T. J., Anderson, J. L., Antman, E. M., Braniff, B. A., Brooks, N. H., Califf, R. M., . . . Weaver, W. D. (1996). ACC/AHA guidelines for the management of patients with acute myocardial infarction: Executive summary: A report of the American College of Cardiology/American Heart Association Task Force on Practice Guidelines (Committee on Management of Acute Myocardial Infarction). *Circulation, 94*(9), 2341–2350.

Winters, M. E., & Katzen, S. M. (2006). Identifying chest pain emergencies in the primary care setting. *Primary Care: Clinics in Office Practice, 33*(3), 625–642. doi:10.1016/j.pop.2006.06.006.

Ziegelstein, R. C. (2001). Depression after myocardial infarction. *Cardiology in Review, 9*(1), 45–51. Retrieved from http://ovidsp.ovid.com/ovidweb.cgi?T=JS&NEWS=N&PAGE=fulltext&AN=00045415-200101000-00009&D=ovfte

ADDITIONAL RESOURCES

Alexander, K. P., Newby, L. K., Cannon, C. P., Armstrong, P. W., Gibler, W. B., Rich, M. W., . . . Ohman, E. M. (2007b). Acute coronary care in the elderly, part I: Non-ST-segment-elevation acute coronary syndromes: A scientific statement for healthcare professionals from the American Heart Association Council on Clinical Cardiology: In collaboration with the Society of Geriatric Cardiology. *Circulation, 115*(19), 2549–2569. doi:10.1161/CIRCULATIONAHA.107.182615.

Alexander, K. P., Newby, L. K., Armstrong, P. W., Cannon, C. P., Gibler, W. B., Rich, M. W., . . . Society of Geriatric, C. (2007a). Acute coronary care in the elderly, part II: ST-segment-elevation myocardial infarction: A scientific statement for healthcare professionals from the American Heart Association Council on Clinical Cardiology: In collaboration with the Society of Geriatric Cardiology. *Circulation, 115*(19), 2570–2589. Retrieved from http://ovidsp. ovid.com/ovidweb.cgi?T=JS&NEWS=N&PAGE=fulltext&AN=17502591& D=medl

Mehta, R. H., Rathore, S. S., Radford, M. J., Wang, Y., Wang, Y., & Krumholz, H. M. (2001). Acute myocardial infarction in the elderly: Differences by age. *Journal of the American College of Cardiology, 38*(3), 736–741. doi:10.1016/ S0735-1097(01)01432-2.

Solomon, C. G., Lee, T. H., Cook, E. F., Weisberg, M. C., Brand, D. A., Rouan, G. W., & Goldman, L. (1989). Comparison of clinical presentation of acute myocardial infarction in patients older than 65 years of age to younger patients: The multicenter chest pain study experience. *American Journal of Cardiology, 63*(12), 772–776. Retrieved from http://ovidsp.ovid.com/ ovidweb.cgi?T=JS&NEWS=N&PAGE=fulltext&AN=2648786&D=med3

Then, K. L., Rankin, J. A., & Fofonoff, D. A. (2001). Atypical presentation of acute myocardial infarction in 3 age groups. *Heart & Lung: The Journal of Acute and Critical Care, 30*(4), 285–293. doi:10.1067/mhl.2001.116010.

Case 2.2 I Have This Thing on My Skin

By Everol M. Ennis, Jr., MSN, APRN, A/GNP-BC

Miss L is a 69-year-old Vietnamese woman who has had a medical home at our primary care center over the past 2 years. Today she is complaining of "back and chest pain with an itchy rash all on my left side" for the past 4 days. She states that the pain and itching lasted all day and night and prevented her from sleeping for the past 2 nights. Miss L describes the pain as "sharp" and "burning" and says that it is aggravated by "anything touching the rash" (e.g., clothes). Miss L has tried no treatment for relief of her signs and symptoms. She denies recent outdoor activities; new purchases; new contacts, foods, or medications; change to her routine; fever; or stressors.

Her previous comprehensive physical exam and lab work approximately 3 months ago had no abnormal findings. Miss L was diagnosed with scoliosis as a child along with several other "childhood illness" that she cannot specifically recall. Miss L had a recent episode of otitis media about 1 month ago that was treated successfully with a course of antibiotics. Overall, Miss L is a healthy woman with essentially no health issues.

Miss L is an unemployed widow, who has no children and lives alone. Her neighbor reports that she checks on her daily and states that Miss L is usually in a good mood; which is consistent with her affect at all of her previous visits. Miss L denies tobacco, alcohol, and illicit drug use. She also denies being sexually active for the past 20 years. Miss L has a third-grade education and spent time in a refugee camp as a young child and then again prior to arriving in the United States 4 years ago. As a result, Miss L speaks very little English. Her neighbor

Case Studies in Gerontological Nursing for the Advanced Practice Nurse, First Edition.
Edited by Meredith Wallace Kazer, Leslie Neal-Boylan.
© 2012 John Wiley & Sons, Inc. Published 2012 by John Wiley & Sons, Inc.

always accompanies her to her office visits and serves as a translator. Due to the language challenges, getting an accurate and detailed history is especially important at Miss L's appointments. Miss L's medications include a daily multivitamin. She has no known allergies to drugs, food, or substances.

OBJECTIVE

Miss L's general appearance reflects that she is well groomed and well nourished. She appears to be uncomfortable and does not have her usual pleasant affect. She is alert and responding appropriately to all questions. Her posture is slighted skewed to the left as a result of her scoliosis but her weight and height are stable at 96 lb and 57 inches for a BMI of 21. Her vital signs are BP: 119/71; P: 72 bpm; RR: 16 bpm; T: 98.1; P: 8/10. Cardiac exam reveals regular rhythm and rate, S1, S2 with no murmurs, gallops, or rubs. Her respiratory rhythm and depth are normal, and her lungs are clear to auscultation bilaterally. On examination of her rash, Miss L has a series of clustered and confluent vesicles on an erythematous base with vesicle colors alternating between red and clear. The vesicles are ipsilateral on her left side running from her sternum just below her breast along her rib cage to the middle of her back in a crescent shape.

ASSESSMENT

Primary varicella (primary chickenpox): Given the prevalence of varicella infection, the vesicular and pruritic nature of the lesions, and the time of year (varicella epidemics occur in winter and spring—Wolff, Johnson, Suurmond, 2005), it is important to differentiate primary varicella from other skin conditions with similar symptoms and presentations.

Contact dermatitis: Miss L's skin infection seems to have taken on a very specific crescent-shaped pattern just below the breast around to the back, similar to that of a brassiere. A new clothing item (e.g., underwear) is often identified as the source of many contact dermatitis rashes.

Impetigo: The most common cause of impetigo is *staphylococcus aureus* which can be present in the natural flora of skin. The blisters and bullae of impetigo are vesicular in nature and similar in appearance to Miss L's skin rash. Patients with impetigo have also reported "itching" and "tenderness" at the center.

Herpes zoster: Herpes zoster has a vesicular appearance similar to varicella and also has painful and pruritic skin lesions.

DIAGNOSTICS

Miss L's, complaint of left-sided chest pain called for an electrocardiogram (EKG) to rule out chest pain related to cardiac disease. Ruling out cardiac chest pain allowed the clinical decision making process to proceed more comfortably. Although it was not utilized in Miss L's case, obtaining blood work and bacterial or viral cultures is an option that also will help to make the diagnosis more definitive. If a viral etiology is suspected as the cause of the rash, there are some additional considerations when contemplating lab work.

Varicella-zoster vaccine (VZV) antigen detection, viral culture, and a Tzanck smear are all available as laboratory options but have some specificity/sensitivity issues (Dworkin et al., 2007). The polymerase chain reaction (PCR) technique is the most sensitive and specific test but availability of the technique may pose a problem (Roxas, 2006). In addition, it is important to consider under what conditions a laboratory examination would be utilized. These decisions are often based on available resources to both the provider and patient and how the findings will impact the decision making and course of treatment. A laboratory workup is rarely needed or utilized for the above diagnosis because patient history and clinical presentation provide sufficient evidence for diagnosis (Wolff et al., 2005). Nevertheless, as a general rule, the more information available to support the diagnosis, the more accurate the clinician will be.

CRITICAL THINKING

What is the most likely differential diagnosis and why?

What are Miss L's risk factors that support the differential diagnosis (DDX)?

What is the most appropriate plan of treatment for Miss L?

What other interventions are important to prevent secondary complications?

What are the plans for follow-up care for Miss L?

Does the patient's psychosocial history impact how the clinician might treat this patient?

What if the patient also had kidney failure?

Considering the differentials listed, what are the best treatment options for this patient?

Are there any standardized guidelines that the clinician should use to assess or treat this patient?

RESOLUTION

What is the most likely differential diagnosis and why?

Contact dermatitis is used to describe the inflammatory reaction that occurs when a substance (i.e., irritant or allergen) comes into contact with the skin (Wolff et al., 2005). In Miss L's case, based on the crescent pattern of the lesions just below the breast, the suspected cause is her brassiere. However, if the lesions were in fact from her undergarment, a bilateral pattern of eruption where the brassiere came into contact with the skin would be expected. In addition, her history does not support the likelihood of an allergic reaction. With the bacterial infection of impetigo, lesions can be widespread and localized. However, impetigo most commonly occurs on the face and intertriginous spaces and is more common in children. There is often the characteristic honey-colored crust that is present with minimal erythema (Habif, Campbell, Chapman, Dinulos, Zug, 2005; Wolff et al., 2005). The absence of these findings lowers the suspicion of impetigo as the cause of Miss L's skin condition. One of the herpes virus infections (varicella vs. herpes zoster) is probably the cause of Miss L's dermatological condition.

Varicella, also known as chickenpox, is the **primary** form of the infection caused by the varicella-zoster virus (VZV). Varicella lesions have vesicular and at times bullous appearances and are described as pruritic and sometimes painful. The distribution of the skin lesions is less localized and more widespread to include the face, trunk, and extremities. Varicella is very common and highly contagious. In fact, over 90% of the adult population has been infected with the varicella virus (Roxas, 2006). However, in 90% of those cases, the infection occurred in children younger than 10 years old; fewer than 5% of the cases occur in persons older than 15 years old (Wolff et al., 2005). This clearly indicates that varicella is an infection that occurs in younger years. Based on Miss L's age and the distribution of her skin lesions, the suspicion for herpes zoster is increased.

Herpes zoster (HZ) or shingles is the **latent** form of the varicella infection. It is a reactivation of varicella after a person has contracted chickenpox previously. Because the virus lies dormant in nerve roots, reactivation of the virus causes a very painful experience. Descriptions such as "burning" or "sharp" are often associated with zoster pain, which is likely due to its innervations of nerve roots. The pain and vesicles often follow a pathway known as dermatomes. Dermatomes are areas of the skin that are supplied with nerves (Reuben, et al., 2007). In the overwhelming majority of the cases, the pain and lesions are almost always unilateral along one or more contiguous dermatomes. The dermatomes from T3 to L3 are most commonly involved in herpes zoster (Roxas, 2006). Eruption along any of those specific dermatomes would explain the unilateral crescent shape of Miss L's skin lesions. Being an older woman can also explain her skin lesions.

What are Miss L's risk factors that support the differential diagnosis (DDX)?

Perhaps the most common risk factor of herpes zoster (HZ) is age. The frequency and severity of HZ go up with increasing age; more than half of all recognized cases of HZ occur in immunocompetent persons older than 60 years of age (Oxman, Levin, & Shingles Prevention Study Group, 2008). Advancing age is often associated with waning of immunity, which can precipitate reactivation of the varicella virus. Precipitating factors of herpes zoster outbreaks have not been clearly identified. Approximately 90% of the adult population has had a primary infection of varicella. It is highly conceivable that the "many childhood illnesses" that Miss L mentioned could have included chickenpox, especially given the health conditions or vectors for infection that one might expect in a refugee camp. Based on Miss L's history, profile, and physical presentation, herpes zoster (shingles) is the most likely diagnosis.

What is the most appropriate plan of treatment for Miss L?

The goals of treatment for Miss L are to control her pain, resolve her rash, and reduce the risk of additional infection. Miss L reported that she has lost sleep on at least two different occasions since she noticed her rash. Her sleep disturbance is likely related to the pain, so adequate pain management will address both her pain and sleep disturbance. Furthermore, by utilizing one medication to address two issues, we reduce the patient's pill burden and reduce the risk of polypharmacy. There are a number of options available to address sleep disturbance (e.g., Ambien or trazadone), but most are very sedating and potentially hazardous to older adults.

Miss L appeared very uncomfortable and reported that her rash was very "itchy" and that the pain was interfering with her sleep. The clinician's relationship with Miss L let her know that the skin condition was seriously impacting the patient's overall wellness; this also highlights the importance of the patient/provider relationship and knowing patients. Miss L was prescribed Percocet, 5/325 one tab 4 times daily #60 as needed. Narcotics are often indicated to manage herpes zoster pain. Starting off with adequate analgesia for pain control and then titrating the medication as needed is an effective and practical approach.

Miss L was informed that over-the-counter topical medication such as calamine, Burow solution, colloid oatmeal, and oral antihistamines (nonsedating, if possible) may help to soothe skin and help with the itch. When in doubt about how much medication to prescribe, use the approach of "start low and go slow." It is very important to **always** inform patients, especially older adults, of the potential side effects of the prescribed medication.

Miss L was also given a prescription for antiviral therapy. Antiviral medications work by inhibiting viral replication and are thought to reduce the neuronal damage caused by the replication process (Dworkin et al., 2007). In Miss L's case, she was given valacyclovir, 1000 mg 3 times daily PO for 7 days. Any of the "clovir" medications (e.g., acyclovir, valacyclovir, famciclovir) are appropriate and very effective in treating herpes zoster. Another antiviral, brivudin, is also effective but less readily available in the United States. Topical antibiotics and antivirals play no role in the management of herpes zoster and should be avoided (Dworkin et al., 2007; Habif et al., 2005). One of the most important factors is starting the medication regimen as soon as the onset of symptoms occurs. Starting the medication in 48 to 72 hours of the onset of symptoms has been shown to lessen pain and speed up healing (Habif et al., 2005). Though Miss L presented to the office after this time frame, antiviral medication was still initiated; and she was told to take the medication as directed.

What other interventions are important to prevent secondary complications?

Miss L must be educated about keeping her rash clean and dry during the expected course of the rash (2–4 weeks) and about her potential for spreading the virus while the lesions are active (Wolff et al., 2005). Miss L was informed that crusted-over lesions are not considered contagious but that she should be mindful in her daily casual contacts. Miss L was further informed that there is a chance of chronic pain associated with herpes zoster, called post herpetic neuralgia (PHN), even after the rash resolves and that it may require long-term medication. Miss L was reassured that resolution of the rash and control of other constitutional symptoms is expected. Lastly, Miss L was encouraged to return to the primary care center if other rashes or intense pain (PHN) develop or if she has any other concerns regarding her skin condition.

What are the plans for follow-up care for Miss L?

Miss L was scheduled for followup in 6 weeks for examination of skin lesions and to receive the varicella vaccine. Vaccines help to boost immunity and help the body fight off infections, reducing the likelihood of recurrent infection. According to Roxas (2006) the elderly and those with compromised immunity are at greater risk for developing herpes zoster. An attack of herpes zoster does not confer lasting immunity, and it is not abnormal to have two or three episodes in a lifetime

(Oxman, Levin, & Shingles Prevention Study Group, 2008). Persons with a reported history of zoster can be vaccinated. Zoster vaccine is recommended for all persons aged >60 years who have no contraindications, including persons who report a previous episode of zoster or who have chronic medical conditions (Oxman, Levin, & Shingles Prevention Study Group, 2008). It is critical that health care providers administer the vaccine under the appropriate guidelines. Zoster vaccination is not indicated to treat acute zoster, to prevent persons with acute zoster from developing PHN, or to treat ongoing PHN (Harpaz, Ortega-Sanchez, Seward, 2008). Miss L received her zoster vaccine, was told to watch for injection site reaction, and was told to call the center or go to the emergency room if she experiences any adverse reactions to the vaccine (e.g., chest pain, SOB, or dizziness). Fortunately, Miss L did not report any signs or symptoms of postherpetic neuralgia (PHN) at her 6-week appointment. Nevertheless, outlined below are some treatment options for the management of PHN:

- Neurologic agents such as Neurontin and Lyrica are indicated for PHN and have shown good effects (Dworkin et al., 2007).
- Low dose tricyclic antidepressants (e.g., amitriptyline) are also used with elderly patients and have very good effects for PHN pain. However, according to Harpaz et al. (2008), elderly persons who already have reduced physiological reserve and typically take multiple medications for pre-existing chronic conditions might be unable to tolerate psychotropic medications for management of PHN pain.
- The use of oral steroids helps to decrease pain and quicken rash resolution with herpes zoster, but it is controversial as to whether this use reduces the incidence of postherpetic neuralgia (Habif et al., 2005; Wolff et al., 2005).
- Topical analgesia such as lidocaine and capsaicin are indicated for postherpetic neuralgia with good effect but should not be used on open uncrusted lesions.
- Use of transcutaneous electrical nerve stimulation (TENS) therapy has been beneficial in the management of PHN. In one review, the use of combination therapy consisting of amitriptyline, capsaicin, and TENS was recommended for treatment of PHN over antiviral therapy (Roxas, 2006).

As always, decision making should be made in the clinical context of the patient; and the medication doses and therapy should be adjusted accordingly.

Does the patient's psychosocial history impact how the clinician might treat this patient?
Miss L's social isolation (i.e., widowed, no children, lives alone, unemployed) may predispose her to depression. Her risk is exacerbated by

the sleep disturbance and pain brought on by herpes zoster. Furthermore, sleep deprivation and pain can also predispose Miss L to delirium (Reuben et al., 2005; Geriatrics at Your Fingertips, 7th ed., 2006). Though marital or family status cannot be changed, Miss L's pain and sleep issues can be managed well. As a result, a more aggressive approach to her pain management could help reduce the list of existing risk factors for depression and delirium. Because Miss L lives alone, it is important to reduce the risk factors and conditions that are more severe and difficult to address in isolation (e.g., pain, sleep disturbance, depression, and delirium).

What if the patient also had kidney failure?
Any patient who has kidney failure should be referred to a specialist (e.g., nephrology) for evaluation and consultation. In Miss L's case, kidney failure would have less of an impact on her course of treatment. Because Miss L is a rather healthy woman, her rash would most likely resolve in 3–4 weeks without the use of any medication. As far as the pain and itch associated with herpes zoster, Miss L's Percocet and topical antipruritics require virtually no adjustment for renal function. In addition, the antiviral medication course is relatively short (7 days) and indicated for use in patients with CrCl of <10 and even for patients on dialysis, with the appropriate dose adjustment (Epocratesonline, 2010). In the management of chronic pain from herpes zoster, PHN can be managed with TCAs (amitriptyline), TENS therapy, and topical analgesia (lidocaine/capsaicin), which also require no dosing adjustment for renal function.

Considering the differentials listed, what are the best treatment options for this patient?
Given the short course and good prognosis of the skin conditions listed (varicella, contact dermatitis, impetigo, and herpes zoster), treatment in the outpatient primary care setting is the best treatment option. Although treating these conditions can be challenging, the treatment regimens are not overly complex. These conditions can be treated with prevention (all of them), analgesia (all of them, as needed), antivirals (varicella and herpes zoster), antibiotics (impetigo), steroids (contact dermatitis and herpes zoster, as needed) and time. Certainly, if more serious complications arise and a specialty consult or hospitalization is required, then the appropriate referral should be made.

Are there any standardized guidelines that the clinician should use to assess or treat this patient?
Recommendations for additional information about herpes zoster are available through the National Center for Immunization and Respiratory Diseases at www.cdc.gov. Also there is the Infectious Diseases Society of America, and information about the zoster vaccine can also be found at www.cdc.gov/vaccines.

REFERENCES

Dworkin, R. H., Johnson, R. W., Breuer, J., Gnann, J. W., Levin, M. J., Backonja, M., . . . Whitley, R.J. (2007). Recommendations for the management of herpes zoster. *Clinical Infectious Diseases, 44,* 145–157. Retrieved July 14, 2010, from http://www.journals.uchicago.edu/Doi/full/1086.html

Epocratesonline. Retrieved July16, 2010 from http://www.epocratesonline. com

Geriatrics at your fingertips (7th ed). 2006. Washington, DC: APA.

Habif, T., Campbell, J. L., Chapman, M., Dinulos, J., & Zug, K. (2005). *Skin disease: diagnosis and treatment* (2nd ed.). Philadelphia, PA: Elsevier Mosby.

Harpaz, R., Ortega-Sanchez, I., & Seward, J. (2008). Prevention of herpes hoster: Recommendations of the advisory committee on immunization practices (ACIP). *PubMed.* Retrieved from http://www.ncbi.nlm.nih.gov/pubmed/18528318.html

Oxman, M., Levin, M. J., & Shingles Prevention Study Group (2008). Vaccination against herpes zoster and post herpetic neuralgia. *Journal of Infectious Diseases, 197,* 228–236. Retrieved July 14, 2010, from http://www.journals. uchicago.edu/doi/full/10.1086.html

Reuben, D., Herr, K., Pacala, J., Pollock, B., Potter, J., & Semla, T. (2005). *Geriatrics at your fingertips* (7th ed.). New York: American Geriatrics Society.

Roxas, M. (2006). Herpes zoster and postherpetic neuralgia: Diagnosis and therapeutic considerations. *Alternative Medicine Review, 10,* 102–113.

Wolff, K., Johnson, R. A., & Suurmond, D. (2005). *Fitzpatrick's color atlas & synopsis of clinical dermatology* (5th ed.). New York: Mcgraw-Hill.

Case 2.3 Why Is My Mother Wearing a Diaper?

By Annemarie Dowling-Castronovo, PhD(c), RN

Mrs. D, a 68-year-old female with early stage Alzheimer disease, presents to the subacute rehabilitation unit of a long-term care institution for short-term rehabilitation. She is 3 days postoperative for an open reduction internal fixation (ORIF) of a left head of femur fracture sustained after she fell down a flight of stairs. Her daughter is at her bedside during the clinician's admission assessment and serves as the primary historian. Her medical and surgical histories are significant for psoriasis, "a touch of" emphysema, Cesarean section, and depression. Mrs. D, a widow and only child, lives in a "mother-daughter" home in a first-floor, 1-bedroom apartment. She is financially "well-off". Her daughter, her only child, lives in the second floor, 3-bedroom apartment with her husband and 3 children all under the age of 12. Mrs. D attends a social adult day care program 3 days a week and is able to prepare light cold meals, such as cereal for breakfast or yogurt for a snack. She has dinner every night with her daughter's family. Prior to her diagnosis of Alzheimer's approximately 2 years prior to this admission, she drank approximately 4 glasses of wine a day. Since diagnosis she has only had glasses of non-alcoholic wine to maintain a social appearance at family functions. Her daughter reports that she was a pack-and-a-half per day smoker for over 40 years. Since her fall she has not asked for a cigarette. She attends Catholic mass weekly. She was able to walk several blocks without fatigue. Her father died of an unknown cancer and had rheumatoid arthritis, and her mother died of a hemorrhagic stroke. At present Mrs. D is resting comfortably in bed, denies pain, and is unable to provide a number on a pain scale of 1–10

Case Studies in Gerontological Nursing for the Advanced Practice Nurse, First Edition.
Edited by Meredith Wallace Kazer, Leslie Neal-Boylan.
© 2012 John Wiley & Sons, Inc. Published 2012 by John Wiley & Sons, Inc.

due to incomprehension (She stated, "no hurt."). Her medications include donepezil (Aricept®), 5 mg daily; multivitamin daily; sertraline (Zoloft®), 25 mg daily; and topical steroid creams for psoriasis. She is allergic to penicillin.

OBJECTIVE

Mrs. D is lying in bed; she is awake, alert, and oriented to person but not to place or time. Her Mini-Mental State Exam (MMSE) is 22/30 with errors in place, year, calculation, recall, and naming. Her BMI is 28, and vital signs are 128/74, 84, and 22. Oxygen saturation is 89% on room air (base line is 88%–91%). Her temperature is 98.4 F orally. Neurological exam reveals no focal deficits. Her head is normocephalic. PERRLA. Tympanic membranes are pearly grey. Breath sounds are diminished throughout with poor inspiratory effort; no adventitious sounds are noted. Heart rate is regular with S1 and S2. Bowel sounds are auscultated in all 4 quadrants; and her abdomen is soft, nontender, and without suprapubic tenderness. There is a vertical surgical incision scar on her abdomen. An indwelling urinary catheter is in place draining clear, yellow urine into a bedside drainage bag. Extremities are without edema, and distal pulses are 2+ palpable. Left hip surgical incision is clean and dry; staples are intact with mild erythema, no warmth or swelling. Otherwise the skin is intact without evidence of tissue damage from pressure. Silvery scales (psoriasis) noted on elbows and lower legs.

The indwelling urinary catheter is removed at midnight. The next afternoon the daughter asks the clinician why her mother is wearing a "diaper" since her mother did not have trouble getting to the bathroom prior to the fall and subsequent hospitalization. The clinician assesses and learns that, after the urinary catheter was removed, Mrs. D did not call for assistance. The nursing assistant found her during 4 a.m. rounds trying to get out of bed, and her bed linens were wet with urine. At that time, the nursing assistant cleaned Mrs. D and applied an absorbent brief. Thereafter, the day nursing assistant performed morning care and, again, placed an absorbent brief on Mrs. D.

ASSESSMENT

Urinary incontinence: established—functional: The fact that the daughter states that Mrs. D has not experienced UI before rules out this type of incontinence, although Mrs. D's limited mobility results in difficulty with activities of daily living, including toileting activity, and is the reason for her admission for rehabilitation.

Urinary incontinence: iatrogenic: Although not well-defined in the literature, this form of incontinence may result from various treatments such as pharmacological therapy (e.g., diuretics). Moreover, as in this case, it may be a catheter-associated urinary tract infection (CA-UTI). A patient with an indwelling urinary catheter is 5 times more likely to experience a UTI (Graves et al., 2007). The older adult often has an atypical presentation, meaning that the older adult will not experience the dysuria and fever that are common clinical manifestations of a UTI. Instead, an older adult will have urinary incontinence.

Urinary incontinence: new-onset: The incidence of new-onset UI in hospitalized older adults ranges from 12%—36% (Kresevic, 1997; Palmer, Myers, & Fedenko, 1997; Sier, Ouslander, & Orzeck, 1987).

DIAGNOSTICS

Mrs. D may benefit from a bladder scan to determine a postvoid residual. She may also benefit from a urine sample for a urinalysis culture and sensitivity test.

CRITICAL THINKING

What is the primary diagnosis for this patient?

How should the clinician respond to the nursing assistants?

Are there any standardized guidelines that should be used to assess and treat this episode of incontinence?

Are any referrals needed?

Does the patient's psychosocial history impact how the clinician might treat this patient?

What if this patient were male?

RESOLUTION

What is the primary diagnosis for this patient?
It is essential for the clinician to recognize that this episode of UI is likely transient UI, which is amenable to treatment (Ding & Jayaratnam, 1994; Jeter & Wagner, 1990; Mitteness & Barker, 1995; Schnelle, Alessi, Al-Samarrai, Fricker & Ouslander, 1999; Skelly & Boblin-Cummings,

1999). According to Kresevic (1997), risk factors for new-onset UI for hospitalized older adults include depression, malnutrition, and dependent ambulation. In the case of Mrs. D, she has history of depression and presently depends on others for ambulation. For women with hip fractures, other factors that significantly increase the odds for development of new incontinence include confusion, use of a wheelchair or assistive device for ambulation, and a prefracture need for ambulation (Palmer, Baumgarten, Langenberg, & Carson, 2002).

The initial nursing assessment should be guided by the mnemonic TOILETED to identify possible reversible causes of new-onset UI.

Thin, dry vaginal and urethral epithelium (atrophic vaginitis)
Obstruction of stool
Infection (e.g., urinary tract infection)
Limited mobility
Emotional
Therapeutic medications (e.g., furosemide)
Endocrine disorders (diabetes)
Delirium.

Specific to Mrs. D's case are the following: inspection of perineum revealed no atrophic vaginitis; digital rectal exam revealed minimal stool; a clean catch urine specimen revealed no UTI; limited mobility was an issue; depression was being treated; no therapeutic medications were noted to have irritating effects on the bladder; and there was no evidence of diabetes or delirium (confusion assessment method). Despite the fact that Mrs. D has dementia of Alzheimer's type (DAT), urinary incontinence is not common during the early stages of DAT (Sakakibara, Uchiyama, Yamanishi, & Masahiko, 2008). Therefore, the UI should not be viewed as an established UI, a consequence of the later stages of Alzheimer disease.

How should the clinician respond to the nursing assistants?

Urinary incontinence is a symptom defined as the involuntary loss of urine sufficient to be a problem (Resnick & Ouslander, 1990; Fantl et al., 1996). Regardless of the setting, containment and concealment strategies are implemented to control incontinence and preserve skin integrity (Tannenbaum, Labrecque, & Lepage, 2004; Wagg, Mian, Lowe, Potter, & Pearson, 2005). Containment and concealment strategies typically include absorbent products such as reusable and disposable adult briefs, perineal pads, and incontinence pads. Typically, routine nighttime nursing rounds in nursing homes are performed to check and change wet and soiled absorbent products on incontinent nursing home residents (Jervis, 2001; Schnelle, Cruise, Alessi, Al-Samarrai & Ouslander, 1998). However, containment and concealment strategies should not be first-line strategies.

Are there any standardized guidelines that should be used to assess and treat this episode of incontinence?

Evidence-based clinical guidelines (Dowling-Castronovo & Bradway, 2008; Fantl et al., 1996; International Consultation on Incontinence, 2000; National Collaborating Centre for Women's and Children's Health, 2006; Scottish Intercollegiate Guidelines Network [SIGN], 2004; The Royal Australian College of General Practitioners, 2002) typically identify the following 2 types of UIs: 1) transient, acute, or new-onset UI and 2) established UI. Transient UI is characterized by the sudden onset of potentially reversible UI symptoms for which the mnemonic TOILETED (Dowling-Castronovo, 2007) may help guide nursing assessment. Generally, it has a duration of less than 6 months (Specht, 2005). However, there may be cases of acute UI that are not transient, such as in the case of acute UI secondary to a spinal cord injury. Lack of assessment and treatment of transient UI may lead to the second type of UI—established UI, such as stress, urge, mixed, or functional.

According to the clinical guidelines, Mrs. D's assessment should determine Mrs. D's voiding habits by using a bladder record or diary (http://consultgerirn.org/uploads/File/trythis/try_this_11_1.pdf; http://kidney.niddk.nih.gov), which revealed that Mrs. D did not always ask for or initiate toileting activity. As a result, the health care team determined that prompted voiding and an individualized toileting schedule would best suit her needs. Mrs. D is currently dependent on adaptive devices (e.g., a walker) and her caregivers for assistance with voiding. In addition, she also has Alzheimer's which may result in the inability to recall voiding times or recognize the need to void. Individualized scheduled toileting programs and prompted voiding are developed based on the results of the bladder record/diary, so that the intervention mimics the patient's normal voiding patterns. Continual assessment and evaluation improves success. For example, if the initial scheduled toileting time is set for 6 a.m., yet at 5:30 a.m. the patient time and again attempts to independently void or is noted to be incontinent, then the toileting time is adjusted to 5:30 a.m. Prompted voiding requires the caregiver to ask if the patient needs to void, offer assistance, and then offer praise for successful voiding (Eustice, Roe, & Paterson, 2005; Colling, Ouslander, Hadley, Eisch, Campbell, 1992; Ostaszkiewicz, Johnston, & Roe, 2004). In addition, diet and fluid interventions are focused on maintaining adequate hydration and fiber intake to avoid bladder irritation and constipation. Other strategies for UI such as pharmacological agents, pelvic floor muscle exercises, and intermittent catheterization were not considered appropriate for Mrs. D. Inclusion of Mrs. D and her daughter in the care planning process resulted in the team's decision not to use absorbent briefs or "diapers". The daughter agreed to provide extra undergarments. In addition, the daughter hired a private nursing assistant to feel "guaranteed" that Mrs. D's individualized toileting needs were met. It is known that inadequate staffing and staff attitudes are barriers to strategies such as prompted voiding and toileting schedules (Dingwall & Mclafferty, 2006; Boblin & Skelly, 1999; Schnelle et al., 2002; Tannenbaum et al., 2005).

Are any referrals needed?

A referral for home care is indicated to ensure Mrs. D's transition back to home.

Does the patient's psychosocial history impact how the clinician might treat this patient?

Mrs. D's Alzheimer's and confusion may have been worsened by her hospitalization and can negatively impact her ability to respond to treatment. Two important aspects from Mrs. D's psychosocial history positively impact her treatment. First, she has a supportive family that is involved in her care. Second, she is financially able to afford private care to ensure that her individual toileting needs are met. Care for UI is known to be a cause of stress for family caregivers (Cassells & Watt, 2003; National Institute of Health, 2008). Therefore, the daughter should be provided with education and support and may benefit from an Alzheimer's support group for family caregivers.

What if this patient were male?

If this patient were an older adult male then there would be the need to consider the normal aging changes of the prostate gland or the risks of prostate cancer.

REFERENCES

Boblin, A., & Skelly, J. (1999). Health-care providers' knowledge, attitudes and decisions about incontinence care. *Clinical Effectiveness in Nursing, 3*, 156–162.

Cassells, C., & Watt, E. (2003). The impact of incontinence on older spousal caregivers. *Journal of Advanced Nursing, 42*, 607–616.

Colling, J., Ouslander, J., Hadley, B. J., Eisch, J., & Campbell, E. (1992). The effects of patterned urge-response toileting (PURT) on urinary incontinence among nursing home residents. *Journal of the American Geriatrics Society, 40*(2), 135–141.

Ding, Y. Y., & Jayaratnam, F. J. (1994). Urinary incontinence in the hospitalized elderly: A largely reversible disorder. *Singapore Medical Journal, 35*, 167–170.

Dingwall, L., & Mclafferty, E. (2006). Do nurses promote urinary continence in hospitalized older people? An exploratory study. *Journal of Clinical Nursing, 15*, 1276–1286.

Dowling-Castronovo, A. (2007). Urinary incontinence assessment in older adults: Part I: Transient urinary incontinence. In M. Boltz (Ed.), *Try this: Best practices in nursing care to older adults from the John A. Hartford foundation institute for geriatric nursing, issue 11.1.* Hartford Institute for Geriatric Nursing, New York University, College of Nursing. Retrieved from http://consultgerirn.org/uploads/File/trythis/try_this_11_1.pdf

Dowling-Castronovo, A., & Bradway, C. (2008). Urinary incontinence. In E. Capezuti, D. Zwicker, M. Mezey, & T. Fulmer (Eds.), *Geriatric nursing protocols* (3rd ed., pp. 309–336). New York: Springer Publishing Company, LLC.

Eustice, S., Roe, B., & Paterson, J. (2005). Prompted voiding for the management of urinary incontinence in adults. *The Cochrane Library*, (4). (ID CD002113).

Fantl, A., Newman, D. K., Colling, J., et al. (1996). *Urinary incontinence in adults: Acute and chronic management.* Rockville, MD: Agency for Health Care Policy and Research. Publication No. 92-0047.

International Consultation of Incontinence (2000). Assessment and treatment of urinary incontinence. *Lancet, 355*, 2153–2158.

Jervis, L. L. (2001). The pollution of incontinence and the dirty work of caregiving in a U.S. nursing home. *Medical Anthropology Quarterly, 15*, 84–99.

Jeter, K. F., & Wagner, D. B. (1990). Incontinence in the American home: A survey of 36,500 people. *Journal of the American Geriatrics Society, 38*, 379–383.

Kresevic, D. M. (1997). New-onset urinary incontinence among hospitalized elders (Doctoral dissertation, Case Western Reserve University, 1997). (UMI No. 9810934).

Mitteness, L. S., & Barker, J. C. (1995). Stigmatizing a "normal" condition: Urinary incontinence in late life. *Medical Anthropology Quarterly, 9*, 188–210.

National Collaborating Centre for Women's and Children's Health (2006). Urinary incontinence: The management of urinary incontinence in women. Retrieved July 10, 2010, from http://www.nice.org.uk/nicemedia/pdf/CG40fullguideline.pdf

National Institutes for Health (2008). National Institutes of Health state-of-the-science statement: Prevention of fecal and urinary incontinence in adults. *Annals of Internal Medicine, 148*(6), 1–10.

Ostaszkiewicz, J., Johnston, L., & Roe, B. (2004). Timed voiding for the management of urinary incontinence in adults. *The Cochrane Database of Systematic Reviews (Protocol)*, (Issue 1). Issue Art. No.: CD002802. doi:10.1002/14651858. CD002802.pub2.

Palmer, M., Baumgarten, M., Langenberg, P., & Carson, J. L. (2002). Risk factors for hospital-acquired incontinence in elderly female hip fracture patients. *Journal of Gerontology., 10*, M672–M677.

Palmer, M. H., Myers, A. H., & Fedenko, K. M. (1997). Urinary continence changes after hip-fracture repair. *Clinical Nursing Research, 6*, 8–24.

Resnick, N. M. & Ouslander, J. G. (1990). Urinary incontinence—Where do we stand and where do we go from here? *Journal of the American Geriatrics Society, 38*, 264–265.

Sakakibara, R., Uchiyama, T., Yamanishi, T., & Masahiko, M. (2008). Dementia and lower urinary dysfunction: With a reference to anticholinergic use in elderly population, *International Journal of Urology, 15*, 778–788.

Schnelle, J. F., Alessi, C. A., Al-Samarrai, N. R., Fricker, R. D., & Ouslander, J. G. (1999). The nursing home at night: Effects of an intervention on noise, light, and sleep. *Journal of the American Geriatrics Society, 47*, 430–438.

Schnelle, J. F., Alessi, C. A., Simmons, S. F., Al-Samarrai, N. R., Beck, J. C., & Ouslander, J. G. (2002). Translating clinical research into practice: A randomized controlled trial of exercise and incontinence care with nursing home residents. *Journal of the American Geriatrics Society, 50*, 1476–1483.

Schnelle, J. F., Cruise, P. A., Alessi, C. A., Al-Samarrai, N., & Ouslander, J. G. (1998). Individualizing nighttime incontinence care in nursing home residents. *Nursing Research, 47*, 197–204.

Scottish Intercollegiate Guidelines Network (SIGN) (2004). Management of urinary incontinence in primary care. A national clinical guideline. Edinburgh (Scotland) Retrieved July 10, 2009, from http://www.sign.ac.uk/pdf/sign79.pdf

Sier, H., Ouslander, J., & Orzeck, S. (1987). Urinary incontinence among geriatric patients in an acute-care hospital. *Journal of the American Medical Association, 257*, 1757–1771.

Skelly, J., & Boblin-Cummings, S. (1999). Promoting seniors' health—Confronting the issue of incontinence. *Canadian Journal of Nursing Leadership, 12*, 13–17.

Specht, J. (2005). 9 Myths of incontinence in older adults: Both clinicians and the over-65 set need to know more. *American Journal of Nursing, 105*(6), 58–68.

Tannenbaum, C., Labrecque, D., & Lepage, C. (2005). Understanding barriers to continence care in institutions. *Canadian Journal on Aging, 24*(2), 151–160.

Tannenbaum, C., Labrecque, D., & Lepage, C. (2004). Understanding barriers to continence care in institutions. *Canadian Journal on Aging, 24*(2), 151–160.

The Royal Australian College of General Practitioners (2002). Managing incontinence in the general practice: Clinical practice guidelines, Retrieved July 10, 2010, from http://www.racgp.org.au/Content/NavigationMenu/ClinicalResources/RACGPGuidelines/Managingincontinence/Management_of_incontinence.pdf

Wagg, A., Mian, S., Lowe, D., Potter, J., & Pearson, M. (2005). National audit of continence care for older people: Results of a pilot study. *Journal of Evaluation in Clinical Practice, 11*, 525–532.

ADDITIONAL RESOURCES

Retrieved June 11, 2011. http://consultgerirn.org/uploads/File/trythis/try_this_11_1.pdf

Retrieved June 11, 2011. http://kidney.niddk.nih.gov

National Institute for Health, http://www.nlm.nih.gov/medlineplus/urinaryincontinence.html

The Simon Foundation for Continence. http://www.simonfoundation.org/index.html

Case 2.4 My Aching Back

By Anne Moore, DNP, RN

Mrs. P is an 80-year-old female who developed significant lower back pain 4 months prior to her initial visit. The patient describes the pain as nearly constant and radiating to the right lower extremity. She describes her pain as moderate to severe and reports that it has caused her to limit her normal activities. She feels as if her leg is going to give out, and she fell in the past week while climbing stairs. She denies any bowel or bladder incontinence but has experienced some increase in urgency. She is independent with basic ADL and mobility. She does not use an assistive device.

The past medical history for Mrs. P is significant for a spinal compression fracture in 1992, coronary artery disease, left lower leg phlebitis post delivering her second child 50 years ago, osteoporosis, status post CABG in 2007, and dyslipidemia. She is unable to do any vigorous activity and experiences mild dyspnea and chest tightness if she walks more than 50 yards quickly.

Mrs. P's mother expired at age 78 of MI; her father died at age 75 of renal disease. This patient has one sister, age 76, who has hypertension but is otherwise in good health. The patient lives with her husband in a private house with interior stairs. She is a retired teacher with 2 adult children. Her husband is in good health but no longer drives. One daughter lives in Connecticut and visits often. She denies any history of smoking or alcohol or drug abuse. She has Medicare and AARP supplemental insurance. She states that she has a reaction to statins, including muscle cramps. She is allergic to morphine, which makes her vomit. Her medications include metoprolol, 12.5 mg PO twice daily;

Case Studies in Gerontological Nursing for the Advanced Practice Nurse, First Edition.
Edited by Meredith Wallace Kazer, Leslie Neal-Boylan.
© 2012 John Wiley & Sons, Inc. Published 2012 by John Wiley & Sons, Inc.

Welchol, 1875 mg PO twice daily; Aclasta IV, once yearly; Cipro, 500 mg PO twice daily; ibuprofen, 400 mg PO every 8 hours; Robaxin, 500 mg PO 3 times daily

OBJECTIVE

Mrs. P is 60 inches, weighs 133 lb, and has a BMI of 26. Her BP is 136/88, pulse is 88, and respirations are 16. The examination reveals the patient as well developed, well nourished, and in moderate distress. There are no skin markings, masses, skin tags, or discoloration on the back. She has mild kyphosis and a normal gait. Range of motion of the lumbar spine is limited with extension exacerbating her pain. Her patellar tendon reflex is absent on the right. She has right-sided decreased sensation on the anteromedial thigh, the lateral and medial aspect of her lower leg, and the dorsum of her foot with some mild weakness in dorsiflexion of the ankle and the leg. Her EKG shows normal sinus rhythm, nonspecific T wave abnormality—no change since 2007.

Labs: INR/PT INR 1, PTT 31, PT 9.8 all within normal range. CBC: normal BUN; Cr, glucose, electrolytes normal. Urinalysis: cloudy, elevated WBC and leukocyte esterase, few bacteria, many calcium oxalate crystals. The patient was put on Cipro, 500 mg twice daily for 7 days.

ASSESSMENT

Herniated disc: More than 90% of lumbar disc herniations occur at L4-L5 or L5-S1 (Seller, 2000). Most patients with a herniated disc have experienced previous less-severe episodes of pain. The pain has a sudden onset and often radiates to the buttock and the posterolateral aspect of the leg and sometimes to the foot. Disc herniation is most common in males with a mean age of 35 years (Spengler & Donatelli, 2005). A herniated disc may result in paresthesia and muscle weakness due to pressure on the nerve root. Intermittent back pain may be caused by a disc that does not produce significant root irritation (Seller). The pain is often exacerbated by coughing, sneezing or hyperextension of the lumbar spine.

Spinal stenosis: Thirty percent of people over 60 years old have spinal stenosis (Spengler & Donatelli, 2005). Back pain is a common symptom but is not often the chief complaint in patients over 50 years old. When it is the chief complaint, it may be a symptom of spinal stenosis (Seller, 2000).In a recent study, Kalichman, et al. (2010) reported that the only correlation of low back pain to a diagnosis that was significant was in patients with spinal stenosis. Spinal stenosis affects males and females alike and often occurs at L4-L5 and L3-L4 (Spengler & Donatelli, 2005). The pain is usually in the buttocks or thighs and worsens with extension. The pain often improves with flexion.

Spinal tumor: Engelhard et al. (2010) reported on the incidence of spinal tumors based on data from a previous study by the Commission on Cancer of the American College of Surgeons using the National Cancer Center database. Of the 430 patients with primary tumors of the spinal cord, meninges, or cauda equine, 56.7% were women and the mean age was 49.3. The most common symptoms were pain and weakness. Spinal tumors may cause pain and neural deficits. The deficits depend on the spinal level involved. The symptoms are caused by compression of the spinal canal and nerve roots. The rate of neurologic dysfunction may progress over weeks or months depending on the aggressiveness of the tumor (Spengler & Donatelli, 2005).

Spondylolisthesis: Spondylolisthesis occurs most frequently in females who are mildly overweight and over the age of 40 (Spengler & Donatelli, 2005). The most common level is L4-L5. Symptoms may include back and radicular leg pain. The back pain may be aggravated by bending, lifting, or twisting. Mrs. P may develop neurogenic claudication and other symptoms similar to spinal stenosis (Spengler & Donatelli).

DIAGNOSTICS

The level of involvement can be evaluated through the physical examination and then confirmed by MRI. Table 2.4.1 lists the myotomes, dermatomes, and usual locations of pain for the associated nerve roots (Cohen, Rowlingson, & Salahadin, 2004; Scifers, 2008). Myotome testing assesses muscle strength for a given motion.

McGee (2007) reports the likelihood ratio (LR) of the associated level of the spine based on findings on physical exam in patients with sciatica and lumbosacral radiculopathy. The following are some of the best predictors based on the LR for the lumbar spine. An abnormal quadriceps reflex or weak knee extension indicates level L3 or L4; sensory loss in the dorsum of the foot indicates level L5. The lateral heel, a reduced Achilles reflex, and ipsilateral calf wasting indicates sensory loss in level S1.

- **Magnetic Resonance Imaging (MRI):** MRI is useful in depicting abnormalities of the anatomy such as herniation or stenosis and tissue abnormalities like disk desiccation and marrow changes.

TABLE 2.4.1. Myotomes, Dermatomes, and Location of Pain.

Nerve Root	Myotome	Dermatomes	Pain
L1	Hip flexion	Superior lateral hip and groin	Low back; groin
L2	Hip flexion	Anterior thigh	Low back; anterior and inner thigh
L3	Knee extension	Patellar region	Low back; upper buttock to anterior thigh; anterior knee; medial lower leg
L4	Ankle dorsiflexion; ankle inversion	Inferior knee; medial lower leg; medial arch	Low back; hip; thigh; anterior leg; inner leg to medial portion of foot
L5	Great toe extension	Dorsum of foot; lateral lower leg	Low back; buttock; hip; posterolateral thigh; lateral aspect of lower leg; dorsum of foot; first 2 toes
S1	Ankle plantarflexion; ankle eversion	Lateral foot; posterior lateral leg	Sacroiliac joint; hip; buttock; posterolateral thigh and leg; lateral edge of foot, heel, sole

MRI of the lumbar spine can be a useful predictor of diagnoses (Carrino et al., 2009).

- **Computed Tomography Imaging (CT scan):** CT scan is often used to provide a detailed image of bony structures. It is often used to depict spinal degenerative changes and provides a clear image of the facet joints (Leone, Guglielme, Casser-Pulicino, & Bonomo, 2007).
- **Flexion/extension radiography:** Flexion/extension radiography is often used to assist in the diagnosis of patients presenting with low back pain. It is a widely available, low cost, and easily administered test. It is the most commonly used test for intervertebral instability (Leone et al., 2007).

The results of Mrs. P's diagnostic tests are as follows: MRI Impression: Disc bulging and facet arthropathy resulting in severe canal stenosis at L2-3, moderate to severe canal stenosis at L3-4, and severe canal stenosis at L4-5 and L5-S1. CT spine impression: Moderate to severe canal stenosis and left neural foramen stenosis at L2-3. Grade 1 anterolisthesis L4 on L5. Flexion/extension radiography impression: Diffuse osteopenia. Grade 1 anterolisthesis L4 on L5 with flexion which reduces with extension. There is degenerative disc disease at L5-S1 and to a lesser extent L1-2 through L3-4. Compression fracture T11; age indeterminate.

CRITICAL THINKING

What is the most likely differential diagnosis and why?

What would have been different if Mrs. P exhibited loss of bowel and bladder control?

What is the plan of treatment?

What evidenced-based practice guidelines or protocols might be implemented during Mrs. P's postoperative course?

What if Mrs. P developed postoperative confusion?

Are any referrals needed?

What would be included in the discharge instructions?

What is the plan for follow-up care?

RESOLUTION

What is the most likely differential diagnosis and why?
As is evidenced in this case study, older adults with back pain may have more than one diagnosis. In addition, one or more levels of the spinal column may be involved. It is imperative that a complete history and physical exam be performed along with the diagnostic tests. The most likely differential diagnosis in this case would be spinal stenosis. The acute onset of the worsening of the symptoms on the right side would lead one to question another event. Combined with findings from the physical exam, level 4–5 would have probable involvement. In this case, the patient was scheduled for a decompressive laminectomy and fusion at L2-S1 with discectomy for herniated disc on the right at L2-3 and the left L5-S1. Her postoperative diagnosis was spondylosis with stenosis, degenerative disc disease with disc herniation.

What would have been different if Mrs. P exhibited loss of bowel and bladder control?
Loss of bowel and bladder control, in addition to her other symptoms of back pain and lower extremity involvement and her history of a fall and previous vertebral fracture, might indicate cauda equina syndrome. Causes for cauda equina syndrome include central disc herniation, epidural abscess or hematoma, trauma to the spine, and vertebral burst fracture (Spengler & Donatelli, 2005). Cauda equina syndrome usually requires emergency surgery.

What is the plan of treatment?

The plan of treatment for Mrs. P should include postoperative management including routine VS and O$_2$ Sat, incentive spirometer, deep breathing and wound care. Foot pumps or a sequential compression device are used while the patient is in bed. Anticoagulants are not routinely used with spinal surgery. PT/PTT and INR were normal in the preoperative period and should be done postoperatively as well especially with this patient's history of CABG and DVT. Pain management with PCA pump and then oral narcotics are planned, along with assessment of all systems on every shift. It is important to assess cardiac, GI, and GU systems in this patient because of her history. The physical therapist will educate the patient about spinal precautions and how to don/doff the brace she will need to wear. They will assist with the first ambulation. Nursing should reinforce spinal precautions and how to don/doff the brace. If Mrs. P becomes confused, interventions for delirium should be implemented in order to prevent falls and ensure safety. A CT scan should be scheduled for postoperative day 2 to check ensure alignment of the spine, the position of the hardware, and any abnormalities.

What evidenced-based practice guidelines or protocols might be implemented during Mrs. P's postoperative course?

Evidenced-based guidelines for fall risk, skin care, and delirium should be implemented. The vertebrae will not fuse for several months, and care must be taken to protect the spine. There are several guidelines with various levels of recommendations for specific treatment modalities published by the National Association of Spine Surgeons (NASS). The most recent appropriate guidelines available are *Antithrombotic Therapies in Spine Surgery* (NASS Evidenced Based Guideline Committee, 2009), *Degenerative Lumbar Spinal Stenosis* (NASS Clinical Guideline Development Committee, 2007), and *Antibiotic Prophylaxis in Spine Surgery* (NASS Evidenced Based Guideline Development Committee, 2007). There is also a practice advisory from the American Society of Anesthesiologists (ASA) task force on perioperative visual loss associated with spinal surgery (American Society of Anesthesiologists Task Force on Perioperative Blindness, 2006).

What if Mrs. P developed postoperative confusion?

Postoperatively Mrs. P was on a patient controlled analgesia (PCA) Dilaudid pump and had foot pumps while in bed. Her wound was intact and the dressing was clean and dry. She had a normal postoperative course on the day of surgery and postoperative day 1. Her postoperative pain was controlled by the PCA pump. Her sciatica was relieved with surgery; she was OOB with assistance and a lumbar sacral orthosis (LSO) brace. VS and blood work were within normal limits. The PCA pump was discontinued in the afternoon of postoperative day 1, and she was placed on Vicodin. On postoperative day 2 she became significantly confused to person, place, and time. At that point all narcotics were discontinued, and she was started on Toradol for pain. Mrs. P continued to be confused. She appeared anxious and was complaining of severe pain. She developed a low grade fever, and her WBC count was 18.3. Vital signs: Temp: 99.7: P: 100; RR: 18; BP: 102/54; O_2 Sat: 93 on room air.

There are a number of potential causes for postoperative confusion among older adults. Pulmonary embolism should be ruled out as Mrs. P is postoperative and on extended periods of bedrest. She appears anxious and is confused. There is a very low rate of thromboembolism following elective spinal surgery done with a posterior approach (NASS Evidenced Based Guideline Committee, 2009). However, the patient has a previous history of DVT, CABG, and dyslipidemia. A urinary tract infection (UTI) is the most common bacterial infection in older persons and may be associated with the use of an indwelling bladder catheter (Yoshikawa, 2006). Mrs. P had a previous UTI, a low grade fever, and a WBC of 18.3. Mrs. P had a urinary catheter for 24 hours postsurgery. Given that Mrs. P is postoperative and on extended periods of bed rest, she also may have pneumonia. Her elevated WBC count and low grade fever support this diagnosis. According to Rosenthal (2006), pneumonia is the most common post-operative complication in the elderly. The patient used her incentive spirometer and followed her deep breathing and coughing routine as ordered before she became confused. Finally, Mrs. P could have drug-/anesthesia-induced confusion. Mrs. P is 80 years old. She was in surgery for 6.5 hours. Anesthesia may have a major effect on mental functioning in the older adult. The metabolic changes associated with surgery as well as the effect on all of the systems of the body can compromise cerebral function and can cause neuropsychiatric disorders. The most common psychiatric problem in this age group in the postoperative period is delirium (Albert, 2006).

The most likely cause of the confusion in Mrs. P could have been any of those listed: drug-/anesthesia-induced, PE, or UTI. However, the immediate intervention was to stop the narcotics and give her Toradol for pain. Controlling the pain is important even if the confusion is thought to be medication induced to prevent further agitation from the pain. Once the narcotics were discontinued, the other possible causes could be determined by the following testing: a urine culture to rule out a UTI; a chest X-ray to detect pneumonia; and a VQ Scan to identify a PE.

Are any referrals needed?
A referral would be made to the patient's cardiologist. Care management would be requested for care postdischarge. Depending on the amount of time it takes the confusion to clear from Mrs. P, she may need to be admitted to a subacute rehabilitation facility. If she is able to be

discharged to home, she will need visiting nurses, physical therapy, and possibly occupational therapy, as well as a referral to social services for community resources if needed. The patient's husband does not drive, and she will need to be seen for followup. Also, the daughter's involvement in assisting her mother with obtaining groceries and cooking will need to be evaluated. If pain is not well controlled prior to discharge, referral to a pain specialist will be appropriate.

What would be included in the discharge instructions?

The discharge instructions would include instructions to the patient on when to call her surgeon including the following: sudden severe pain in the back or leg that pain medication does not control; pain, swelling, or redness in the lower part of the leg; inability to move the leg(s) as well as she could move it when she left the hospital; bright redness, warmth, swelling, or pain around the incision; bleeding or drainage from the incision; fever over 101° or chills. The patient would be instructed to call 911 for chest pain or difficulty breathing. She would also be instructed on incision care, exercise, spine precautions, pain management, and managing constipation. She would be given instructions to follow up with her physician in 2 weeks when the staples would be removed.

What is the plan for follow-up care?

The patient would be instructed to see her surgeon in 2 weeks. Visiting nurses will monitor the wound and do a complete assessment of all systems. The physical therapist will reinforce spine precautions and evaluate the home for safety. The primary therapy for spinal surgery is ambulation. Once the spine is fused, core strengthening exercises may be added. At 3 months, a CT scan would be taken to monitor the progress of the fusion. If rehab is progressing as it should, the patient would be then seen 6 months and 1 year postsurgery. At each visit, Mrs. P will be given a complete exam with a neural assessment. Many spine physicians and nurse practitioners use a functional assessment tool, such as the SF36, to monitor their patient's progress and quality of life.

REFERENCES

Albert, M. S. (2006). Neuropsychological testing. In C. K. Cassel, R. M. Leipzig, H. J. Cohen, E. B. Larson, & D. E. Meier (Eds.), *Geriatric medicine* (4th ed.). New York: Springer Science & Business Media, LLC.

American Society of Anesthesiologists Task Force on Perioperative Blindness (2006). Practice advisory for perioperative visual loss associated with spine surgery. *Anesthesiology, 104,* 1319–1328.

Carrino, J. A., Lurie, J. D., Tosteson, A. N., Tosteson, T. D., Carragee, E. J., Kaiser, J., . . . Herzog, R. (2009). Lumbar spine: Reliability of MR imaging findings. *Radiology, 250*(1), 161–170.

Cohen, S. P., Rowlingson, J., & Salahadin, A. (2004). Low back pain. In C. A. Warfield, Z. H. Bajwa (Eds.), *Principles and practice of pain management*. New York: McGraw-Hill.

Engelhard, H. H., Villano, J. L., Porter, K. R., Stewart, A. K., Barker, F. G., & Newton, H. B. (2010). Clinical presentation, histology, and treatment in 430 patients with primary tumors of the spinal cord, spinal meninges, or cauda equina. *Journal of Neurosurgery: Spine, 13*(1), 67–77.

Leone, A., Guglielme, G., Casser-Pulicino, V. N., & Bonomo, L. (2007). Lumbar intervertebral instability: A review. *Radiology, 245*(1), 62–77.

Kalichman, L., Kim, D.H., Li, L., Guermazi, A., Hunter, D.J., Spine, J. (2010). Computed tomography–evaluated features of spinal degeneration: Prevalence, intercorrelation, and association with self-reported low back pain. Mar 10(3):200–8. Epub 2009 Dec 16.

McGee, S. (2007). *Evidenced based physical diagnosis* (2nd ed.). St. Louis, MI: Saunders Elsevier.

NASS Clinical Guideline Development Committee (2007). Degenerative lumbar spinal stenosis. Retrieved September 1, 2010, from http://www.spine.org/Documents/NASSCG_Stenosis.pdf

NASS Evidenced Based Guideline Committee (2009). Antithrombotic therapies in spine surgery. Retrieved September 1, 2010, from http://www.spine.org/Documents/Antithrombotic_Therapies_ClinicalGuidelines.pdf

NASS Evidenced Based Guideline Development Committee (2007). Antibiotic prophylaxis in spine surgery. Retrieved September 1, 2010, from http://www.spine.org/Documents/Antibiotic_Prophylaxis_Web.pdf

Rosenthal, R. A. (2006). Surgical approaches to the geriatric patient. In C. K. Cassel, R. M. Leipzig, H. J. Cohen, E. B. Larson, & D. E. Meier (Eds.), *Geriatric medicine* (4th ed.). New York: Springer Science & Business Media, LLC.

Scifers, J. R. (2008). *Special tests for neurological examination*. Thorofare, NJ: SLACK Incorporated.

Seller, R. H. (2000). *Differential diagnosis of common complaints* (4th ed.). Philadelphia, PA: W.B. Saunders Company.

Spengler, D., & Donatelli, R. (2005). Spine (Section Eds.). In L. Y. Griffin (Ed.), *Essentials of musculoskeletal care* (3rd ed.). Rosemont, IL: American Academy of Orthopaedic Surgeons.

Yoshikawa, T. T. (2006). Infectious disease. In C. K. Cassel, R. M. Leipzig, H. J. Cohen, E. B. Larson, & D. E. Meier (Eds.), *Geriatric medicine* (4th ed.). New York: Springer Science & Business Media, LLC.

Case 2.5 More Than Just Constipation

By Frieda R. Butler, PhD, MPH, FAAN, FGSA

Ms. Z is a 67-year-old retired physical education teacher in a local high school. She is a widow and lives at home with her son and grandson. Ms. Z presented to her primary care practitioner with a chief complaint of chronic lower abdominal pain, lack of energy, abdominal bloating, and constipation alternating with diarrhea. She has had significant changes in her bowel habits, including difficulty moving her bowels, but has bouts of frequent soft stools. She denies nausea and vomiting, but has occasional fevers and believes she may have caught a virus from a student. Ms. Z visited a gastroenterologist for complaints of lower abdominal pain 3 months ago, which seems worse on the lower left side. The gastroenterologist ordered a barium enema, which was negative except for diverticulosis. Her last colonoscopy was 4 years ago. It, too, was negative except for moderate diverticulosis. She is being treated for hypertension and arthritis, which are well managed with medication. Ms. Z visits her primary care practitioner every 4 months for followup of hypertension; otherwise, she is in very good health. She admits to being overweight and plans to manage her diet and nutrition better. Ms. Z has an occasional glass of wine with her meals and perhaps 1–2 drinks at social events, and does not smoke. She has a surgical history of a knee replacement 2 years ago and is ambulating well now. She travels frequently and has an active social life. Her last trip was to Eastern Europe, where she visited several countries for about a week. She attends a nearby church occasionally and is active in civic groups. Ms. Z works part-time as a basketball

Case Studies in Gerontological Nursing for the Advanced Practice Nurse, First Edition.
Edited by Meredith Wallace Kazer, Leslie Neal-Boylan.
© 2012 John Wiley & Sons, Inc. Published 2012 by John Wiley & Sons, Inc.

coach and substitute teacher which, along with her pension, is more than adequate for her financial support. Both of her parents are deceased, with her father having died of a stroke at the age of 72. Her mother passed away at the age of 56 with a diagnosis of colon cancer.

The review of systems is negative for any other complaints except for arthritis of her knees and back. She denies headaches, dizziness, and problems with vision, but has mild hearing loss. No complaints of chest pains, palpitations, shortness of breath on exertion, or cough. She has no problems with urination. She is 16 years postmenopausal and denies any vaginal bleeding. She has no problems with gait or balance and denies frequent falls. She states that she has had several bone density scans and was told she had mild osteopenia in her right hip. Ms. Z has had several colonoscopies; the last was 4 years ago and was negative for cancerous growths or polyps (see Figure 2.5.1). She was told she had diverticulosis throughout her colon. No history of diabetes or other endocrine problems. She denies having emotional or mental problems; she occasionally experiences bouts of anxiety which may interfere with sleeping. Ms. Z has experienced intermittent abdominal cramping, bloating, flatulence, and constipation over the past 4 months. Sometimes she has a constant ache, which is relieved by evacuation. Lately she has experienced increased pain in her lower

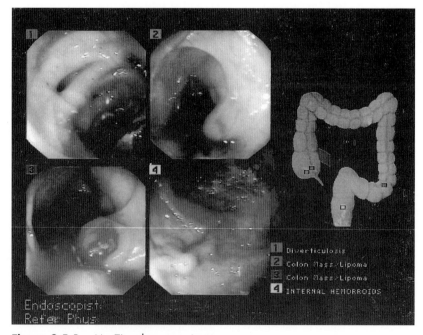

Figure 2.5.1. Ms. Z's colonoscopy image.

left side. She has frequent constipation alternating with diarrhea. Usually symptoms appear several hours after eating and upon awakening in the morning. She has not observed any blood in her stools and denies any nausea and/or vomiting. Her medications include Norvasc, 5 mg per day; hydrochlorothiazide, 25 mg per day; Celebrex, 200 mg per day; and alendronate, 75 mg 1 tab per week. She has no known allergies (NKA).

OBJECTIVE

Ms. Z is conscious, alert, and oriented, but appears listless at times. She responds well to questions. Vitals are temp: 100; heart rate: 92; BP: 132/80. HEENT: Mild hearing loss, otherwise negative. Chest: Heart and lungs are negative. GI: Skin clear with no scars or lesions on observation; umbilicus in midline; abdomen soft, palpable; tenderness on palpation LLQ; no rebound tenderness RLQ; diminished bowel sounds in LLQ; no masses on palpation. GU and GYN: Negative for urinary and gynecologic problems. Musculoskeletal/neurological: Normal gait and balance; normal ROM; moderate crepitations in right knee.

ASSESSMENT

Diverticulosis: Ms. Z's abdominal complaints are consistent with her earlier diagnosis of diverticulosis on a previous colonoscopy and barium enema; however, her low-grade fever may be indicative of an infectious process. To avoid complications such as perforated diverticula, the practitioner should avoid a repeat colonoscopy and/or barium enema at this time.

Arthritis: Although unrelated to her diverticulosis, any joint pain may indirectly affect her mobility and proper meal preparation.

DIAGNOSTICS

- Vital signs, CBC, urinalysis, sedimentation rate, serum electrolytes
- Stool for occult blood, bacteria, ova, and parasites
- Contrast enhanced CT scan (CT colonography)
- Transabdominal ultrasound

Usually a colonoscopy and /or a barium enema are recommended for suspected diverticulosis for differentiation from diseases with similar symptoms; however, because diverticulitis is suspected, these tests should be avoided due to the danger of perforation (Interpretations, 2009; Jacobs, 2007). CT scanning with contrast and ultrasound are the recommended diagnostic tests for diverticulitis (Kang, Melville, & Maxwell, 2004; Lameris et al., 2008; Sartelli, 2010). It is important to rule out peritonitis, as this is an acute condition and requires immediate care. If peritonitis is suspected, call a physician immediately. Laboratory tests include a complete blood count to determine a low red cell count and elevated white cell count. In diverticulitis, the white cell count is elevated with a shift to the left. Stool tests for occult blood will help to determine hemorrhaging; however if guaiac is positive, further testing is necessary to determine if cause is perforated diverticula. Since Ms. Z has a history of travel outside of the U.S, stool testing for ova and parasites will determine whether there is a presence of parasites in her intestines. She has a low grade fever (99°F); however, older adults may not present with an elevated temperature in the presence of infection. Urinalysis and culture and sensitivity tests can be ordered to determine the presence of a UTI. A diagnosis of uterine or ovarian tumors or cancer can be verified on ultrasound; however, no masses were detected. Serum electrolytes will determine if the patient is dehydrated.

The primary care practitioner obtained a copy of Ms. Z's last colonoscopy. One can see the areas of diverticula in all 4 segments of the large intestine.

CBC revealed an elevated white cell count of 15,000 with a shift to the left; however, sedimentation rate and C-reactive protein were within normal limits. The urinalysis was negative for white cells and bacteria. Stools were negative for blood, ova, and parasites. Ultrasound for abdominal and uterine masses was negative. CT colonography revealed severe diverticulosis throughout the colon with no evidence of perforation.

CRITICAL THINKING

Considering Ms. Z's symptoms, the assessment, and the test results, what is the most likely differential diagnosis?

Is there a need for further study? If so, why?

What would be the most likely differential?

Can Ms. Z be managed on an outpatient basis?

What is the plan of treatment?

Describe the plan for follow-up care.

Does Ms. Z's psychosocial history impact how the clinician might treat her?

Are there any factors, such as environmental, family, psychosocial, or other elements that may impact the treatment plan and follow-up care? If so, describe those factors and their potential impact.

RESOLUTION

Considering Ms. Z's symptoms, the assessment, and the test results, what is the most likely differential diagnosis?

Many of the signs and symptoms evident in Ms. Z's case can be seen in a variety of diseases and conditions. The major disorders the practitioner should keep in mind when diagnosing Ms. Z's condition are inflammatory bowel disease, diverticulosis, uncomplicated diverticulitis, complicated diverticulitis, Crohn disease, appendicitis, cystitis, parasites, PID, bowel obstruction, peritonitis, gynecologic disorders, and medication side effects.

Diverticulosis is more prevalent in developed areas such as the United States, Europe, and Australia and is increasing in Western nations (Marris, 2006). It is believed that the advent of processed foods during the twentieth century is strongly related to the increase in this disease. It affects approximately 5%–10% of the population over 45 and 80% of the population over 80 (Ferzoco, Raptopoulos, & Silen, 1998). It is more common in women than in men and in people over the age of 50; and it increases with advancing age, with about half of the population over 60 having the disease (Cramer, 2002).

Diverticula are small pouches that develop in the walls of the intestine, and they are more likely to develop in the large intestine. Diverticula can develop where a blood vessel enters the wall of the colon. Increased pressure within the colon creates a weak spot and may allow the inner lining (mucosa and submucosa membranes) to herniate into the muscular wall. When many pouches are present, the condition is called diverticulosis, with the sigmoid and distal descending colon being most affected (Kang et al., 2004). Many patients have no symptoms, but some experience abdominal discomfort, such as bloating, cramping, constipation and/or diarrhea. Constipation is reported more often than diarrhea. Colicky abdominal cramping frequently occurs after eating and may be relieved by passing stools or flatulence. There may be changes in stool consistency, and these may be flat or ribbon-like. According to recent research studies, 10%–30% of patients with diverticulosis will go on to develop diverticulitis or painful diverticular disease (Lyon & Clark 2006).

Is there a need for further study? If so, why?
In light of the test results, especially the CT scan, negative guaiac stools, and the lack of outstanding findings on physical examination, there are no indications for further testing at this time. The age and history of the patient and the lack of signs and symptoms that are indicative of a more acute or severe diagnosis lead the practitioner to focus on a more benign condition. Even though a diagnosis can be made with confidence by a clinical examination (Ferzoco et al., 1998), the clinician should collaborate with the physician to confirm the absence of more severe diverticular disease. Following resolution of the acute phase, the practitioner should order a colonoscopy and barium enema after 6–8 weeks to rule out cancer and to further validate the diverticulitis diagnosis.

What would be the most likely differential?
Uncomplicated diverticulitis is the most likely differential. Ms. Z had typical signs of diverticulitis, and diagnostic tests revealed no perforation, abscess, fistula formation, or obstruction. For these reasons, she was diagnosed with uncomplicated diverticulitis and could be managed on an outpatient basis. The pathogenesis of diverticulitis is unclear; however, it is believed that stasis or obstruction in the diverticulum may result in bacterial overgrowth and bowel obstruction (Jacobs, 2007; Marchiondo, 1994). First, due to the side effects of Alendronate, this medication was reduced to 5 mg per day; and her abdominal pain was decreased, but not resolved. CT scanning, usually the test of choice for this disease, confirmed the diagnosis of uncomplicated diverticulitis. This test is crucial to avoid an incorrect diagnosis of complicated diverticulosis, possibly resulting in unnecessary emergency surgery.

Complicated diverticulitis (with perforation) and peritonitis are the next differentials. Given Ms. Z's history of diverticulosis, her abdominal symptoms, elevated temperature, and her age, a perforated diverticulum would mean a diagnosis of complicated diverticulitis, perhaps with peritonitis. Between 1% and 3% of older patients with diverticulosis will experience at least 1 episode of diverticulitis; and 15%–30% of these will be complicated, which may include perforation, peritonitis, or bowel obstruction. Perforated diverticula with peritonitis could be ruled out on physical exam with negative findings of (1) a board-like abdomen, (2) left shoulder tip pain (Kehr sign), (3) rebound tenderness (Blumberg sign), and (4) pain in the RLQ following palpation (Rovsing sign). The position of the patient also suggests a negative abdomen since she did not try to minimize pain by lying perfectly still, guarding, or displaying obvious signs of pain on palpation. These findings also rule out a perforated appendix. She was negative for cutaneous hyperesthesia and psoas sign (RLQ pain with right leg lift), Aaron sign (pain on palpation of McBurney point, and Markle sign (heel jar/heel tap).

The third differential would be irritable bowel syndrome (IBS). IBS is a common condition among many Americans, with 20% reporting symptoms similar to diverticula disease. The etiology of IBS is unknown; however, researchers, scientists, and geneticists continue to look for possible causes.

This disorder also presents with abdominal complaints such as abdominal cramping, bloating and changes in bowel habits. Again the disease occurs in women more than in men and typically shows up in middle age. Researchers are investigating an intriguing mind-body connection and have had favorable results when treating depression, anxiety, and stress (Cramer, 2002).

Can Ms. Z be managed on an outpatient basis?

Since perforation and peritonitis have been ruled out and this first attack appears to be mild, it is likely that Ms. Z can be managed on an outpatient basis. After it was determined that she could tolerate oral hydration, the decision was made to carefully manage her through the primary care clinic.

What is the plan of treatment?

Ms. Z has had an extended period of diarrhea alternating with constipation; therefore, she may lack sufficient hydration. The first step is to rehydrate her and to rest the bowel with a liquid diet for 7 days. In addition, she will be given a regimen of broad spectrum antibiotics, such as ciprofloxacin and metronidazole, for 7–10 days to cover against anerobic microorganisms; this is the standard of care for uncomplicated diverticulitis (Ferzoco et al., 1998; McCafferty, Roth, & Jorden, 2008; Sartelli, 2010). Often in diverticulitis, there is the possibility of microperforation (Ferzoco et al., 1998). Patients who cannot tolerate fluids or experience acute pain should be hospitalized. Following the initial treatment and resolution of the acute phase, Ms. Z will be placed on a high fiber diet.

The role of dietary fiber in the pathogenesis of diverticular disease has been documented in the literature. Low dietary fiber intake results in increased intraluminal pressure which, along with weakened colonic wall structure and abnormal colonic activity, leads to diverticula in the colon. Dietary fiber will increase stool bulk, which leads to increased gastrointestinal transit time and to decreased colonic pressure (Mann & Seo, 2010; Ferzoco et al., 1998). The research has shown that dietary fiber supplements increases stool weight, alters gastrointestinal transit time, decreases intraluminal pressures and as a result, relieves pain, nausea and vomiting, and flatulence. In addition, she will be given a regimen of regular physical exercise. Strate, Liu, Aldoori, & Giovannucci (2009) showed that vigorous physical activity can reduce diverticulitis and the risk of diverticular bleeding by more than a third.

Describe the plan for follow-up care.

Strict adherence to a high fiber diet may help to avoid unnecessary emergency surgery; therefore, the practitioner will reassess the patient in 1 month and every 3 months after that, paying particular attention to Ms. Z's dietary history. A follow-up colonoscopy to further rule out polyps or cancerous growths is planned following resolution of the acute condition.

Does Ms. Z's psychosocial history impact how the clinician might treat her?

Anxiety has been studied as a possible factor in diverticulosis and other bowel diseases. For this reason, it would be wise for the practitioner to investigate Ms. Z's anxiety, including possible causes, precipitating factors, and what brings relief. Depending on the severity and frequency of anxiety attacks, a relationship may be established between that and her diverticulosis.

Are there any factors, such as environmental, family, psychosocial, or other elements that may impact the treatment plan and follow-up care? If so, describe those factors and their potential impact.

Ms. Z should be instructed to discuss her diet with her family members so that all will be informed regarding the need for careful meal planning that will be acceptable to all members. Since a high fiber diet is an important element in maintaining optimal wellness for all, and not just the affected member, perhaps the family should have input in the planning process.

Diagnosing abdominal complaints can be a complex process and requires thoughtful and sound clinical judgment in collaboration with the gastroenterologist. Acute diverticulitis can be a dangerous complication of diverticulosis if not diagnosed and treated promptly. When treating uncomplicated diverticulitis on an outpatient basis, be sure that the patient is able to comply and has good family support. Lack of systemic toxicity, the ability to tolerate clear liquids, no associated immunocompromising conditions, and open communication channels (patient, NP, and physician) are important factors in outpatient treatment and followup of these patients.

Bowel rest and prompt antibiotic therapy usually clear up the condition without further complication. If left without adequate treatment, it can progress to perforations, abscess formations, intestinal blockages, and life-threatening peritonitis. It is recommended that a colonoscopy be performed 6–8 weeks after the acute episode (depending on the date of the last colonoscopy) to exclude the presence of cancer or Crohn disease and any later perforation (McCafferty et al., 2008). In addition, a barium enema should be ordered to determine the extent of the diverticular disease. Continuing dietary education of the patient and family by the NP and encouraging regular exercise are crucial elements in the treatment and recovery of the patient.

REFERENCES

Cramer, D. (2002). Understanding bowel disorders. *Research watch*. Retrieved on June 6, 2010, from http://www.alive.com/6640a17a2.php?subject_bread_cramb=390

Ferzoco, L. B., Raptopoulos, V., & Silen, W. (1998). Acute diverticulitis. *New England Journal of Medicine, 338*(21), 1521–1526.

Interpretations (2009). Transabdominal ultrasound in the initial assessment of adult bowel disease. *British Journal of Hospital Medicine, 70*(12), M182–M185.

Jacobs, D. O. (2007). Clinical practice: Diverticulitis. *New England Journal of Medicine, 357*(20), 2057–2056.

Kang, J., Melville, D., & Maxwell, D. (2004). Epidemiology and management of diverticular disease of the colon. *Drugs and Aging, 21*(4), 211–228.

Lameris, W., van Randen, A., Bipat, S., Bossuyt, P., Boermeester, M., & Stoker, J. (2008). Graded compression ultrasonography and computed tomography in acute colonic diverticulitis: Meta-analysis of test accuracy. *European Radiology, 18*, 2498–2511.

Lyon, C., & Clark, D. (2006). Diagnosis of acute abdominal pain in older patients. *American Family Physician, 74*(9), 1537–1544.

Mann, N., & Seo, S. (2010). Views and practice of gastroenterologists regarding diet modification in patients with colonic diverticulosis. *International Medical Journal, 17*(2), 83–85.

Marchiondo, K. (1994). When the diagnosis is diverticular disease. *RN, 57*(2), 42–47.

Marris, J. A. (2006). Abdominal complaints. *Clinical Journal of Oncology Nursing, 10*(2), 155–157.

McCafferty, M. H., Roth, L., & Jorden, J. (2008). Current management of diverticulosis. *The American Surgeon, 74*, 1041–1049.

Sartelli, M. (2010). A focus on intra-abdominal infections. *World Journal of Emergency Surgery, 5*(9), 1–20. Retrieved from on June 1, 2010, http://www.wjes.org/content/5/1/9

Strate, L. L., Liu, Y. L., Aldoori, W. H., & Giovannucci, E. L. (2009). Physical activities reduce diverticular complications. *American Journal of Gastroenterology, 104*, 1221–1230.

Case 2.6 Are You in the Hospital Again?

By Kimberly O. Lacey, DNSc, MSN, CNS

Mr. T, a 75-year-old man, presents to the cardiologist's office with increasing dyspnea on exertion (DOE), orthopnea, weakness, and new onset cough. He was recently discharged from the hospital after his third inpatient stay within the past 9 months for exacerbation of congestive heart failure (CHF). Mr. T has a history of hypertension (HTN) and Type 2 diabetes mellitus. Prior to his diagnosis with CHF approximately 1 year ago, he was in relatively good health with his HTN well controlled with Monopril, 10 mg daily. His diabetes was well controlled with diet and exercise. Surgical history includes cataract removal bilaterally and appendectomy several years ago. He drinks alcohol socially and has never smoked. He lives alone in his own home in a small suburban town. His wife passed away 5 years ago after a 2-year battle with cancer. He has 2 sons. One is a bartender in a local restaurant and lives locally with his wife, who is an office manager for a local law firm; he occasionally visits his father. Mr. T's eldest son, an architect, lives 2 hours away with his wife and 4 young children; he visits when he can, usually about once a month. Since retiring at 65 years old from his high school teaching job, Mr. T has enjoyed golfing, walking, reading, crossword puzzles, and volunteering at the local food bank. He participates in community events such as planning and attending parades, town concerts, and other celebrations, as well as local political events. He has several friends with whom he spends time socially and has a circle of professional friends with whom he goes out to dinner monthly. He attends church each Sunday after which he visits his wife's grave to

Case Studies in Gerontological Nursing for the Advanced Practice Nurse, First Edition.
Edited by Meredith Wallace Kazer, Leslie Neal-Boylan.
© 2012 John Wiley & Sons, Inc. Published 2012 by John Wiley & Sons, Inc.

pay his respects; then he enjoys breakfast with friends at a café. He is financially secure with a hefty pension from his teaching job, his social security, and income from investments. His parents both lived to be in their eighties. His mother died of "old age;" she had no significant health problems. His father died of "lung disease." He remembers his father as being "generally" healthy. Although for most of his life he has been diligent about seeking health care and preventing illness, he did not do so consistently for a period of approximately 2 years after his wife's death. His HTN and diabetes were both diagnosed when he resumed regular medical followup approximately 3 years ago. Today Mr. T presents with DOE, orthopnea, weakness, and a cough, all of which he reports have been increasing over the past 3 days. On review of systems, he has no other complaints. He denies headache, vision changes, numbness, tingling, chest pain, nausea, edema, vomiting, or changes in bowel or urinary habits. His medications include metformin, 500 mg twice a day; Monopril, 20 mg every morning; and HCTZ, 25 mg every morning. He has no known allergies (NKA).

OBJECTIVE

Mr. T is alert, oriented, and well groomed, but seems to be less spirited than usual. His posture is somewhat slouched, and his gait slow but steady. He is 5 ft 8 inches tall and 175 lb. BP: 185/92; P: 114; RR: 24 at rest; O_2 Sat 91%. He is afebrile with a temperature of 98.2. Lungs: Basilar rales bilaterally. Cardiac exam reveals tachycardia but regular rate and rhythm with S1, S2. No adventitious sounds are noted. DOE with ambulation 25 feet from waiting room to exam room, resolved with rest. Abdomen is soft, nontender with positive bowels sounds in all 4 quadrants. Skin is dry and intact; no lesions or scars noted. There is no pedal edema, and positive (+2) pulses are present bilaterally. Eyes appear normal without clouding or jaundice; PERRLA. Hearing is intact, and ears appear normal without extensive wax buildup. Random fingerstick glucose was 130 mg/dl.

ASSESSMENT

Hypertension: Mr. T's blood pressure is elevated at this office visit. This may be a true exacerbation, or it may be the result of his heart failure symptoms. It may also be related to stress brought on by concerns about his health, in general. A noncritical, one-time elevation does not necessarily require immediate changes in treatment, but it does warrant further monitoring. Hypertension is one of the major causes of heart failure (Heart Failure Society of America, 2010).

Diabetes: Appears to be well controlled with current therapy. Stress related to illness, as well as changes in illness management, can contribute to elevations in blood glucose levels; so continued monitoring will be necessary (American Diabetes Association, 2010).

Risk for depression: Mr. T is less spirited today suggesting that he may be depressed or may be having difficulty coping with his illness. Self-care is a critical aspect of the management of heart failure as well as diabetes. This can present a significant challenge, particularly for older adults. Difficulty coping with heart failure and the associated self-care requirements is associated with depression, which may result in poor disease management (Allman, Berry, & Nasir, 2009; Lin, et al., 2004)

Congestive heart failure: Heart failure is common, but unrecognized and often misdiagnosed. It affects nearly 5 million Americans. Heart failure is the only major cardiovascular disorder on the rise. An estimated 400,000–700,000 new cases of heart failure are diagnosed each year and the number of deaths in the United States from this condition has more than doubled since 1979, averaging 250,000 annually. It is a progressive and debilitating chronic condition (Heart Failure Society of America, 2010).

DIAGNOSTICS

Several issues need to be addressed in this patient. The most straightforward of these is his diabetes. A random fingerstick glucose of 130 mg/dl suggests that Mr. T's diabetes is well controlled. Monitoring daily fasting, postprandial, and random fingersticks is one way to further assess this, as a one-time limited test does not truly reflect diabetes control. Stress related to 3 recent hospitalizations and the possibility of depression or poor coping may be affecting his diabetes management. A more reliable assessment is warranted. Ordering a hemoglobin A1c (HbA1c) and laboratory fasting blood sugar (FBS) is indicated (American Diabetes Association, 2010). The elevation in blood pressure may be related to stress, medication adherence, diet, or current illness. It is important to remember that a single elevation in blood pressure does not warrant an immediate change in therapy. HTN is diagnosed and therapy modified when there is evidence over time that the blood pressure is consistently elevated (American Heart Association, 2011). Additionally, in the case of the patient who has diabetes, a blood pressure above 130/80 is considered hypertensive

(American Diabetes Association, 2010). Chronic illnesses in the elderly, particularly CHF, can result in poor coping and depression. As with diabetes, CHF management warrants a significant amount of self-care and commitment on the part of the patient. For many, particularly the elderly, this care is overwhelming; and in the case of illness exacerbations it becomes even more difficult to follow prescribed therapy. Although alert, oriented, and well groomed, Mr. T is noted to have an altered mood; "He is less spirited." Therefore, the possibility of depression and/or poor coping must be considered. At a minimum, a discussion with Mr. T regarding his mood, coping, and ability to manage his illnesses is necessary. Finally, CHF is the most acute concern for this patient who presents with progressive DOE, orthopnea, cough, tachycardia, reduced O_2 Sat, and rales. An electrocardiogram (EKG) and echocardiogram are both warranted. These tests will provide data to determine if there have been changes in heart function or further damage to the heart muscle. Additional necessary blood work includes a CBC with differential, LFTs, and a metabolic panel.

The results of the diagnostic tests are as follows: FBS: 90; HbA1c: 7.2; CBC, LFTs, and metabolic panel are all within normal limits. EKG is unchanged from the previous one 3 months ago, and results of the echocardiogram indicate an ejection fraction (which indicates pumping ability of the heart [Heart Failure Society of America, 2010]) of 50% which is also unchanged from the last hospitalization.

Understanding that recurrent hospitalization can be discouraging to a patient, after review of the diagnostics, the cardiologist determines that Mr. T has reported his symptoms early enough to avoid hospitalization. However, he must have support and is therefore referred for home care services with a follow-up appointment scheduled with the cardiologist in 2 weeks. The goals of therapy are to improve the management of Mr. T's heart failure and to keep him out of the hospital.

CRITICAL THINKING

Explain the need for and the results of the laboratory FBS and HbA1c.

How will the clinician address the concerns of poor coping and possible depression?

What interventions will the clinician initiate specific to the management of Mr. T's CHF?

What type of heart failure does Mr. T have?

What adjustments in therapy, if any, would the clinician make?

Are there any standardized guidelines that the clinician would use to assess and treat this patient?

RESOLUTION

Explain the need for and the results of the laboratory FBS and HbA1c.
Laboratory FBS is a more reliable and accurate measure of blood glucose when compared to the home FBS, while the HbA1c indicates blood glucose control over time. Mr. T's FBS is acceptable and within the recommended range of 70–130 mg/dl. His HbA1c is just above the recommended level of <7% (American Diabetes Association, 2010). Overall, these data suggest that Mr. T has been able to keep his diabetes controlled despite frequent hospitalizations and CHF exacerbations. However, given his current health status, it will be important to continue to have him monitor his FBS, post-prandial blood sugar, and random blood sugars. By doing this, the clinician can get a clearer picture of how his diabetes is being managed on a day-to-day basis and whether any medication adjustments are necessary. In addition, it can help Mr. T determine how he might be able to keep his diabetes under the best possible control through diet and exercise. Tight control of blood glucose levels prevents and slows the progression of diabetes complications such as heart disease, nephropathy, retinopathy, and neuropathy (Diabetes Control and Complications Trial Research Group, 1993). For Mr. T, while tight control will reduce his risk for developing these complications, specific to his heart failure, it is important to reduce further heart muscle damage.

How will the clinician address the concerns of poor coping and possible depression?
The risk of depression in older adults increases with other illnesses including CHF and when their ability to function becomes limited. Estimates of major depression in older people living in the community range from less than 1% to about 5%, but this rises to 13.5% in those who require home health care and to 11.5% in elderly hospital patients. In addition, an estimated 5 million older adults have subsyndromal depression, symptoms that fall short of meeting the full diagnostic criteria for a disorder (National Institute of Mental Health, 2010). Although the prevalence rates for depression in patients who have heart failure vary between 60% and 95% data have shown that depression in heart failure is associated with poorer outcomes (Rutledge et al., 2006) and reduced ability to cope with management and medication regimens (Morgan et al., 2006). In the case of Mr. T, his change in "spirit" and slouched posture suggest that he may be experiencing depressive symptoms, poor coping, and difficulty with managing his health, which are contributing to his current CHF exacerbation. Mr. T should be screened for depressive symptoms using a validated instrument such as the Center for Epidemiologic Studies Depression Scale (CES-D) (Radloff, 1977). If the results suggest depressive symptoms and/or risk for depression, a referral to a counselor or social worker

may be appropriate; but spending time talking with Mr. T to learn more about how he is feeling will be helpful in determining the next step. Beginning the patient on antidepressant therapy, such as a serotonin reuptake inhibitor (SSRI), may also be appropriate.

What interventions will the clinician initiate specific to the management of Mr. T's CHF?

First and foremost, a comprehensive assessment of Mr. T's physical and emotional health is necessary, as well as determining his current and previous levels of functioning. Taking the time to perform a detailed assessment will provide valuable information that will be useful in developing his plan of care. With the assistance of telemonitoring, BP, along with apical heart rate, RR, weight, and O_2 Sat to monitor level of oxygenation will be taken daily for the next 2 weeks and reported to the clinician. A blood pressure that continues to be elevated above 130/80 in the context of medication adherence and support will serve as a prompt for further assessment and possible changes in his HTN medications. Apical heart rate provides information on the rate and rhythm and heart sounds. Changes in these may indicate worsening CHF, heart muscle damage, valve disorders (which may result from HTN), and arrhythmias. Daily weights will be monitored so that early fluid retention can be identified. Lungs will be auscultated and the presence of edema will be assessed 3 times a week during a nursing visit. Medication adherence will be monitored at each home visit. The importance of adherence will be emphasized, and problems with adherence will be discussed with the patient so that more effective strategies can be implemented. Dietary restrictions for sodium will be discussed, and strategies for identifying and avoiding high sodium foods will be implemented. Using a telemonitoring system Mr. T will transmit data on vital signs, weight, presence of edema, SOB, DOE, and cough each morning. He will also be asked to provide subjective data on how he feels and his functional status. The data will be reviewed by the clinician who will look for trends suggesting improvement or decline in status. Identifying early symptoms of worsening heart failure is critical if rehospitalization is to be avoided. Providing up-front intensive support for Mr. T will strengthen his chances of successfully managing his CHF. In addition, a psychosocial assessment to determine available resources for Mr. T is necessary. Having a solid support system whether it is family, friends, or other services can have a positive impact on chronic illness management, rehospitalization, and quality of life (Phillips et al., 2004).

What type of heart failure does Mr. T have?

Based on Mr. T's known diagnosis of HTN, lack of other cardiac history (infarction or arrhythmia), his symptoms of DOE, orthopnea, tachycardia, weakness, and rales, and the absence of edema or distended neck veins, it makes sense that Mr. T suffers from left-sided heart failure.

Heart failure occurs when the heart is unable to pump sufficient amounts of blood to meet the metabolic needs of the body. HTN causes left ventricular hypertrophy (enlargement) which results in inefficient heart muscle pumping and subsequent fluid backup and CHF (Heart Failure Society of America, 2010).

What adjustments in therapy, if any, would the clinician make?
The first goal is to stabilize Mr. T so that his symptoms can be improved and hospitalization can be avoided. He is already taking an ACE inhibitor (Monopril) and a thiazide diuretic, both of which are recommended first lines of therapy for treating patients who have HTN and CHF. ACE inhibitors work by blocking the conversion of angiotensin I to angiotensin II, thereby reducing vascular resistance and aldosterone secretion (which reduces sodium and water retention) in turn decreasing blood pressure and improving cardiac output by reducing fluid backup. ACE inhibitors are also effective in reducing nephropathy in patients with diabetes. Thiazides are mild diuretics that remove excess sodium and water from the body by preventing reabsorption of water and sodium in the kidneys. With a plan in place for Mr. T to receive supportive care and close monitoring over the next 2 weeks, a conservative approach would be to increase his HCTZ daily for 3 days to draw off extra fluid and sodium with subsequent evaluation of clinical data and telemonitoring trends to assess effectiveness and the need for additional changes. A second option would be to leave the HCTZ alone and increase the Monopril to 30 mg (Caboral, Salak, & Mitchell, 2009; Grady, 2006; Gould and Dyer, 2006; Heart Failure Society of America, 2010). Electrolytes should be carefully evaluated during this diuretic therapy.

Are there any standardized guidelines that the clinician would use to assess and treat this patient?
The American College of Cardiology Foundation/American Heart Association Task Force has developed practice guidelines for the diagnosis and management of heart failure in adults. A focused update developed in collaboration with the International Society for Heart and Lung Transplantation was published in 2009. This is available at http://content.onlinejacc.org/cgi/content/full/53/15/1343.

REFERENCES

Allman, E., Berry, D., & Nasir, L. (2009). Depression and coping in heart failure patients: A review of the literature. *Journal of Cardiovascular Nursing, 24*(2), 106–117.

American Diabetes Association (2010). Standards of medical care in diabetes—2010. *Diabetes Care, 33*(Suppl. 1), S11–S61.

American Heart Association (2011). http://www.heart.org/HEARTORG/Conditions/HighBloodPressure/High-Blood-Pressure_UCM_002020_SubHomePage.jsp

Caboral, M. F., Salak, K., & Mitchell, J. (2009). Are you up to date with heart failure? *Nursing 2009 Critical Care*, 4(6), 36–41.

Gould, B. E. and Dyer, R. M. (Eds.) (2006). Cardiovascular Disorders. In: *Pathophysiology for the health professions* (4th ed.), pp. 271–322. St. Louis, MO: Saunders; Elsevier.

Diabetes Control and Complications Trial Research Group (1993). The effect of intensive treatment of diabetes on the development and progression of long-term complications in insulin-dependent diabetes mellitus. *NEJM*, 329(14), 977–986.

Grady, K. (2006). Management of heart failure in older adults. *Journal of Cardiovascular Nursing*, 21(55), 510–514.

Heart Failure Society of America (2010). *Quick facts and questions about heart failure*. Retrieved from http://www.hfsa.org/heart_failure_facts.asp

Lin, E. H., Katon, W., Von Korff, M., Rutter, C., Simon, G. E., Oliver, M., Ciechanowski, P., . . . Young, B. (2004). Relationship of depression and diabetes self-care, medication adherence, and preventive care. *Diabetes Care*, 27(9), 2154–2160.

Morgan, A. L., Masoudi, F. A., Havranek, E. P., Jones, P. G., Peterson, P. N., Krumholz, H. M., . . . Rumsfeld, J. S. (2006). Difficulty taking medications, depression, and health status in heart failure patients. *J. Card. Fail.*, 12(1), 54–60.

National Institute of Mental Health (2010). *Older Adults and Mental Health*. Retrieved from http://www.nimh.nih.gov/health/topics/older-adults-and-mental-health/index.shtml

Phillips, C. O., Wright, S. M., Kern, D. E., Singa, R.M., Shepperd, S. & Rubin, H.R. (2004). Comprehensive discharge planning with post-discharge support for older patients with congestive heart failure: A meta-analysis. *JAMA*, 291(11), 1358–1367. Retrieved from http://jama.ama-assn.org/cgi/content/full/291/11/1358.

Radloff, L. S. (1977). The CES-D scale: A self report depression scale for research in the general population. *Applied Psychological Measurement*, 1, 385–401.

Rutledge, T., Reis, V. A., Linke, S. E., Greenberg, B. H., & Mills, P. J. (2006). Depression in heart failure a meta-analytic review of prevalence, intervention effects, and associations with clinical outcomes. *J. Am. Coll. Cardiol.*, 48(8), 1527–1537.

ADDITIONAL RESOURCES

Moser, D. K. and Watkins, J. F. (2008). Conceptualizing self care in heart failure: A life course model of patient characteristics. *Journal of Cardiovascular Nursing*, 23(3), 205–218.

Naylor, M. and Keating, S. A. (2008). Transitional care. *AJN*, 108(9) *Supplement*, 58–63.

Case 2.7 It Hurts When I Pee

By Rebecca Herter, MSN, RN

Mrs. J presented to the primary care office today with complaints of acute onset low fever, lower abdominal pain, and urinary frequency and pain, which she has been experiencing for 4 days. Mrs. J is an 86-year-old woman whose past medical history includes hypertension, hyperlipidemia, COPD, and a long history of smoking. She has been seen regularly here for 26 years and is also followed by a cardiologist. Her past surgical history includes left breast biopsy at age 75, L4-5 disc fusion at age 79, and total abdominal hysterectomy and bilateral salpingo oophorectomy (TAH BSO) at age 54 for persistent vaginal bleeding. Mrs. J is married and lives at home with her husband. She is a retired high school teacher. She has 2 sons who do not live in the area and 3 grandchildren. Mrs. J drinks socially, generally 1–2 glasses of red wine every other week. She currently smokes 1 pack of cigarettes per day and has done so for 50 years. She generally feels well. She walks 20 minutes a day, 3 days per week, and gardens in the spring and summer. Both of her parents are deceased. Her father died at 54 of colon cancer, and her mother died in her 90s of "old age". She has no siblings. One of her sons is 60 and has hypertension and hyperlipidemia. Her other son is 57 and is healthy. During this visit, she denies cough, chest pain, shortness of breath, nausea, vomiting, change in bowel patterns, and vaginal discharge. She reports that she is generally continent but has occasional stress incontinence with coughing. She also reports that she moves her bowels regularly and does not require any laxatives. She had a colonoscopy 2 years ago that indicated

Case Studies in Gerontological Nursing for the Advanced Practice Nurse, First Edition.
Edited by Meredith Wallace Kazer, Leslie Neal-Boylan.
© 2012 John Wiley & Sons, Inc. Published 2012 by John Wiley & Sons, Inc.

significant sigmoid diverticulosis. Her medications include lisinopril, 20 mg PO daily; Lipitor, 20 mg PO daily; Spiriva HandiHaler, 18 mcg/cap DPI 1 cap inhaled daily; HCTZ, 25 mg PO daily; and Cardizem, 240 mg PO daily. She is allergic to sulfa.

OBJECTIVE

Mrs. J is awake, alert, and oriented. She appears clean, and her attire is appropriate. She is an obese woman in mild distress. She appears acutely ill. She is 5 ft 5 inches and weighs 190 lb. Temp: 99.8°F (baseline temp 97.4°F); BP: 160/90; HR: 110; RR: 20; O_2 Sat: 95% RA. Her lungs are clear to auscultation in all lung fields. Cardiac exam reveals regular heart rate, S1, S2 with no S3, S4 murmurs, gallops, clicks, or rubs. Her abdomen is soft and nondistended with mild suprapubic tenderness. Bowel sounds are present in all 4 quadrants. No CVA tenderness. She has no edema in her extremities. A bimanual pelvic exam reveals no masses or tenderness. Her rectal exam is heme negative with no tenderness.

ASSESSMENT

Urinary Tract Infection (UTI): Acute onset fever, lower abdominal pain, and urinary frequency suggest a possible UTI. A postmenopausal woman is at high risk for UTI because of the estrogen deficiency that results from normal aging. This estrogen deficiency causes the normally acidic pH of the vagina to become more alkaline, consequently suppressing the growth of predominantly gram positive normal flora and potentially allowing more pathogenic enteric gram negative bacilli to populate. In addition, estrogen decline in older women may also lead to atrophy of the vaginal epithelium which when inflamed may add to symptoms of urinary frequency, urgency, dysuria, and incontinence (Nicolle, 2001).

Diverticulitis: In a woman with known diverticulosis by colonoscopy, acute onset fever and tenderness in the lower abdomen could signal diverticulitis. With her history of TAH BSO, an inflamed bowel could irritate the bladder, accounting for the urinary frequency reported by the patient.

Bladder cancer: With Mrs. J's age and long smoking history, a diagnosis of bladder cancer could explain her abdominal discomfort and urinary frequency. Smoking increases the risk of bladder cancer 2- to 4-fold, and the risk increases with the amount of tobacco use and the duration of smoking (Morrison et al., 1984). Most patients with bladder cancer also present after the age of 60 years (Lynch & Cohen, 1995).

DIAGNOSTICS

Considering Mrs. J's symptoms and exam findings, appropriate initial diagnostic tests should include urine dip and culture and sensitivity (C & S), as well as complete blood count (CBC) with differential. A urine dip is important to determine if there is pyuria or hematuria. The presence of leukocyte esterase (indicating the presence of pyuria or white blood cells in the urine) and the presence of nitrites (generated from urinary nitrate reducing the activity of bacteria) are highly suggestive of UTI. These 2 tests can be misleading at times though. UTI may be present in patients with below-threshold numbers of WBCs in the urine when accompanied by symptoms referable to the urinary tract and thus a urine C & S should still be performed. Further, the nitrite test does not detect bacteriuria caused by *Pseudomonas*, *Staphylococcus*, or *Enterococcus* species. Hematuria, as indicated by a urine dip, is not very specific and could be present with either UTI or bladder cancer. Urine C & S would confirm the presence of bacteria and indicate which antibiotics would be appropriate choices for treatment based on antimicrobial sensitivities. A CBC with differential could also reveal an infectious process. A more elevated WBC count may be more indicative of diverticulitis than UTI.

Urine dipstick is positive for leukocyte esterase, nitrites, and protein and negative for hematuria. Urine C & S reveals the presence of greater than 100,000 CFU/mL of *E. coli* and shows sensitivities to trimethoprim/sulfamethoxazole, nitrofurantoin, ciprofloxacin, and fosfomycin. CBC with differential indicates a WBC count of 9000/mcL with 80% granulocytes.

CRITICAL THINKING

What is the most likely differential diagnosis and why?

What is the plan for treatment?

What is the plan for follow-up care?

How might the presentation of UTI in older adults differ from that in younger, healthier adults?

If Mrs. J had come in for her annual complete physical exam and routine urinalysis revealed significant pyuria, yet she was completely asymptomatic, should the clinician treat her for a UTI?

What aspects of the history, physical exam, diagnostics, and treatment plan are important to consider in an older male with possible UTI?

How would the treatment plan change in a patient with an indwelling urinary catheter?

What measures can be taken to help Mrs. J avoid future UTIs?

RESOLUTION

What is the most likely differential diagnosis and why?
Given Mrs. J's presentation with fever (in older adults, baseline temperatures may be lower than in younger adults), urinary frequency, and lower abdominal pain, slight abdominal tenderness to palpation on physical exam, and the fact that UTI is the most common infection seen in older adults across all care settings, a likely diagnosis is UTI. Combined with a urine dip positive for leukocyte esterase and nitrites, a urine C & S indicating the presence of greater than 100,000 CFU/ml of *E. coli*, and CBC with slightly elevated WBC count, the most likely diagnosis for Mrs. J is UTI. In almost all cases, hematuria would be present on urine dip in a patient with bladder cancer; and CBC with differential would be normal. In addition, if Mrs. J had diverticulitis, her CBC with differential would most likely indicate a more elevated WBC count.

What is the plan for treatment?
The treatment plan for UTI should almost always be based on the urine C & S. Exceptions in which the infection should be treated empirically with antibiotics include patients with severe urinary tract symptoms of dysuria or impending sepsis syndrome and febrile nursing home patients who meet the Diagnostic and Statistical Manual of Mental Disorders (DSM-IV) criteria for delirium (Nicolle, 2001). In all other cases, empirical treatment for an unclear diagnosis of UTI may obscure the diagnosis of other infections. Mrs. J's urine C & S indicates that trimethoprim/sulfamethoxazole, nitrofurantoin, ciprofloxacin, and fosfomycin would be appropriate choices for treatment. However, since she has an allergy to sulfa medications, trimethoprim/sulfamethoxazole would not be an option. The optimal duration for antibiotic therapy in older women has yet to be determined. At least 7 days of treatment is recommended, as relapse is a common occurrence with only 3 days of therapy (Nicolle, 2001). It is also important to find a recent serum creatinine level and calculate creatinine clearance to determine if renal dosage adjustment is necessary. In addition, phenazopyridine (Pyridium) is not appropriate for use in older patients to reduce bladder spasm caused by UTI.

What is the plan for follow-up care?
Unless symptoms persist after the antibiotics course, there is no need for follow-up care. If symptoms of infection persist, a repeat urine culture should be performed to determine if a secondary infection with a new organism resistant to the chosen antibiotic therapy has emerged. Signs and symptoms of infection recurring within 2 weeks of treatment indicate a UTI relapse, and the relapse will most likely be caused by the same strain of bacteria that caused the initial infection. Signs and symptoms of infection recurring 4 weeks after the completion of treatment signify a recurrent UTI that may be caused by a different bacterial strain than that which caused the initial infection (Nicolle, 2001).

How might the presentation of UTI in older adults differ from that in younger, healthier adults?
Older patients may not present with the classic signs and symptoms that often accompany UTI in younger, healthier patients such as urinary frequency, burning, dysuria, urgency, or suprapubic discomfort. At any age, UTI usually has acute onset. Unlike in younger patients, older patients with UTI commonly present with fever, urinary frequency, incontinence, nausea and/or vomiting. Although not specific to UTI, falls, increased or new urinary incontinence, changes in mental or functional status, hematuria, and anorexia and/or vomiting in older adults signify the need for further investigation (Duthie, Katz, & Malone, 2007).

If Mrs. J had come in for her annual complete physical exam and routine urinalysis revealed significant pyuria, yet she was completely asymptomatic, should the clinician treat her for a UTI?
No. The likelihood of significant bacteriuria (more than 10^5 CFU/mL) increases with age and debility. Using routine screening of asymptomatic community dwelling older adults, studies have revealed that 5%–15% of older men and 15%–20% of older women have significant bacteriuria. These rates increase in nursing home residents and patients with long-term indwelling urinary catheters. Asymptomatic bacteriuria is considered a benign condition and does not necessitate treatment. Treatment of asymptomatic bacteriuria has been shown to confer no benefit to patients in terms of well-being or morbidity and mortality. In most patients, symptomatic bacteriuria clears spontaneously or occurs intermittently. In addition, antibiotic treatment of asymptomatic bacteriuria promotes antibiotic resistance. Thus, antibiotic therapy is only indicated for patients without an indwelling urinary catheter if they have significant bacteriuria in addition to 3 of the following: dysuria, fever>100°F (or 2.4°F above baseline), hematuria, frequency, new or increased urgency or incontinence, suprapubic discomfort, or CVA tenderness (Nicolle, Bradley, & Colgan, 2005).

What aspects of the history, physical exam, diagnostics, and treatment plan are important to consider in an older male with possible UTI?

In almost all cases, UTIs in men are complicated by structural or functional abnormalities. Normal aging processes lead to obstructive prostatic hypertrophy and large post void residuals (PVR), allowing greater opportunity for bacteriuria and UTI. In addition, neoplasms and stones occurring through the urinary tract become more common as a person ages and cause obstruction. When taking the history for a man presenting with possible UTI, questions about history of benign prostatic hypertrophy (BPH), prostate cancer, and renal stones should be included. Physical exam in such a patient should include a rectal exam monitoring for impaction and prostate tenderness, masses, or enlargement. Diagnostics in men with suspected obstructive uropathy should include ultrasound or CT scan, and a urology referral is recommended. First line treatment for men with UTI is ciprofloxacin. Because of concerns about associated prostatitis, β-lactam antibiotics and nitrofurantoin should be avoided in older men with UTI. The length of treatment for UTI in men should be longer than in women, typically 10–14 days (Nicolle, 2001).

How would the treatment plan change in a patient with an indwelling urinary catheter?

Urinary devices such as indwelling urinary catheters can directly introduce bacteria into the bladder or allow bacteria to migrate into the bladder along the external surfaces of the catheter. Within 30 days, all patients with indwelling urinary catheters will become bacteriuric. Around 3% of catheterized patients who develop symptomatic bacteriuria will go on to develop bacteremia (Parker et al., 2009). Treatment of bacteriuria related to chronic indwelling urinary devices should only be considered in patients with significant bacteriuria and 2 of the following: fever >100°F (or 2.4°F above baseline) and new onset CVA tenderness, chills, or delirium. These patients should be treated for complicated UTI and such treatment entails IV antibiotic therapy with a 3rd generation cephalosporin or a fluoroquinolone. The recommended treatment course is 14 days, but IV antibiotics should not be discontinued until the patient is afebrile for at least 48 hours and is able to tolerate oral medications and adequate amounts of fluid. Additionally, indications for urinary catheter usage should be reviewed; and if the indications are appropriate, the catheter system should be changed at the first signs and symptoms of UTI (Nicolle, 2001).

What measures can be taken to help Mrs. J avoid future UTIs?

In older patients with recurrent UTI (more than 3 episodes per year), several strategies may be effective in preventing future UTIs. In patients with reversible obstruction and urinary stasis, surgical or pharmacologic measures may be a good option. In women, the use of topical estrogen may help normalize vaginal flora and pH, thus reducing the frequency of episodes. Additionally, cranberry juice may reduce pyuria and significant bacteriuria as it inhibits the binding of gram negative bacilli to uroepithelial cells. Finally, some studies have indicated success with prophylaxis of recurrent UTI with postcoital or once-daily low doses of trimethoprim/sulfamethizole, quinolones, or nitrofurantoin (Nicolle, 2001; Sen, Middleton, & Perez, 1994; Terpenning & Bradley, 1991).

REFERENCES

Duthie, E. H., Katz, P. R., & Malone, M. L. (2007). *Practice of geriatrics* (4th ed.). Philadelphia, PA: Saunders.

Lynch, C. F., & Cohen, M. B. (1995). Urinary system. *Cancer, 75*(Suppl. 1), 316–329.

Morrison, A. S., Buring, J. E., Verhoek, W. G., Aoki, K., Leck, I., Ohno, Y., & Obata, K. (1984). An international study of smoking and bladder cancer. *The Journal of Urology, 131*(4), 650–654.

Nicolle, L. E. (2001). Urinary tract infections. In T. T. Yoshikawa, D. C. Norman (Eds.), *Infectious disease in the aging* (pp. 99–112). Totowa, NJ: Humana Press.

Nicolle, L. E., Bradley, S., & Colgan, R. (2005). Infectious Disease Society of America guideline for the diagnosis and treatment of asymptomatic bacteriuria in adults. *Clinical Infection and Disease, 40,* 643–654.

Parker, D., Callan, L., Harwood, J., Thompson, D., Webb, M. L., & Wilde, M. (2009). Catheter-associated urinary tract infections: Fact sheet. *Journal of Wound, Ostomy, & Continence Nursing, 36*(2), 156–159.

Sen, P., Middleton, J. R., & Perez, G. (1994). Host defense abnormalities and infections in older persons. *Infection and Medicine, 11,* 34–37.

Terpenning, M. S., & Bradley, S. F. (1991). Aging and host resistance to infection. *Geriatrics, 46,* 77–80.

Case 2.8 The History Reveals All

By Devon Kwassman, MSN, RN

Mrs. K, a 72-year-old woman, presents to the primary care clinic complaining of fatigue, shortness of breath, and a nonproductive cough x10 days. She has a past medical history significant for Type 2 diabetes and hypertension, which have been adequately controlled with medications. She visits the clinic annually, but has not been to the office yet this year. Her immunizations are up-to-date, and she receives a flu shot annually. Her surgical history is significant for a tonsillectomy at age 15. She had no complications from this procedure and no history of past trauma/injury. Mrs. K is a retired administrative assistant who was widowed 7 years ago. She has no children and lives alone in a second-story apartment. Her father died of a stroke at age 79, and her mother died of "unknown causes" at age 88. She has 1 living sister who was diagnosed with breast cancer at age 55. Her sister lives in the same apartment building, and Mrs. K describes their relationship as "very close". Her sexual history includes unprotected vaginal intercourse with 3 male partners over the past 10 months. She is satisfied with her level of sexual activity and function. She drinks 1–2 glasses of red wine a week and denies the use of any tobacco products or recreational drug use. Her review of systems is positive for an unintentional weight loss of 25 lb over the past 6 months, as well as frequent painful "canker sores" inside her mouth for the past 2–3 months. Remaining review of systems is negative. She denies fever, night sweats, chills, changes in appetite, weakness, nausea, vomiting, diarrhea, constipation, discharge, chest pain, wheezing, hemoptysis, paroxysmal nocturnal dyspnea, palpitations, joint stiffness/swelling, sore throat, insomnia,

Case Studies in Gerontological Nursing for the Advanced Practice Nurse, First Edition.
Edited by Meredith Wallace Kazer, Leslie Neal-Boylan.
© 2012 John Wiley & Sons, Inc. Published 2012 by John Wiley & Sons, Inc.

skin rashes, and changes in memory/cognition. Her medications are Starlix, 60 mg 3 times daily, and captopril, 25 mg/HCTZ 15 mg once daily. She has no known allergies (NKA).

OBJECTIVE

Mrs. K is alert and oriented to person, place, and time. She ambulates without difficulty, is well-groomed, and is appropriately dressed. She appears to be in slight respiratory distress with open-mouth breathing. She is 5 ft 3 inches and 117 lb. BP: 118/72; HR: 112; RR 26; T: 99.1; O_2 Sat 92% at rest; 88% on exertion. Her skin is warm and dry to the touch, with no clubbing or cyanosis. Her head is normocephalic with symmetrical facial features. Her eyes exhibit PERRLA bilaterally. EOMs are intact; optic disc margins are sharp and clear. Her ears are nontender; canals are clear. The TM is pearly gray with landmarks intact. Her nares are patent with nose and septum midline. She exhibits no nasal flaring, frontal/maxillary sinus tenderness, or discharge. The oral mucosa is pink with dry mucous membranes. Her uvula rises midline and symmetrically on phonation. Tonsils are 2+, and her pharynx is pink without exudates. Oral lesions are present on the buccal mucosa. Her neck is supple with FROM. The trachea is midline, and the thyroid is nonpalpable. She has positive generalized lymphadenopathy. Cardiac exam reveals tachycardia; S1 and S2 present with regular rhythm. No S3, S4, or other adventitious sounds are heard. AP: Transverse diameter is 1:2. Audible crackles are present at the base of the lungs bilaterally, with dullness to percussion in the lower lobes. Her abdomen is soft, nontender, and nondistended. Bowel sounds are auscultated in all 4 quadrants. Tympany is heard throughout her abdomen with no bruits, masses, or hernias. All 4 of her extremities have FROM, with 4+ muscle strength throughout. Deep tendon reflexes are 2+ bilaterally, with CN II–XII grossly intact. She has a steady, even gait. Gynecological exam is unremarkable.

ASSESSMENT

Viral pneumonia: Mrs. K's complaints of shortness of breath, fatigue, and a nonproductive cough may be suggestive of viral pneumonia. Her abnormal vital signs, in particular the tachypnea and O_2 Sat, as well as the bilateral crackles and dullness in the lungs, point toward this diagnosis. It is important to note that advanced age is associated with a poorer prognosis in individuals diagnosed with pneumonia (Goroll & Mulley, 2009).

Chronic Obstructive Pulmonary Disease: COPD is a progressive disease characterized by shortness of breath and a productive cough. According to the National Heart Lung and Blood Institute (NHLBI), this disease has been identified as the fourth leading cause of death in older adults age 65 and over (2010). Therefore, it is important to consider COPD as a possible diagnosis for Mrs. K's symptomatology. However, the acute nature of her symptoms makes COPD an unlikely diagnosis. Furthermore, the central cause of COPD is cigarette smoking, which is inconsistent with her history (NHLBI, 2010).

Pneumocystis Jiroveci **Pneumonia (PCP) secondary to HIV infection:** PCP is the most frequently diagnosed pulmonary opportunistic infection in adults with HIV/AIDS (Goroll & Mulley, 2009). The classic presentation of PCP includes fever, a nonproductive cough, and dyspnea noted particularly on exertion (Goroll & Mulley, 2009). PCP is an opportunistic infection associated with a later stage of HIV infection. Though the occurrence of HIV/AIDS does not discriminate between age groups, the diagnosis is often delayed among the geriatric population, with symptoms falsely attributed to comorbid conditions more commonly found among older adults (Jedlovsky & Fleischman, 2000). Therefore, a large number of geriatric patients are first diagnosed with HIV/AIDS at the time of an opportunistic event, such as PCP (Jedlovsky & Fleischman, 2000).

DIAGNOSTICS

In this case, laboratory testing will be the most essential component of the diagnosis, as well as the development of the treatment plan. An induced sputum sample should be ordered to test for pneumonia secondary to HIV infection. It is important to obtain an induced sample, as a spontaneous sample has low sensitivity for the diagnosis of PCP (CDC, 2009). The clinician sends Mrs. K for a posteroanterior and lateral chest radiography to determine not only the severity of a suspected pneumonia, but also to check for complications, such as a pleural effusion (Goroll & Mulley, 2009). The clinician also orders arterial blood gases (ABGs) to supplement these pulmonary procedures. At this visit, Mrs. K should also receive a routine HIV test due to the nature of her presenting symptoms and her high-risk sexual history. The clinician then orders an enzyme-linked immunosorbent assay (ELISA) test that will detect the presence of HIV antibodies in the blood. However, the diagnosis of HIV can only be confirmed with a follow-up Western blot test. In the event of a positive ELISA, a Western blot test to confirm the diagnosis will be conducted, followed by a CD4 cell count and test for HIV viral load. A CD4 cell count measures the number of CD4 cells, or T-cells, that are available in the blood. A low level of CD4 cells in the blood indicates a weaker immune system and subsequently increased risk of infection. A test for viral load reveals the amount of the virus that is present in the blood. There is an inverse relationship between CD4 cell count and viral load, so that when viral load is high, CD4 cell count will be low. The Health Resources and Services Administration (HRSA) HIV/AIDS Bureau states that the ultimate goal of treatment for HIV is to decrease the viral load until it is no longer measurable in the blood at approximately 50 copies/mL (2004).

The sputum culture reveals the presence of the organism *P. jiroveci*. The results of the chest radiography demonstrate a bilateral interstitial infiltrate. Results of the ABGs show a PaO_2 of 73 mmHg and an A-a O_2 gradient of 32 mmHg. The results of the ELISA test are positive for HIV antibodies. The Western blot test is also positive for HIV. Her CD4 cell count is <200/mm^3, and her viral load is 80,000 copies/mL.

CRITICAL THINKING

Given these results, what is the most likely differential diagnosis and why?

What other laboratory tests and diagnostics would be most appropriate to order next?

What is the plan of treatment?

What other disciplines or referrals would be important to include in her management of care?

What would the clinician suspect if the patient also reported a recent decline in memory or cognition?

What aspects of patient history are most important to include when screening for HIV?

Are there any standardized guidelines for HIV testing among older adults?

RESOLUTION

Given these results, what is the most likely differential diagnosis and why?

P. jiroveci pneumonia secondary to HIV infection is the most likely differential diagnosis given the test results and nature of the patient's symptoms. Her report of unprotected sexual intercourse with 3 male partners over the past 10 months alerts us immediately to behaviors that place her at high risk for contracting HIV. Her physical exam findings of oral lesions, lymphadenopathy, and crackles in the lungs, along with her report of a 25 lb unintentional weight loss over the past 6 months also heighten suspicion for an opportunistic infection related to HIV. The results of her sputum culture identified the causative organism to be *P. jiroveci*, and the chest radiography demonstrated the most common presentation in patients with this type of pneumonia (Khan, Irion, MacDonald, Allen, 2008). Though her ELISA test was positive, a Western blot test was needed to confirm the diagnosis of HIV. Currently, the ELISA test followed by the Western blot is considered the gold standard for the detection of HIV/AIDS (CDC, 2001). The positive results from both tests confidently point toward the diagnosis of HIV infection. Furthermore, normal CD4 counts are $>500/$ mm^3; values less than or equal to 200 are indicative of high risk for opportunistic infections (HRSA, 2004). Her CD4 cell count of $<200/$ mm^3 thereby indicates that she is at an increased risk for an infection such as PCP. The average viral load in an individual with HIV is 30,000 copies/mL (HRSA, 2004). Mrs. K's viral load of 80,000 indicates the need to rapidly initiate treatment for HIV. It is evident from the multiple factors included in Mrs. K's history, physical exam findings, and test results that this is a case of *P. jiroveci* pneumonia secondary to HIV infection.

What other laboratory tests and diagnostics would be most appropriate to order next?

As a newly diagnosed HIV patient, several other laboratory and diagnostic tests should be ordered to thoroughly evaluate her health status. A CBC is an essential test that will determine if Mrs. K is facing any additional complications associated with HIV infection, such as thrombocytopenia and anemia of chronic disease (Goroll & Mulley, 2009; Nguyen & Holodniy, 2008). A CMP and lipid profile should also be performed to obtain a baseline evaluation prior to the initiation of drug treatment and to detect any comorbid conditions that may be further affected by therapy (Goroll & Mulley, 2009; Nguyen & Holodniy, 2008). HIV resistance testing is necessary to determine the presence of drug-resistant HIV-1, which requires alterations in treatment options (Nguyen & Holodniy, 2008). Beyond these baseline tests, serology tests should be performed for other diseases that are transmitted through the same avenues as HIV, such as syphilis and hepatitis (Nguyen & Holodniy, 2008). A purified protein derivative (PPD) tuberculin skin test is needed to assess for tuberculosis if the patient has no previous history of TB or has had a previous positive test result (Goroll & Mulley, 2009; Nguyen & Holodniy, 2008). It is also important for Mrs. K to be screened for pelvic and cervical conditions with a thorough examination and Pap smear (HRSA, 2004; Nguyen & Holodniy, 2008). Neuropsychiatric testing may be considered to identify the occurrence of HIV-associated dementia (HAD) (Goroll & Mulley, 2009).

What is the plan of treatment?

The advent of antiretroviral therapy (ART) has transformed HIV into chronic disease management often spearheaded by the primary care practitioner. In the case of Mrs. K, her opportunistic infection becomes the immediate priority of the treatment plan. According to the HRSA HIV/AIDS Bureau (2004), if $PaO_2 > 70$ mmHg and A-a O_2 gradient < 35 mmHg, this is classified as mild-moderate PCP. Severe disease is noted to be $PaO_2 < 70$ mmHg with an A-a O_2 gradient > 35 mmHg (HRSA, 2004). Therefore, Mrs. K falls into the range of mild-moderate severity with her PaO_2 of 73 mmHg and an A-a O_2 of 32 mmHg. First-line treatment of mild-moderate PCP includes an outpatient regimen of oral trimethoprim-sulfamethoxazole (TMS) at a dose of 15 mg/kg per day by trimethoprim content, in 3–4 divided doses (CDC, 2009; Goroll & Mulley, 2009). It is important to test for renal function and adjust the dose accordingly before initiating therapy with TMS. Alternative treatment options are available and may be accessed at: http://www.cdc.gov/mmwr/preview/mmwrhtml/rr5804a1.htm?s_cid=rr5804a1_e

As the clinician is managing this infection on an outpatient basis, it is essential to provide close follow-up care and be prepared to hospitalize this patient should the clinical picture worsen.

Once her condition has stabilized, a treatment plan for HIV can commence. With a CD4 count of <200/mm^3 and viral load of 80,000 copies/mL, Mrs. K needs to be started on highly active antiretroviral therapy (HART). As her primary care provider, the management of human immunodeficiency virus (HIV) must be integrated into that of her other comorbid conditions of hypertension (HTN) and noninsulin dependent diabetes mellitus (NIDDM). The initial drug regimen for HIV typically includes a combination of 3 drugs consisting of either 2 nucleosides and a protease inhibitor (PI) or 2 nucleosides and a non-nucleoside reverse transcriptase inhibitor (NNRTI) (HRSA, 2004). These drugs have several adverse effects and toxicities that may be more pronounced in older adults due to such factors as decreased bioavailability and an increased risk of polypharmacy among older individuals taking several other medications (Manfredi, 2004). There is no one standard of treatment for HIV, and no current guidelines exist for specifically targeting the care of HIV-infected older adults (Nguyen & Holodniy, 2008). Therapy must be individualized for each patient, and Mrs. K may need to be referred to an HIV specialist for the development of her initial treatment plan. Adherence to ART is paramount and education must be provided concerning this issue, as well as education on drug toxicities, the disease process, and how to prevent transmission. Frequent followup will be necessary after treatment initiation to monitor disease status, adherence, and potential adverse effects and drug interactions. Additional information on the use of antiretrovirals can be found at: http://aidsinfo.nih.gov/contentfiles/ AdultandAdolescentGL.pdf

What other disciplines or referrals would be important to include in her management of care?

Due to the complex nature of HIV, a multidisciplinary approach is the best technique for management of care (HRSA, 2004). An HIV specialist should be included in the case management once a diagnosis of the virus has been established (Goroll & Mulley, 2009). Mrs. K may also need a referral to a psychologist to help her cope with the shock of this diagnosis. Referral to community resources is necessary for such aspects as social and financial support. Additional medical professionals that would be important to consult for this case include an endocrinologist, cardiologist, and registered dietician.

What would the clinician suspect if the patient also reported a recent decline in memory or cognition?

The HIV virus has the potential to cause cognitive impairment known as HIV-associated dementia (HAD). HAD typically begins when a patient notices subtle difficulties with reading, math, comprehension, or memory (HRSA, 2004). Eventually, HAD becomes advanced dementia, affecting widespread areas of the brain (HRSA, 2004). Older adults with HIV may present atypically, with dementia as the sole symptom of the virus (Tangredi, Danvers, Molony, Williams, 2008). Therefore, it is important to include HAD as a differential diagnosis for an older adult presenting with cognitive symptoms similar to Alzheimer or Parkinson diseases (Tangredi et al., 2008).

What aspects of patient history are most important to include when screening for HIV?

When screening for HIV infection among older adults, a thorough history remains the key component in identifying high-risk behaviors that will prompt early testing, diagnosis, and access to treatment. A health risk assessment that addresses such aspects as sexual history and substance use should be performed (Tangredi et al., 2008). Specifically, providers should be sure to assess type of sexual practices, number of sexual partners and encounters, sexual preferences, use of protection, known risk of partners, past history of STDs, type of substances used (how often, routes of administration), and past history of drug treatment (HRSA, 2004; Tangredi et al., 2008). These questions should be a routine part of the visit, facilitating an open discussion and opportunity for education (Tangredi et al., 2008). It is important to note that many older adults have not received proper education about HIV transmission and prevention compared to their younger counterparts

(Tangredi et al., 2008). Therefore, education plays an integral role in screening for HIV among older adults.

Are there any standardized guidelines for HIV testing among older adults?

The CDC has released new guidelines providing recommendations for HIV testing in older adults. These guidelines are available at: http://www.cdc.gov/mmwr/preview/mmwrhtml/rr5514a1.htm

REFERENCES

CDC (2001). *HIV testing implementation guidance for correctional settings*. Retrieved June 23, 2010, from http://www.cdc.gov/hiv/topics/testing/resources/guidelines/correctional-settings/section4.htm

CDC (2009). *Guidelines for prevention and treatment of opportunistic infections in HIV-infected adults and adolescents*. Retrieved June 10, 2010, from http://www.cdc.gov/mmwr/preview/mmwrhtml/rr5804a1.htm?s_cid=rr5804a1_e

Goroll, A. H., & Mulley, A. G. (2009). *Primary care medicine: Office evaluation and management of the adult patient* (6th ed.). Philadelphia, PA: Lippincott Williams & Wilkins.

HRSA HIV/AIDS Bureau: HRSA (2004). HIV/AIDS Bureau. Retrieved from http://www.hrsa.gov/about/organization/bureaus/hab/

HRSA (2004). *A guide to primary care for people with HIV/AIDS, 2004 edition*. Retrieved June 23, 2010, from http://hab.hrsa.gov/tools/primarycare-guide/index.htm

Jedlovsky, V., & Fleischman, J. K. (2000). Pneumocystis carinii pneumonia as the first presentation of HIV infection in patients older than fifty. *AIDS Patient Care STDS, 14*, 247–249.

Khan, A. N., Irion, K. L., MacDonald, S., & Allen, C. M. (2008). *Pneumonia, pneumocystis carinii*. Retrieved June 10, 2010, from http://emedicine.medscape.com/article/359972-overview

Manfredi, R. (2004). HIV infection and advanced age: Emerging epidemiological, clinical, and management issues. *Aging Research Reviews, 3*, 31–54.

Nguyen, N., & Holodniy, M. (2008). HIV infection in the elderly. *Clinical Interventions in Aging, 3*, 453–472.

NHLBI (2010). *COPD*. Retrieved July 1, 2010, from http://www.nhlbi.nih.gov/health/dci/Diseases/Copd/Copd_WhatIs.html

Tangredi, L. A., Danvers, K., Molony, S. L., & Williams, A. (2008). New CDC recommendations for HIV testing in older adults. *The Nurse Practitioner, 33*, 37–44.

ADDITIONAL RESOURCES

Bhavan, K. P., Kampalath, V. N., Overton, E. T. (2008). The aging of the HIV epidemic. *Current HIV/AIDS Reports, 5*, 150–158.

Centers for Disease Control (2006). Revised recommendations for HIV Testing of adults, adolescents, and pregnant women in health-care settings. MMWR 55(No. RR-14): 1–17. Retrieved from http://www.cdc.gov/mmwr/preview/mmwrhtml/rr5514a1.htm

DHHS (2011). Guidelines for the use of antiretroviral agents in HIV-1–infected adults and adolescents. Retrieved from http://aidsinfo.nih.gov/contentfiles/AdultandAdolescentGL.pdf

Case 2.9 *Kneedless* Pain

By Maureen E. O'Rourke, RN, PhD, and Kenneth S. O'Rourke, MD

Mrs. G is a 70-year-old female, new patient, with a chief complaint of hand and knee pain. She is a retired broker, who 6 months prior moved to the area to take advantage of the warmer weather and extensive cooking classes offered by the local culinary institute. She describes a 2-year history of hand pain and stiffness, initially intermittent, but now daily over the past 5 months. Her symptoms are predominately in the middle- and end-finger joints and the thumb side of the wrists. These joints are stiff for 15–20 minutes upon awakening. Her pain is exacerbated by typing, gardening, and working in her pastry and bread-making class; but it improves with rest. The affected finger joints have been swollen "for years," without appreciable change in size; but they have limited her fine finger dexterity and grip strength. Her left knee has been intermittently painful for over 5 years. There has been no knee locking or giving away, although on occasion it is mildly swollen when painful. Knee pain is worse with squatting, going both up and down stairs, and after prolonged walking or standing. At least once she has had to leave cooking class early due to weight-bearing knee pain.

Mrs. G's past medical history includes essential hypertension (HTN) for 9 years and gastroesophageal reflux disease (GERD) for 5 years. Her family history includes her mother's history of "crippling" arthritis of the hands. Her medications include hydrochlorothiazide, 25 mg daily; metoprolol, 25 mg twice daily; ranitidine, 75 mg once daily as needed.

Case Studies in Gerontological Nursing for the Advanced Practice Nurse, First Edition.
Edited by Meredith Wallace Kazer, Leslie Neal-Boylan.
© 2012 John Wiley & Sons, Inc. Published 2012 by John Wiley & Sons, Inc.

She has taken over-the-counter acetaminophen, 500 mg 1 tab per dose, on an as-needed basis, with mild pain relief.

OBJECTIVE

Mrs. G presents with stable vital signs (VS) as follows: BP: 150/86; pulse: 64; afebrile; body mass index (BMI): 32. She is overweight and is in no distress at rest. The remainder of the exam is unremarkable except for symmetric bony hypertrophy of the proximal interphalangeal (PIP) and distal interphalangeal (DIP) joints of the fingers in each hand. A few of the joints are tender to palpation; none are inflamed. There is similar bony ridging but with moderate tenderness to palpation over each first carpometacarpal (CMC) joint. The metacarpophalangeal (MCP) joints are normal. The fingertips are a full fingerbreadth from the palm with maximum active finger curl/flexion. Passive wrist motion is full and painless bilaterally, and there is no dorsal wrist tenderness. The knees are cool to touch. The left knee has a subtle varus deformity that can be passively reduced. There is tenderness to palpation in the middle and posterior aspects of the left medial tibiofemoral joint line. Each knee has palpable crepitus over the patellofemoral joint lines with passive motion, and neither knee demonstrates ligamental laxity with stress testing or an effusion. Leg lengths are equal. Gait is without limp.

DIAGNOSTICS

Labs were performed 7 months prior by her last provider and include the following: Erythrocyte sedimentation rate (ESR): 41 mm/h; rheumatoid factor (RF): 18 IU (normal $\leq$ 13.9); anti-cyclic citrullinated peptide antibody (anti-CCP antibody): negative; antinuclear antibody (ANA): 1:80 in a diffuse pattern; uric acid: 7.9 (normal < 7); and anti-streptolysin O titre (ASO titre) negative.

ASSESSMENT

Gouty arthritis: Gouty arthritis usually presents as an acute, very painful mono- or oligoarticular arthritis, although in the elderly it may be more commonly polyarticular than in younger adults. Gout in the elderly is highly associated with diuretic use and renal insufficiency.

Osteoarthritis (OA): OA is the most common chronic illness among older adults. The diagnosis is principally a clinical one (as opposed to laboratory confirmation) and follows interpretation of a thorough patient history and diligent physical examination.

Rheumatoid Arthritis (RA): RA is a chronic systemic inflammatory disease affecting diarthrodial joints that is 2.5 times more likely in young adult women, but it affects genders nearly equally in the elderly. While the subjective and objective findings in the assessment do not fully support RA, it is a possibility in Mrs. G's case.

CRITICAL THINKING QUESTIONS

What is the most likely diagnosis for her joint complaints? How is the diagnosis supported by the findings noted above?

What is the significance of the test results for ESR, RF, ANA, and anti-CCP?

How should her elevated uric acid level be interpreted?

What nonpharmacologic and pharmacologic measures should be implemented to treat her symptoms?

Are there any published guidelines to assist in the formulation of the treatment plans?

How would medical management change if she were on warfarin?

What additional tests, if any, should be ordered?

RESOLUTION

What is the most likely diagnosis for her joint complaints? How is the diagnosis supported by the findings noted above?
Arriving at the diagnosis in a patient presenting with musculoskeletal complaints is dependent primarily on the information derived from a thorough history and examination. One approach to differentiating joint diseases is to distill the information from such an evaluation into three clinical questions: Is the problem localized to the joint or joints (intraarticular) or originating from periarticular tissues (extraarticular); is it inflammatory or noninflammatory; and is there a recognizable pattern of distribution?

Patient descriptors and the elicitation of pain and inflammatory signs during the musculoskeletal exam together can distinguish the site of symptoms as from within or external to a joint. Pain from an articular source is often described by the patient as generalized or encompassing the entire joint region whereas extraarticular pain is more often localized to an area within a joint region or described as superficial. On examination, pain elicited during passive joint motion implies an intraarticular source, but extraarticular pain generators are painful with active or resisted active motion. When present, inflammatory signs (e.g., warmth, swelling, or tenderness) are often noted diffusely about the joint circumference in an articular problem; but they are only localized when the problem is extraarticular.

Further clues from the history that support an inflammatory etiology of disease are the presence of prolonged (generally >60 minutes) morning joint stiffness, constitutional symptoms (e.g., fever or weight loss), increased symptoms after long periods of inactivity, and commonly a responsiveness to corticosteroids. Noninflammatory conditions may be associated with brief (<20–30 minutes) morning joint stiffness, are painful with or after use, but are not associated with constitutional symptoms and fail to improve following steroid therapy.

Finally, recognizing clinical patterns of distribution principally in exam findings is critical to reaching an appropriate diagnosis (American College of Rheumatology Ad Hoc Committee on Clinical Guidelines, 1996; Dao & Cush, 2006; Pinals, 1994; Revaz, Dudler, & Kai-Lik So, 2006). The common inflammatory (rheumatoid arthritis) and noninflammatory (osteoarthritis) arthritides have characteristic distributions of joint involvement (Table 2.9.1). There are a number of non-mutually exclusive ways to categorize clinical patterns of joint distribution, including presentation (acute vs. insidious), duration (brief [less than 4–6 weeks] vs. chronic), number of joints involved (monoarticular vs. oligoarticular [2–4 joints] vs. polyarticular), and overall distribution (symmetric vs. asymmetric, axial vs. extremity vs. combination). Table 2.9.2 summarizes how a musculoskeletal diagnosis can be considered

TABLE 2.9.1.   Typical Joint Distribution in Patients with Osteoarthritis or Rheumatoid Arthritis.

Arthritis	Characteristic Joint Distribution	Joints Not Involved
Osteoarthritis	AC, PIP, DIP, 1st CMC, hips, knees, midfoot, 1st MTP, mid-to-low cervical spine, lumbar spine	MCP, elbow
Rheumatoid arthritis	Elbow, wrist, MCP, PIP, knee, ankle, MTP, upper cervical spine	DIP, lumbar spine

Abbreviations: AC, acromioclavicular; CMC, carpometacarpal; DIP, distal interphalangeal; MCP, metacarpophalangeal; MTP, metatarsophalangeal; PIP, proximal interphalangeal.

TABLE 2.9.2. Initial Differential Diagnosis of Musculoskeletal Complaints Based on the Number of Joint Regions Involved and Whether the Etiology Is within or outside of the Joint.

Site	Number of Joint Regions Involved	
	Mono-Regional	**Poly-Regional**
Intraarticular	Septic arthritis Crystalline arthritis Hemarthrosis (trauma, tumor, coagulopathy) Monoarticular onset of polyarticular disease	*Bony enlargement:* Osteoarthritis *Synovitis, asymmetric:* spondyloarthropathy *Synovitis, symmetric, acute*:* viral, serum sickness *Synovitis, symmetric, chronic:* connective tissue disease (e.g., rheumatoid arthritis, systemic lupus erythematosus)
Extraarticular	Bursitis Myofascial pain Tendinitis	Fibromyalgia syndrome Myopathy Polymyalgia rheumatica

*Less than 4–6 weeks' duration.

based on the number of joints involved and whether the etiology is intraarticular or extraarticular.

Mrs. G presents with findings typical for osteoarthritis (Felson, 2006). She has symmetric polyarthritis with symptoms exacerbated by use (e.g., kneading dough and prolonged weight bearing) in association with minimal morning stiffness and lack of constitutional symptoms. She has bony enlargement in characteristic hand joints for osteoarthritis and involvement of the left knee, in the major weight-bearing (medial) compartment as well as patellofemoral crepitus (consistent with her expressed difficulties in activities associated with deep-knee bending, such as squatting and stair use). The varus left knee deformity implies a reduction in the medial knee joint space, likely from a reduction in the depth of her articular cartilage and/or meniscus from the chronicity of the osteoarthritic involvement. Joint effusions may accompany knee involvement; and when not associated with an overlapping crystalline arthritis, they typically will demonstrate a synovial white blood cell (WBC) count of less than 2000 cells per mL.

Her years of finger joint swelling, accompanied by reduced joint motion, reflect the bony enlargements (osteophytes) palpable on her exam. Most patients with osteoarthritis of the fingers may have only bony enlargement for months to years prior to the development of activity-limiting pain. CMC joint pain can be interpreted by the patient as coming from the wrist, as in this patient. However, there is no synovitis on exam that would suggest an inflammatory arthritis such as rheumatoid arthritis (RA); and the distribution of joint involvement is not typical for RA. The lack of inflammatory signs and the chronic polyarticular course makes gouty arthritis unlikely.

What is the significance of the test results for ESR, RF, ANA, and anti-CCP?

The results of autoantibody testing alone rarely provide a diagnosis in a patient with musculoskeletal complaints. Individual tests should be ordered only to refute or support an established diagnostic suspicion (pre-test probability) formed after a thorough history and physical exam, and not as a panel of tests (as was performed in this patient) to screen for rheumatic disease (Colglazier & Sutej, 2005). The prevalence of false positive tests for either an RF or ANA test is estimated to be as high as 10% of the general population, and their low sensitivity in early disease makes them a poor choice for screening. The elderly is one population for whom the prevalence of false positive autoantibody tests is well established. Such results are usually of low titre; and in the case of a positive ANA, the fluorescent pattern is usually reported as homogeneous (also called diffuse), the most nonspecific pattern (Solomon, Kavanaugh, & Schur, 2002). The anti-CCP antibody is more specific than RF when considering a diagnosis of RA. Thus, in our patient the negative anti-CCP is consistent with her diagnosis of osteoarthritis. However, osteoarthritis is a clinical diagnosis; and under the best circumstances the diagnosis of our patient's noninflammatory arthritis could have been made in the absence of any autoantibody testing.

The ESR and C-reactive protein are nonspecific measurements of the acute phase response, which is the change in hepatic production of plasma proteins (usually an increased production) as a response to inflammation or tissue necrosis (Gabay & Kushner, 1999). This response is driven by cytokines released from the site of inflammation into the systemic circulation and is primarily driven by the effect of interleukin-6 (IL-6) on hepatocytes. Mean levels of IL-6 in the elderly are higher than in younger adults, and IL-6 is likely the major contributing factor that results in the mean ESR for older adults being higher. Our patient's ESR of 41 mm/h is normal for her age. A normal ESR for a patient's age may be estimated by the equations of age/2 for men or (age + 10)/2 for women (Griffiths et al., 1984).

How should her elevated uric acid level be interpreted?

Serum urate levels reflect the body's balance between supply (diet, cellular/tissue degradation, new purine synthesis) and excretion (one-third through alimentary elimination and the remainder mainly by urinary excretion) (Terkeltaub, Bushinsky, & Becker, 2006). In isolation, an elevated uric acid level in the presence of joint pain does not justify the diagnosis of gouty arthritis. Gouty arthritis is best diagnosed by the demonstration of monosodium urate crystals in synovial fluid taken from a symptomatic joint. Uric acid levels may be elevated due to an increase in production (only 10% of those with hyperuricemia) (Terkeltaub et al., 2006), a decrease in excretion, or their combination. Underexcretion of uric acid may be the consequence of a primary renal disorder in urate transport or secondary to impaired renal function (with associated decreased urate transport) or drug-induced renal toxicity. Our patient's elevated uric acid level is due to the effects of her diuretic on the kidney. Increased renal reabsorption of urate back into the systemic circulation from diuretics is due to volume depletion and likely from a direct effect of the drug to stimulate the renal urate transporter.

What nonpharmacologic and pharmacologic measures should be implemented to treat her symptoms?
The overall goals of therapy are to relieve pain, preserve function, and prevent progression. The best outcomes occur when an individualize treatment plan includes not only medical therapies but also nonpharmacologic measures that work to either correct and/or prevent joint malalignment, instability, and their consequences (Felson, 2006).

There is a growing body of literature supporting the use of varied nonpharmacologic augmentative therapies in the treatment of OA. Patient and family education related to risk factors and prognosis is critical to ensuring an understanding of the rationale for the therapeutic plan. The importance of weight loss to decrease mechanical load across the hips and knees cannot be underestimated, and it may decrease disease progression in affected joints. Standard physical and occupational treatment options include the use of thermal modalities (e.g., ultrasound, paraffin baths), splinting and bracing (e.g., thumb spica splint for the 1st CMC joint, unloader knee braces and/or wedged shoe insoles for knee pain in the presence of reducible knee deformity, canes and other assistive devices to off-load painful hips and knees) (Gross, 2010), and exercise therapy (Latham & Chiung-ju, 2010; Messier, 2010).

Alternative therapies to reduce pain, as reviewed in recent meta-analyses, may include tai chi (TC) (Lee, Pittler, & Ernst, 2008) and acupuncture (Kwon, Pittler, & Ernst, 2006). TC involves mild aerobic activity combined with relaxation techniques, deep and regulated breathing, and slow controlled movement. Purported physical benefits include diminished joint pain and improvements in balance, flexibility, joint stability, strength and coordination, which are all beneficial with the added gain of the potential for reduction of falls in a vulnerable elderly population. Both TC and acupuncture have favorable safety profiles but deserve further extensive study. The combination of oral glucosamine and chondroitin sulphate was postulated to provide an analgesic effect; but the results of a 2-year randomized, double-blind, and Celebrex- and placebo-controlled trial showed no statistical benefits in pain or function over placebo (Sawitzke et al., 2010).

Conventional pharmacologic therapies have focused on pain control (Harvey & Hunter, 2010), as to date there is no medication shown to reverse the process of articular cartilage degeneration or to inhibit the formation of bony enlargement at the joint line. Acetaminophen is the initial analgesic of choice, given its excellent safety profile and reasonable efficacy. Efficacy is maximized when acetaminophen is taken on a regular basis in divided doses up to the maximum daily amount as allowed by the patient's renal and hepatic function. Should further analgesia be required then options for the addition or substitution of an as-needed or regularly dosed analgesic commonly include tramadol or a nonsteroidal antiinflammatory drug (NSAID). Each of these medications is to be used cautiously in the elderly. Tramadol (and opiate medications) may cause dizziness or light-headedness predisposing falls, while NSAIDs (particularly indomethacin) are associated with a higher prevalence of central nervous side effects in addition to their better-known risks to the gastrointestinal tract (Towheed et al., 2006) and blood pressure control (Chobanian, 2003; Cooney & Pascuzzi, 2009) (Table 2.9.3). Systemic side effects are reduced with the use of topical NSAIDs or analgesics (e.g., capsaicin) but are limited by practical concerns for the number of joints to be treated and frequency of daily application, which may be required for efficacy.

TABLE 2.9.3.   Selected Gastrointestinal and Hypertensive Risks of NSAIDs.

Target Side Effect	Effect of NSAID Therapy in Elderly
Upper gastrointestinal bleeding	Increased risk in setting of low albumin (increased free drug level) and decreased hepatic and/or renal function (increases drug half-life)
	When used with warfarin: 12.7-fold increased risk*
	When used with corticosteroids: 4.4-fold increased risk†
Hypertension	Normotensive patient: Average increased blood pressure of 8–10 mmHg due to sodium and fluid retention and the renal effects of decreased prostaglandin production
	Hypertensive patient: Reduces the antihypertensive effect of beta-blockers, angiotensin converting enzyme inhibitors (ACEI) and angiotensin receptor blockers (ARB), diuretics, and alpha-blockers

*Shorr, Ray, Daugherty, & Griffin, 1993.
†Piper, Ray, Daugherty, & Griffin, 1991.

Intraarticular (IA) injection therapy may provide short-term benefits with minimal risk for systemic side effects. Corticosteroid preparations and hyaluronic acid derivatives may be considered for adjunctive treatment, but for a specific joint there are insufficient data for either of these two groups of agents to accurately predict which joint characteristics are associated with long-term efficacy.

In Mrs. G, whose medical comorbidities and medications pose significant risks for gastrointestinal and hypertensive side effects, an initial therapeutic plan (in addition to patient education) would include regularly scheduled doses of acetaminophen and directed weight loss. Additional interventions would include referral to a therapist for the construction of thumb splints to wear regularly during sleep and as needed during the day, accompanied by specific instructions on lower-extremity strengthening exercises and home options for thermal treatments for the hands.

Are there any published guidelines to assist in the formulation of the treatment plans?
As the number of published clinical trials of pharmacologic and non-pharmacologic therapies have grown, so have the number of publications that provide evidence-based treatment guidelines based on an analysis of available data mixed with expert opinion when evidence does not exist. These guidelines—the products of professional societies or health care organizations—are meant to improve the quality of care by promoting proven therapies and discouraging unnecessary or ineffective practices. However, guidelines are single-disease focused and do not always take into account comorbidities; thus all recommendations must be individualized to the patient. Published guidelines for the management of OA are very consistent across a broad range of recommendations, yet are frequently not implemented (particularly nonpharmacologic measures) in clinical practice (Hunter, 2010). Adherence to analogous quality indicators, measures of provider accountability not uncommonly tied to compensation and/or certification, has been used as one strategy to improve the implementation of specific guideline recommendations. To date there are only a small number of adequately developed and validated quality indicators, and not all of those have been associated with documented improvements in patient care over time. A list of representative osteoarthritis clinical guidelines and quality indicators are summarized in Table 2.9.4.

How would medical management change if she were on warfarin?
The presence of warfarin therapy would alter choices for potential analgesic or anti-inflammatory medication and/or their dosing. Acetaminophen may potentiate the anticoagulant effect of warfarin, although the effect is inconsistent. The International Normalized Ratio (INR) should be more closely monitored in those patients on warfarin therapy who are also taking a cumulative daily dose of 2g of

TABLE 2.9.4. Selected Published Guidelines and Quality Indicators for the Management of Osteoarthritis.

Author or Organization (Year)	Summary	Reference
Clinical guidelines		
American Academy of Orthopaedic Surgeons (2010)	Management of the knee	*J Bone Joint Surg Am, 92,* 990–993
American College of Rheumatology (2001, 2011 in press)	Management of the hip, knee, and hand	*Arthritis Rheum, 43,* 1905–1915
European League against Rheumatism (2003, 2005, 2007)	Management of knee (2003), hip (2005), and hand (2007)	*Ann Rheum Dis, 62,* 1145–1155; *64, 669–681; 66, 377–388*
National Institute of Health and Clinical Excellence (2008)	Management not limited to specific joint	* and *BMJ, 336,* 502–503
Osteoarthritis Research Society International (2007)	Management of the hip and knee	*Osteoarthritis Cartilage 15,* 981–1000
Quality indicators		
Arthritis Foundation (2004)	14 focusing on exam, pain and function assessment, nonpharmacologic treatment, acetaminophen, surgery, and radiographs	*Arthritis Rheum, 51,* 538–548
Centers for Medicare and Medicaid Services Physician Quality Reporting Initiative (PQRI) (updated annually)	Measure 142: Assessing for use of antiinflammatory or analgesic over-the-counter medications	†
ACOVE (Assessing Care of Vulnerable Elders) (2007)	11 focusing on pain and function, acetaminophen use, nonpharmacologic therapy, and surgery	† and *J Am Geriatr Soc,* *55 suppl. 2,* S383–391

*http://www.nice.org.uk/CG059.
†http://www.cms.gov/pqri/.
‡http://www.rand.org/health/projects/acove/acove3.

acetaminophen for more than a few days (Med Lett Drugs Ther, 2008; Dharmarajan& Sajjad, 2007). Regular dosing of acetaminophen, as contrasted to intermittent therapy, may minimize great swings that might otherwise occur in the INR in a patient concomitantly on warfarin.

The reversible inhibition of platelet function induced by standard NSAID therapies (e.g., ibuprofen and naproxen) may prolong bleeding from minor trauma. When these medications are used simultaneously with warfarin, the risk for serious bleeding is markedly increased because both pathways for acquiring hemostasis—the coagulation cascade and platelet-associated thrombosis—are blocked by the warfarin and the NSAID respectfully. For patients on warfarin who absolutely require an NSAID, the best choice would be one with little-to-no antiplatelet effect, either a cyclooxygenase-2 (COX-2) inhibitor (celecoxib) or a non-acetylated salicylate (e.g., salsalate or choline magnesium trisalicylate). The INR should be monitored closely given the case reports that describe elevation of the INR in anticoagulated patients given COX-2 inhibitors.

What additional tests, if any, should be ordered?
As the diagnosis of osteoarthritis is made on clinical grounds, tests are not required to make a diagnosis. Rather, tests are more appropriately used to adjust medication doses and to monitor for toxicity or severity. Initial laboratory tests would include a serum creatinine and hepatic function tests as bases for proper instruction of the patient regarding maximum allowable doses of acetaminophen. NSAID therapy requires baseline complete blood count, serum creatinine, and hepatic function tests; and repeats of these labs at a minimum of every 6 months to survey for evidence of subclinical drug-induced toxicity (gastrointestinal bleeding, renal insufficiency, and hepatic dysfunction, respectfully) is recommended.

While knee radiographs are not indicated to establish the diagnosis of osteoarthritis, they should be ordered to assess the severity of disease in the patient with persistent symptoms despite appropriate therapy, as well as to exclude other causes of knee pain. The order for knee radiographs should include anteroposterior (AP) and lateral views in the standing position and views of the patella with the knee flexed ("skyline", or "sunrise", views). Radiographs are indicated in the patient with hand osteoarthritis and persistent symptoms (including degrees of joint swelling and redness) despite therapy to evaluate for either erosive osteoarthritis or superimposed gouty arthritis.

Erosive osteoarthritis is a more severe variant of osteoarthritis, is seen more commonly in older women and typically in the PIP and DIP joints of the fingers, and is identified radiographically by the presence of subchondral, "seagull shaped" erosions in the center of the joint. Gouty arthritis in the elderly has been described as occurring in a similar finger joint distribution and has a different, yet characteristic, pattern to the radiographic appearance of the joint and/or bony erosion. The crystal etiology is proven by arthrocentesis to demonstrate the presence of the typical negatively birefringent crystals.

Joint aspiration for synovial fluid gram stain, culture, WBC count and differential, and crystal analysis should be performed in the patient with an acute-to-subacute symptomatic swollen joint to exclude infection and/or a crystalline arthritis. A crystalline arthritis from monosodium urate (gout), calcium pyrophosphate dihydrate (pseudogout), or basic calcium phosphate crystals may mimic a flare of knee osteoarthritis.

REFERENCES

American College of Rheumatology Ad Hoc Committee on Clinical Guidelines (1996). Guidelines for the initial evaluation of the adult patient with acute musculoskeletal symptoms. *Arthritis and Rheumatism, 39*, 1.

American College of Rheumatology Subcommittee on Osteoarthritis Guidelines (2001). Recommendations for the medical management of osteoarthritis of the hip and knee: 2000 update. *Arthritis Rheum, 43*, 1905–1915.

Chobanian, A. V., Bakris, G. L., Black, H. R., Cushman, W. C., Green, L. A., Izzo, J. L. Jr, . . . Roccella, E. J. (2003). The seventh report of the Joint National Committee on Prevention, Detection, Evaluation, and Treatment of High Blood Pressure: The JNC 7 report. *The Journal of the American Medical Association, 289*, 2560–2572.

Colglazier, C. L., & Sutej, P. G. (2005). Laboratory testing in the rheumatic diseases: A practical review. *Southern Medical Journal, 98*, 185–191.

Conaghan, P. G., Dickson, J., Grant, R. L., on behalf of the Guideline Development Group. (2008) Guidelines: Care and management of osteoarthritis in adults: Summary of NICE guidance. *BMJ, 336*, 502–503.

Cooney, D., & Pascuzzi, K. (2009). Polypharmacy in the elderly: Focus on drug interactions and adherence in hypertension. *Clinics in Geriatric Medicine, 25*, 221–233.

Dao, K., & Cush, J. J. (2006). Acute polyarthritis. *Best Practice & Research in Clinical Rheumatology, 20*, 653–672.

Dharmarajan, L., & Sajjad, W. (2007). Potentially lethal acetaminophen-warfarin interaction in an older adult: An under-recognized phenomenon? *Journal of the American Medical Directors Association, 8*, 545–547.

Felson, D. T. (2006). Osteoarthritis of the knee. *The New England Journal of Medicine, 354*, 841–848.

Gabay, C., & Kushner, I. (1999). Acute-phase proteins and other responses to inflammation. *The New England Journal of Medicine, 340*, 448–454.

Griffiths, R. A., Good, W. R., Watson, N. P., O'Donnell, H. F., Fell, P. J., & Shakespeare, J. M. (1984). Normal erythrocyte sedimentation rate in the elderly. *British Medical Journal (Clinical Research Edition.), 289*, 724–725.

Gross, K. D. (2010). Device use: Walking aids, braces, and orthoses for symptomatic knee osteoarthritis. *Clinics in Geriatric Medicine, 26*, 479–502.

Harvey, W. F., & Hunter, D. J. (2010). Pharmacologic intervention for osteoarthritis in older adults. *Clinics in Geriatric Medicine, 26*, 503–515.

Hunter, D. J. (2010). Quality of osteoarthritis care for community-dwelling older adults. *Clinics in Geriatric Medicine, 26*, 401–417.

Jordan, K. M., Arden, N. K., Doherty, M., Bannwarth, B., Bijlsma, J. W. J., Dieppe, P., Gunther, K., . . . Dougados, M. (2003). European League against Rheumatism. EULAR recommendations 2003: An evidence based approach to the management of knee osteoarthritis: Report of a task force of the

Standing Committee for International Clinical Studies Including Therapeutic Trials (ESCISIT) *Ann Rheum Dis*, *62*, 1145–1155.

Kwon, Y. D., Pittler, M. H., & Ernst, E. (2006). Acupuncture for peripheral joint osteoarthritis: A systematic review and meta-analysis. *Rheumatology*, *45*, 1331–1337.

Latham, N., & Chiung-ju, L. (2010). Strength training in older adults: The benefits for osteoarthritis. *Clinics in Geriatric Medicine*, *26*, 445–459.

Lee, M. S., Pittler, M. H., & Ernst, E. (2008). Tai chi for osteoarthritis: A systematic review. *Clinical Rheumatology*, *27*, 211–218.

MacLean, C. H., Pencharz, J. N., & Saag, K. G. (2007). quality indicators for the care of osteoarthritis in vulnerable elders. *J Am Geriatr Soc*, *55* suppl. 2, S383–S391.

Messier, S. P. (2010). Diet and exercise for obese adults with knee osteoarthritis. *Clinics in Geriatric Medicine*, *26*, 461–477.

Pencharz, J. N. & MacLean, C. H. (2004) Measuring quality in arthritis care: The Arthritis Foundation's quality indicator set for osteoarthritis. *Arthritis Rheum*, *51*, 538–548.

Pinals, R. S. (1994). Polyarthritis and fever. *The New England Journal of Medicine*, *330*, 769–774.

Piper, J. M., Ray, W. A., Daugherty, J. R., & Griffin, M. R. (1991). Corticosteroid use and peptic ulcer disease: Role of nonsteroidal anti-inflammatory drugs. *Annals of Internal Medicine*, *114*, 735–740.

Revaz, S., Dudler, J., & Kai-Lik So, A. (2006). Fever and musculoskeletal symptoms in an adult: Differential diagnosis and management. *Best Practice & Research in Clinical Rheumatology*, *20*, 641–651.

Richmond, J., Hunter, D., Irrgang, J., Jones, M. H., Snyder-Mackler, L., Van Durme, D., Rubin, C., . . . McGowan, R. (2010).American Academy of Orthopaedic Surgeons clinical practice guideline on the treatment of osteoarthritis (OA) of the knee. *J Bone Joint Surg Am*, *92*, 990–993.

Sawitzke, A. D., Shi, H., Finco, M. F., Dunlop, D. D., Harris, C. L., Singer, N. G., . . . Clegg, D. O. (2010). Clinical efficacy and safety of glucosamine, chondroitin sulphate, their combination, celecoxib or placebo taken to treat osteoarthritis of the knee: 2-year results from GAIT. *Annals of the Rheumatic Diseases*, *69*, 1459–1464.

Shorr, R. I., Ray, W. A., Daugherty, J. R., & Griffin, M. R. (1993). Concurrent use of nonsteroidal anti-inflammatory drugs and oral anticoagulants places elderly persons at high risk for hemorrhagic peptic ulcer disease. *Archives of Internal Medicine*, *153*, 1665–1670.

Solomon, D. H., Kavanaugh, A. J., & Schur, P. H. (2002). Evidenced-based guidelines for the use of immunologic tests: Antinuclear antibody testing. *Arthritis and Rheumatism*, *47*, 434–444.

Terkeltaub, R., Bushinsky, D. A., & Becker, M. A. (2006). Recent developments in our understanding of the renal basis of hyperuricemia and the development of novel antihyperuricemic therapeutics. *Arthritis Research and Therapy*, *8*(Suppl. 1), S4–S12.

Towheed, T. E., Maxwell, L., Judd, M. G., Catton, M., Hochberg, M. C., & Wells, G. (2006). Acetaminophen for osteoarthritis. *Cochrane Database of Systematic Reviews*, (1), CD004257.

Warfarin-acetaminophen interaction. (2008). *The Medical Letter on Drugs and Therapeutics*, *50*(1288), 45.

Zhang, W., Doherty, M., Arden, N., Bannwarth, B., Bijlsma, J., Gunther, K-P., Hauselmann, H. J., . . . Dougados, M. (2005) EULAR evidence based recommendations for the management of hip osteoarthritis: Report of a task force of the EULAR Standing Committee for International Clinical Studies Including Therapeutics (ESCISIT). *Ann Rheum Dis, 64,* 669–681.

Zhang, W., Doherty, M., Leeb, B. F., Alekseeva, L., Arden, N. K., Bijlsma, J. W., Dinçer, F., . . . Zimmermann-Górska, I. (2007) EULAR evidence based recommendations for the management of hand osteoarthritis: Report of a Task Force of the EULAR Standing Committee for International Clinical Studies Including Therapeutics (ESCISIT). *Ann Rheum Dis 66,* 377–388.

Zhang, W., Moskowitz, R. W., Nuki, G., Abramson, S., Altman, R. D., Arden, N., Bierma-Zeinstra, S., . . . Tugwell, P. (2007) OARSI recommendations for the management of hip and knee osteoarthritis, Part I: Critical appraisal of existing treatment guidelines and systematic review of current research evidence. *Osteoarthritis Cartilage 15,* 981–1000.

Case 2.10 Life after a Right CVA

By Cynthia S. Jacelon, PhD, RN, CRRN, FAAN

Mr. W is a 78-year-old white male. He is married and lives in New England with his wife of 51 years. They have 3 grown children, 6 grandchildren, and 8 great grandchildren living throughout the United States. No children or grandchildren live near the Ws. in New England. Since Mr. W retired from teaching high school geometry several years ago, he and his wife have spent approximately 6 months of every year touring the country in their RV and visiting their children. Mrs. W does not drive and did not work outside the home. The W's live in a 2-story farmhouse; and when at home, Mr. W enjoys working in his wood shop. He has a small business designing and making wood puzzles. He is proud of his collection of power tools.

While on a trip 6 weeks ago, Mr. W experienced a transient ischemic attack (TIA) consisting of blindness and mild left-sided weakness and numbness lasting for a few minutes. (For more information on TIAs, see http://www.talkabouttia.com/.) Mr. and Mrs. W left the RV with their son and flew home so that Mr. W could go to his own clinician. Mr. W and his wife described themselves as having good health prior to the TIA. Mr. W took daily medication to manage his blood pressure and was mildly concerned about his cholesterol level. His medications include Lasix, 40 mg by mouth every day; Zestril, 10 mg by mouth every day; Simvastatin, 10 mg by mouth every day at bedtime. He has no known allergies (NKA).

Case Studies in Gerontological Nursing for the Advanced Practice Nurse, First Edition.
Edited by Meredith Wallace Kazer, Leslie Neal-Boylan.
© 2012 John Wiley & Sons, Inc. Published 2012 by John Wiley & Sons, Inc.

OBJECTIVE

Mr. W is 6 ft 1 inch tall and weighs 225 lb. Mrs. W is 5 ft 2 inches tall and weighs 125 lb. Upon examination, the clinician found an elevated cholesterol level of 347, no carotid sounds on the left side, but a pronounced bruit over the right carotid artery. The clinician ordered carotid Doppler ultrasound studies. The studies revealed 90% occlusion of the left carotid, and 70% occlusion of the right. The clinician referred Mr. W to a vascular specialist who recommended a right carotid endarterectomy to be performed as soon as possible. (For more information, see http://www.stroke.org/site/PageServer?pagename=carotid.)

After discussing the risks and benefits of the procedure with the specialist, Mr. and Mrs. W spoke with their children by telephone and explained the procedure and risks to each of them. The decision was made to proceed with the surgery, consent forms were signed, Mr. W was admitted to the hospital, and he was prepared for surgery. In addition to the consent forms, Mr. W designated his wife as his health care proxy.

The surgery proceeded as planned, and the first 10 hours postoperatively were uneventful. When the nurse made rounds late on the day of surgery, Mr. W. was found to be paralyzed on the left side; his gaze was to the right; and his eyes could not cross midline. When spoken to from the left side, he searched for the speaker on his right. He was unable to find objects placed in front of him to the left of midline. Although Mr. W had no difficulty with language, he seemed confused at times; and he did not seem to recognize people he knew well, such as his physician. It was determined that Mr. W had suffered a right cerebrovascular accident (CVA) with left hemiparesis and profound left neglect, probably embolic in origin. Subsequent treatment with thrombolytics did not affect Mr. W's symptoms. Mr. W's condition stabilized, and the remainder of his acute stay in the hospital was medically unremarkable.

However, Mr. W. presented several challenges for nursing care. He was difficult to position and tended to reposition himself to lie with his head facing to the right. His left heel was constantly on the sheets, and he preferred to lie on his back. He was difficult to position in a chair and accused the staff of trying to push him over when they tried to transfer him. Mr. W had one fall while he was in the acute unit. He was found on the floor on the right side of bed. When asked what happened, he stated, "What is the matter with this place? There is already someone in that bed. I am not sharing a bed with a stranger!" He was NPO initially, then found to have an incompetent swallow and referred to the speech pathologist for further evaluation and an eating plan. On the fifth day postoperatively, he was transferred to the acute rehabilitation unit.

Upon admission to the rehabilitation unit, the clinician introduced herself to Mr. W and his wife. She asked Mr. W why he was admitted to rehabilitation; and he replied, "I was discharged from the hospital and needed a place to stay." When she asked about his paralyzed left side, he raised his right hand and said, "They tell me I had a shock, but I don't believe it. See? I can move my arm." The clinician notes that Mr. W's gaze is to the right and that he is craning his neck to attempt to look over his right shoulder to see from where the voice is originating. He is dependent for all purposeful mobility and activities of daily living. He is incontinent of the bladder. The speech pathologist recommended thickened liquids, mechanical soft diet, and a swallowing protocol of chin tuck and turn to the left for each swallow, which Mr. W was unable to do without assistance. Upon discharge to home, Mr. W was prescribed Coumadin 2.5 mg by mouth every day; measurement of INR every 3 days until stable; Lasix, 40 mg by mouth every day; Zestril, 10 mg by mouth every day; and Simvastatin, 10 mg by mouth every day at bedtime.

ASSESSMENT

Altered self-management of health status: Mr. W's stroke caused anosognosia, which is a lack of awareness of one's own disabilities. Therefore, Mr. W was not able to participate in his care because he failed to understand the need for the care.

Altered eating ability: The swallowing deficit combined with impulsiveness and other perceptual problems associated with a right CVA combine to make administering a safe eating program very challenging.

Urinary incontinence: Urinary incontinence is a common sequela to CVA. In this case Mr. W likely has an uninhibited neurogenic bladder. This type of incontinence is characterized by urgency, frequency, nocturia, small or absent postvoid residual, and intact "anal wink" reflex.

Altered mobility (hemiparesis): Contralateral hemiparesis is a common sequela of CVA. The most common area for an embolic stroke is branches of the middle cerebral artery. This artery supplies blood to the motor strip of the frontal lobe, the sensory strip of the parietal lobe, and the sensory integration areas of the parietal lobe. If Mr. W's CVA had been on the left side, in all likelihood he would have expressive aphasia, receptive aphasia, or both. It is likely that Mr. W also has a left hemianopsia. That is a visual field deficit in which the left half of the visual field of each eye is damaged.

Altered role function: Currently Mr. W is dependent for all ADL and unable to perform many usual life roles. He is the sole driver in the family, and there is a large size difference between Mr. and Mrs. W. His hobby of woodworking may not be viable based on his deficits.

Altered cognitive processes (anosognosia): A right CVA can affect a number of cognitive processes including comprehension of the CVA itself. A right CVA can also affect an individual's ability to identify certain types of faces (such as the faces of people one knows well). In addition, an individual with right CVA may exhibit impulsiveness and disinhibition; the individual does not screen their verbal comments and often says rude and inappropriate things.

Altered perception (unilateral neglect). Damage to the right parietal lobe of the brain has a profound effect on a person's perception. Unilateral neglect is not a deficit of seeing, hearing, or moving, but one of looking, listening, or touching. It is a deficit that is most dramatic early in the recovery period, but residual neglect can continue for extended periods.

Altered judgment. Impulsivity and poor judgment are characteristics of individuals with RCVAs. The combination of anosognosia, perceptual alterations, disinhibition, and impulsivity all contribute to impaired judgment.

CRITICAL THINKING

What was the reasoning behind the decision to do a right endarterectomy rather than a left?

What is the plan of treatment for each of the problems listed above?

What is the plan for follow-up care?

How will the clinician include Mrs. W in the plan of care?

How does Mr. W's psychosocial history affect the treatment plan?

RESOLUTION

What was the reasoning behind the decision to do a right endarterectomy rather than a left?
Approximately 85% of CVAs are ischemic in origin (Mauk, 2007, 157). The flow in the right carotid was at 30%. With a 70% blockage and an audible bruit, the turbulence in the artery is such that it increases the

likelihood of clot formation. The flow in the left side was so diminished that there is likely insufficient turbulence to be at high risk for clot formation.

What is the plan of treatment for each of the problems listed above? In order to effectively help Mr. W rehabilitate from his stroke, he will need the services of an interdisciplinary team. An interdisciplinary team is a team of health care providers in which the providers (registered nurse, physical therapist, occupational therapist, speech and language pathologist, physiatrist, and a variety of others) work with the patient and family to set realistic patient goals (Mauk, 2007). The team works together in a matrix to help the patient achieve the goals. It is estimated that Mr. W will be in a rehabilitation unit for approximately 3 weeks; then he will likely need visiting nurse support at home.

Altered self-management of health status: Mr. W will need a lot of support for self-management as he learns to live with the deficits from his CVA. He will need to learn to manage his medications, and adjust to his new physical status. Mrs. W will be an important member of the rehabilitation team as she will have the primary responsibility for supporting Mr. W at home.

Long-term goal: Adjustment to disability as demonstrated by verbalization of the disease process and demonstration of compensatory techniques by D/C.

Short-term goals:
1. Mr. W will actively participate in therapies and his rehabilitation program by 3 days following admission.
2. His wife will attend scheduled sessions beginning 1 week after admission.
3. Mr. and Mrs. W will discuss diagnosis with clinician by 2 weeks after admission.
4. Mr. and Mrs. W will demonstrate safe medication management by discharge.

Teaching needs: Medical diagnosis, health maintenance, and medication management.

Staff involved in meeting goals: RN, MD, pharmacist, psychologist, other staff as support

Interventions:
1. Monitor vital signs as per protocol.
2. Administer medications.
3. Implement self-/wife medication management.
4. Implement psychosocial adaptation skills.
5. Implement and evaluate a rehabilitation program.

Altered eating ability: Following a videofluoroscopy swallowing study (Logemann, 1994), the speech-language pathologist recommended a swallowing protocol for meals. Because of Mr. W's left neglect, he was prone to reaching for the tray of the person sitting on his right. The nurse had to position Mr. W and his meal in such a way as to maximize Mr. W's ability to focus on his meal. Often Mr. W would eat only the food from the right side of his tray. In addition, Mr. W's cholesterol is high, so the dietician will meet with Mr. and Mrs. W to discuss nutritional intake.

Long-term goal: Maintain well balanced diet without aspiration

Short-term goals:
1. Mr. W should demonstrate swallowing protocols with supervision by 2 weeks after admission.
2. Mr. W. should demonstrate an understanding of diet restrictions by discharge.

Teaching needs: There should be education on swallowing protocols and a low cholesterol diet.

Staff involved in meeting goals: RN, SLP, OT, RD.

Interventions:
1. Swallow evaluation
2. Weekly weighing
3. 1:1 supervision during meals
4. Calorie counting
5. Menu planning

Urinary incontinence: Following an assessment of Mr. W's 24-hour voiding pattern, including postvoid residual, a bladder management program was instituted. Because of the anticipated home situation, it was decided that continence at night would not be a focus of rehabilitation.

Long-term goal: Urinary continence during the day by discharge.

Short-term goals:
1. Void on request by day 3.
2. Identify the need to void by day 8.
3. Void with assistance by day 15.

Teaching needs: Educate on the causes and management of incontinence.

Staff involved in meeting goals: RN.

Interventions:
1. Implement continence protocol.
   - Fluid intake
     - 1500–2000 mL
     - Limit fluids after 6 p.m.

- Toilet every 2 hours
- Assess postvoid residual.

Altered mobility: The physical therapist conducted an assessment of Mr. W's mobility on admission to rehabilitation. Based on his admission status and mobility needs for discharge, the following plan was created.

Long-term goals:
1. Independent transfers by day 10.
2. Ambulate with supervision and device with minimal cues by day 20.
3. Independent with wheelchair. Mobility 150 ft on all surfaces by discharge.

Short-term goals:
1. Transfers with occasional cues by day 7.
2. Propels wheelchair 75 ft independently over even surfaces day 15.
3. Will ambulate with straight cane, contact guard, and moderate cues by 15.

Teaching Needs: Bed, W/C, car transfers; family training

Staff Involved in Meeting Goals: Mr. W is supported by all staff.

Interventions:
1. For 5–6x/wk for 1–1½ hours, Mr. W will have stretching, gait, W/C mobility, and transfer training, and participate in community outings.
2. Reinforce teaching.

Altered role function: Dependent for ADL; impaired leisure activities.

Long-term goals:
1. Self care with minimal assist by discharge.
2. Develop new leisure activities by 1 month post discharge.

Short-term goals:
1. Will complete bathing tasks with <3 verbal cues and close supervision by week 2.
2. Will complete oral hygiene with minimal assistance by week 2.
3. Will dress himself with moderate cues by week 2.
4. Will perform tub-seat transfer with contact guard by day 10.

Teaching needs:
1. Patient training in ADL skills.
2. Family training on how to assist patient.

Staff involved in meeting goals: OT, RN, all staff.

Interventions:
1. OT 5–6x/week for 1–1 1/2 hours/day for ADL training, passive range of motion, motor facilitation, and exploration of leisure activities.
2. Home evaluation.
3. Reinforce training.

Altered cognitive processes:
1. Left neglect
2. Cognition/problem solving.

Long-term goals:
1. Compensate for neglect by increasing to left hemisphere evidenced by attending to left with minimal verbal cues by D/C.
2. Orientation to person, place, and time 100% of time by D/C.
3. Functional problem solving using compensatory techniques, such as self-correcting and environmental cues.

Short-term goals:
1. Locate items on the left side during ADL with <4 verbal cues during a 1-hour session by week 2.
2. Attend to objects on the left side with moderate cues by week 2.
3. Identify the time of day 75% of the time with minimal cues by week 1.
4. Use environmental cues to problem solve 40% of the time by week 3.

Teaching needs:
1. Causes of left neglect.
2. Safety r/t left neglect.
3. Teach Mrs. W how to cue Mr. W to attend.

Staff involved in meeting goals: PT, OT, and RN.

Interventions
1. Therapeutic exercises to improve scanning.
2. Activities to make Mr. W look left.
3. Approach Mr. W from the left side; cue as needed.
4. Verbal and visual cues for sequencing.
5. Encourage participation in decision making.

What is the plan for follow-up care?
Mr. W will likely need continued rehabilitation after he is discharged. Ideally he could attend a day rehabilitation program. There are two barriers to this plan. First, Mrs. W does not have a driver's license. She will not be able to drive Mr. W to therapy appointments, so he will need some sort of public transportation to get to appointments. The second problem is that Mr. and Mrs. W live in a rural area. Day rehabilitation programs may not be available in the area.

A second possibility for follow-up for Mr. W is visiting nurse services. In this case, therapists and nurses will come to Mr. W's home for therapy. He will also likely need INR testing to regulate his Coumadin dosage.

Mr. and Mrs. W's house will need some reorganizing. Mr. W will not be able to climb the stairs in their home. Fortunately, the bathroom is on the first floor; but Mr. W's bedroom will need to be moved downstairs.

Mr. W will not be able to pursue his puzzle business for some time. Because of his perceptual problems, he may not be safe with power tools. An occupational therapist will need to evaluate his safety.

How will the clinician include Mrs. W in the plan of care?

Mrs. W is integral to the plan of care. Because Mr. W's perception and judgment is impaired, Mrs. W is going to have to learn all of Mr. W's needs and supervise and assist with his care. Throughout the rehabilitation stay, Mrs. W should be included in all therapy sessions. After discharge, Mr. and Mrs. W will likely need some support as they adjust to their new lifestyle. Community support groups could be beneficial.

How does Mr. W's psychosocial history affect the treatment plan?

Mr. W has a background that was based on his perceptual awareness. Geometry is focused on spatial relationships, and his love of puzzles is also based on spatial relationships. Mr. W's current disabilities may be particularly frustrating based on this background. It will be a challenge to find activities that are of interest to him now that he will not be able to drive the RV or work in his shop.

There are no children or grandchildren living near Mr. and Mrs. W. They will need support from neighbors, friends, and others in their community. The health care team may need to suggest strategies for Mr. and Mrs. W to reconnect with their community in Vermont.

REFERENCES

Logemann, J. A. (1994). Evaluation and treatment of swallowing disorders. *American Journal of Speech-Language Pathology, 3*, 41–44.

Mauk, K. L. (Ed.). (2007). *The specialty practice of rehabilitation nursing: A core curriculum* (5th ed.). Glenview, IL: Association of Rehabilitation Nursing.

Talk about TIA. Retrieved July 30, 2010, from Web site http://www.talkabout-tia.com/

Case 2.11 It Takes My Breath Away

By Kathy Murphy, RN, BA, DipN, RNT, MSc, PhD,
Dympna Casey, RGN, BA, MA, PhD,
and Bernard McCarthy, MSc

Mrs. H, a 65-year-old woman with a history of hypertension, presents to the clinician with a continued complaint of a cough. She has been to the office 3 times over the last 6 months with the same troublesome cough. She has had 2 chest infections, 1 of which resulted in an admission to the hospital. She reports that she has been feeling increasingly fatigued and breathless on exertion over the past few weeks. She had a hysterectomy 20 years ago and an appendectomy when she was a child. She lives on her own in a rural area. Her husband died when she was in her 40s. She has 4 children, 2 living nearby and 2 in the UK. She has an occasional social drink, does not currently smoke, but has a smoking history of 15–20 cigarettes per day for 45 years. She stopped smoking 4 years ago. Her income comes primarily from social security and a small widow's pension. She is very involved with her family and attends Catholic services weekly.

Recently she feels that her health is declining, and she finds that she is able to do less and less. In particular, she finds housework almost impossible; and she has just moved her bedroom to the ground floor as she finds it very difficult to climb stairs. She is having some problems with bathing and dressing, and she finds these to be increasing struggles. She visits her clinician every month for repeat prescriptions and, when needed, follow-up of her hypertension. Her children are healthy. Both of her parents are deceased. Her father died in his sixties of chronic bronchitis. Her mother died of cancer at 66. On review it is

Case Studies in Gerontological Nursing for the Advanced Practice Nurse, First Edition.
Edited by Meredith Wallace Kazer, Leslie Neal-Boylan.

evident that she is experiencing increasing shortness of breath (SOB), dyspnea on exertion (DOE), difficulty in undertaking household tasks, and disturbed sleep due to coughing. She is also experiencing fatigue and is worried about her capacity to manage her home tasks. Her medications include Spiriva, 500 mcg once daily; Seretide, 200 mcg twice daily; Ventolin, 200 mcg as needed; and Exforge, 100 mg once daily. She has no known allergies (NKA).

OBJECTIVE

Mrs. H is awake, alert, and oriented. She appears breathless on exertion. Her oxygen saturation levels are 93%, dropping to 90% following exertion. She appears clean and well kept. Her clothes are appropriate. She is 5 ft 2 inches and weighs 180 lb. Her vital signs are BP: 164/92; P: 110; respirations: 25 per minute. She is afebrile with a temperature of 97.8. There is hyperinflation of the chest, some use of accessory muscles of respiration, crackles, and an occasional audible wheeze. Cardiac exam reveals a regular heart rate, S1, S2, and no abnormal sounds. Her abdomen is soft and nontender, and her bowel sounds are present in all 4 quadrants.

She has a small scar as a result of an appendectomy as a child. Her skin is dry and intact, and there is some dehydration evident. She has slight pedal edema and positive pedal pulses. Her eyes reveal clear normal sclerae with PERRLA. Her ears reveal heavy wax buildup and normal tympanic membranes bilaterally. Her mouth is dry; oral mucosa is spotted with possible thrush present. Neurological exam reveals 2+ deep tendon reflexes bilaterally and equal strength. Her gait is normal, and she has full range of motion of all extremities.

ASSESSMENT

Asthma: Asthma is becoming increasingly more common among older adults. However, the patient with asthma is typically under the age of 35, has a history of waking in the nighttime breathless or experiencing wheezing, rarely experiences a productive cough, and has symptoms that vary from day to day. However, asthma can usually be distinguished on clinical presentation and by the patient's history.

Cor pulmonale: Mrs. H complains of dyspnea, wheeze, and an inability to undertake tasks that require physical exertion; and she has pedal edema. However, she does not have any evidence of cyanosis or pulmonary hypertension.

Emphysema: Emphysema is a chronic obstructive pulmonary disease (COPD), an umbrella term used to describe chronic lung diseases that cause obstruction in airflow. Globally, COPD is considered a major cause of chronic morbidity (NHLB, 2005). It is projected that by 2030 COPD will rank seventh in the worldwide burden of disease (Mathers & Loncar, 2006) and will be the third most frequent cause of death (World Health Organisation, 2008).

DIAGNOSTICS

An important point to consider is how spirometry is performed and how the results are interpreted. It is common to take a pre-bronchodilator measurement and a post-bronchodilator measurement using spirometry. Controversy exists as to whether reversibility using bronchodilators should be used to confirm diagnosis. The recent Global Initiative for Chronic Obstructive Lung Disease Guidelines (2009) does not support reversibility. The test results reveal pre-bronchodilator: FVC 1.64, FEV1 .98, FEV1% predicted 47%, FEV1/FVC ratio 60%. Post-bronchodilator: FEV1 .96, FEV1% predicted 55%, FVC 1.62, FEV1/FVC 59%.

CRITICAL THINKING

What is causing Mrs. H's dyspnea and fatigue, and how is a diagnosis best made?

What is the most likely differential diagnosis and why?

What is the plan of care?

What is the plan for follow-up care?

Does the patient's psychosocial history impact how the clinician might treat this patient?

What if the patient also had asthma?

What if the patient had cor pulmonale?

Considering the differentials listed, what are the best treatment options for this patient?

Are there any standardized guidelines that the clinician should use to assess or treat this case?

RESOLUTION

What is causing Mrs. H's dyspnea and fatigue, and how is a diagnosis best made?
Breathlessness is a common feature of acute respiratory infective exacerbations, but breathlessness during normal everyday activity develops insidiously over many years. Most patients will have lost more than 50% of their predicted FEV1 by the time that breathlessness becomes a problem. The BORG dyspnea scale (Table 2.11.1) outlined below is commonly used to assess breathlessness in patients with COPD (Borg, 1982).

Key Point

When assessing symptoms such as cough and breathlessness, use objective measures to assess the patient. The Borg dyspnea scale is a useful measurement for breathlessness.

Wheeze is often an accompanying feature of breathlessness and may be erroneously attributed to asthma. There may be signs of hyperinflation of the chest which include a barrel-shaped chest (increased antero-posterior diameter), use of accessory muscles of respiration, reduction of the cricosternal distance, paradoxical in drawing of the lower ribs on inspiration, intercostal recession, hollowing out of the supraclavicular fossae, pursed-lip breathing, and reduced expansion. These signs are highly suggestive of emphysema. Other features of emphysema are

TABLE 2.11.1. Borg Dyspnea Scale.

Which of the following best describes your breathlessness now?	
0	No Breathlessness At All
0.5	Very, Very Slight (Just Noticeable)
1	Very Slight
2	Slight Breathlessness
3	Moderate
4	Somewhat Severe
5	Severe Breathlessness
6	
7	Very Severe Breathlessness
8	
9	Very, Very Severe (Almost Maximum)
10	Maximum

prolonged expiration, especially forced expiration which can be greater than 5 seconds, frequent fine crackles, and an occasional audible wheeze. On percussion, the patient may present with hyperresonant lung fields. None of these signs are specific to emphysema and do not correlate very well with the severity of the disease, both of which emphasize the need for objective assessment.

The cough is usually worse in the mornings but bears no relationship to the severity of the disease. A hacking, rasping cough with associated volumes of thick mucoid sputum may be suggestive of bronchiectasis. Hemoptysis should alert the clinician to an infective exacerbation or the presence of a carcinoma of the bronchus, which is a common comorbidity in patients with emphysema. With progression of the condition, signs of right ventricular dysfunction may develop (cor pulmonale) because of the effects of chronic hypoxemia and hypercapnia. Presenting signs of cor pulmonale might include peripheral edema, raised jugular venous pressure, hepatic congestion, and the presence of metabolic flapping tremor. Clubbing of the fingers is a common feature and may be indicative of chronic long-term disease, not just respiratory diseases.

Diagnosis of emphysema has become a topic of current debate within both health care and health economists' spheres as early diagnosis combined with early intervention is known to have major health and cost implications. In most countries little proactive diagnosis of emphysema is undertaken. For those countries proactive in diagnosis the current debate is on, whether to mass screen the entire population or target screen the at-risk population that match predetermined phenotypes. The latter approach is the option which appears to have the greater support due to its pragmatic approach, especially in the area of cost and implementation.

An appropriate history, in conjunction with an objective confirmation of airway obstruction using spirometry, may be used to confirm a diagnosis of COPD (National Institute for Health and Clinical Excellence [NICE], 2010; Global Initiative for Chronic Obstructive Lung Disease, 2009; ATS/ERS, 2004). Diagnosis of COPD is confirmed as a post-bronchodilator forced expiratory volume in 1 second (FEV1)/forced vital capacity (FVC) of <70%, with the severity of the COPD being determined by the measured post-bronchodilator FEV1 as a percent of predicted FEV1 (National Institute for Health and Clinical Excellence [NICE], 2010; Global Initiative for Chronic Obstructive Lung Disease, 2009; ATS/ERS, 2004). However, the table does not differentiate between the two main conditions associated with COPD, emphysema and bronchitis.

Despite expert international agreement on the above criteria for diagnosis, a major debate is ongoing among the experts as to its accuracy. Many reports in the literature now recommend diagnosing obstruction using the statistically derived lower limit of normal (LLN), which varies for each person according to age, height, ethnicity, and gender. While the use of an FVC 70% ratio is less complicated, it has been shown to result in underdiagnoses of airflow obstruction in younger people and overdiagnoses in the elderly. This is particularly important as older people may be most sensitive to many of the adverse effects of medications used in the treatment of emphysema, including corticosteroids and anticholinergic bronchodilators.

What is the most likely differential diagnosis and why?

Emphysema is an obvious differential diagnosis given the symptoms with which Mrs. H presented. With Mrs. H's clinical history and her spirometry results, she has stage II, moderate emphysema as the post-bronchodilator FEV1% of 55 is between the 50% and 79% predicted (Global Initiative for Chronic Obstructive Lung Disease, 2009).

What is the plan of care?

Medications to manage the airway obstruction, including bronchodilators and steroid therapy, are essential; but the main focus is on enrolling Mrs. H in a pulmonary rehabilitation program. One of the key strategies in improving care for people with emphysema is the provision of pulmonary rehabilitation (PR) programs. PR programs utilize a multidisciplinary approach and usually consist of a patient assessment, exercise training, education, and psychosocial support (Nici, 2006). PR programs have been successful in reducing patients' sense of dyspnea and enhancing health related quality of life (HRQOL) (Effing et al., 2007; Lacasse, Goldstein, Lasserson, & Martin, 2006; Troosters, Casaburi, Gosselink, & Decramer, 2005). PR programs focus on self-care and self-management. Both the National Institute for Health and Clinical Excellence (NICE) guidelines for the management of COPD (2004, 2010) and the Global Initiative for Chronic Obstructive Lung Disease (2006, 2009) endorse the use of PR for patients with emphysema and chronic bronchitis.

Mrs. H will be asked to attend the next 8-week PR run in primary care for 2 hours per week. The focus will be on empowering Mrs. H to self-manage her emphysema by learning breathing techniques such as pursed-lip breathing, the huff coughing technique, and diaphragmatic breathing. These should help to lessen her experience of dyspnea. To learn more about pursed-lip and diaphragmatic breathing, refer to the following Web site http://www.youtube.com/watch?v=pte_GGQb1_4.The clinician can help by checking Mrs. H's inhalation technique, by reinforcing good technique, and by checking her medications. Her dehydration may indicate that she is restricting her fluid intake because she is experiencing difficulty in walking to the toilet. Medications with steroids can lead to oral thrush; and following treatment for her thrush, Mrs. H should be taught to rinse her mouth after medications and should be advised to clean dispensers after each use.

What is the plan for follow-up care?

Assessing and monitoring Mrs. H's emphysema over time through the use of spirometry, oxygen saturation, and symptom measurements (for example, using the BORG breathlessness scale) are important. Over time, as emphysema increases, patients become more hypoxic. Once oxygen saturation levels at rest fall below 90% or PaO_2 falls below 8 kPa, patients start to develop signs of cor pulmonale, in particular peripheral edema. For now Mrs. H should be reviewed by her primary care clinician at least annually and referred to a pulmonary specialist. Repeated lung infections will have a detrimental effect on long-term vital capacity and early intervention is necessary. For this reason many guidelines recommend that a person with emphysema should have antibiotics and steroids prescribed for home storage so that treatment can be started as soon as the person recognizes the onset of an infection. Mrs. H should also be offered the influenza vaccination prior to the onset of winter each year. Breathlessness, lack of absorption due to hypoxia, and increased expenditure of energy due to having to work harder to breathe may lead to weight loss. Mrs. H should have her BMI monitored (normal 20–25). Should her BMI become too high or low, referral to a dietician would be required. During her visits to the clinician, Mrs. H should be questioned and encouraged to continue the activities introduced and covered in the PR program to ensure that exercise, breathing techniques, and good diet and lifestyle changes are embedded into her daily life. Lifestyle changes are not easy, and the clinician has a key role in trying to encourage and motivate Mrs. H. While PR will not improve lung capacity, it may help to prevent acute exacerbations and to improve quality of life.

Does the patient's psychosocial history impact how the clinician might treat this patient?

The facts that Mrs. H is widowed and that she is living alone underscore the need to maintain her ability to undertake activities of independent living for as long as possible. Emphysema can be very disabling, and frequently patients become socially isolated as they relinquish activities they once enjoyed. Therefore, depression may develop. It is estimated that 40% of patients with COPD suffer from depression that is frequently untreated (Yohannes, Baldwin, & Connolly, 2006). Because of this, the primary care providers need to be alert to the existence of depression.

What if the patient also had asthma?

It is not unusual for a patient to have asthma, as well as emphysema. It is essential, therefore, to understand the differences and similarities between the diagnoses and treatments of asthma and emphysema. With asthma, improvement in lung function is anticipated when the inflammation that caused the asthmatic attack is reduced; but in emphysema the lung damage is permanent and irreversible.

What if the patient had cor pulmonale?

It is not unusual for a person with a long-standing history of hypertension and emphysema to develop cor pulmonale. It would be important that this be identified and treated, but remember that a person experiencing dyspnea on exertion may take diuretics only reluctantly as they will result in more frequent trips to the toilet. Therefore, good patient education is an essential element of management.

Considering the differentials listed, what are the best treatment options for this patient?

Treatment for asthma focuses on controlling and eliminating the triggers that lead to inflammation of the airways, for example, controlling allergies. Bronchodilators and antiinflammatories, such as inhaled corticosteroids, are typical treatment options. In cor pulmonale, treatment focuses on identifying and treating the underlying cause.

Following the completion of the PR program, it is important that Mrs. H's care is carefully managed by her primary care clinician. Motivation is essential if a person is to make the lifestyle changes required to make a difference to the experience of dyspnea. Joining a COPD support group may also help maintain motivation.

Are there any standardized guidelines that the clinician should use to assess or treat this case?

There are three main international COPD guidelines: ATS/ERS, Gold, and NICE. A URL link to each of the guidelines is below.

- National Institute for Health and Clinical Excellence (NICE) (2010) http://guidance.nice.org.uk/CG101
- Global Initiative for Chronic Obstructive Lung Disease (Gold) (2009) http://www.goldcopd.com/Guidelineitem.asp?l1=2&l2=1&intId=2003
- ATS/ERS (2004) Standards for the Diagnosis and Management of Patients with COPD http://www.thoracic.org/clinical/copd-guidelines/resources/copddoc.pdf

REFERENCES

ATS/ERS (2004). *Standards for the Diagnosis and Management of Patients with COPD*. Retrieved July 9, 2010, from http://www.thoracic.org/clinical/copd-guidelines/resources/copddoc.pdf

Borg, G. A. (1982). Psychophysical bases of perceived exertion. *Medicine and Science in Sports and Exercise, 14*, 377–381.

Effing, T., Monninkhof, E., van der Valk, P., Zielhuis, G., Walters, E., van der Palen, J. J., et al. (2007). Self-management education for patients with chronic obstructive pulmonary disease. *Cochrane Database of Systematic Reviews*, (4), Art. No.: CD002990.

Global Initiative for Chronic Obstructive Lung Disease (2006). *Global Strategy for Diagnosis, Management, and Prevention of COPD: Update 2006*. Retrieved March 5, 2008, from http://www.goldcopd.org

Global Initiative for Chronic Obstructive Lung Disease (2009). *Global Strategy for Diagnosis, Management, and Prevention of COPD: Update 2009*. Retrieved July 9, 2010, from http://www.goldcopd.org

Lacasse, Y., Goldstein, R., Lasserson, T. J., & Martin, S. (2006). Pulmonary rehabilitation for chronic obstructive pulmonary disease. *Cochrane Database of Systematic Reviews*, (4), Art. No.: CD003793.

Mathers, C. D., & Loncar, D. (2006). Projections of global mortality and burden of disease from 2002 to 2030. *PLoS Medicine*, 3(11), e442.

National Institute for Health and Clinical Excellence (NICE) (2004). *Chronic Obstructive Pulmonary Disease: Management of chronic obstructive pulmonary disease in adults in primary and secondary care*. Retrieved October 8, 2008, from http://guidance.nice.org.uk/CG101

National Institute for Health and Clinical Excellence (NICE) (2010). *Chronic Obstructive Pulmonary Disease: Management of chronic obstructive pulmonary disease in adults in primary and secondary care (Clinical guidelines CG101)*. Retrieved July 20, 2010, from http://guidance.nice.org.uk/CG101.

NHLB (2005). *WHO Global Initiative for Chronic Obstructive Lung Disease (GOLD) workshop report*. Retrieved July 7, 2010, from http://www.goldcopd.com

Nici, L., Donner, C., Wouters, E., Zuwallack, R., Ambrosino, N., Bourbeau, J., Carone, M., . . . Troosters, T. (2006). American Thoracic Society/European Respiratory Society Statement on Pulmonary Rehabilitation. *American Journal of Respiratory and Critical Care Medicine*. 173, 1390–1413. doi: 10.1164/rccm.200508–1211ST.

Troosters, T., Casaburi, R., Gosselink, R., & Decramer, M. (2005). Pulmonary rehabilitation in chronic obstructive pulmonary disease. *American Journal of Respiratory and Critical Care Medicine*, 172(1), 19–38.

World Health Organisation (2008). *The Global Burden of Disease: 2004 update*. Retrieved July 17, 2010, from http://www.who.int/healthinfo/global_burden_disease/GBD_report_2004update_full.pdf

Yohannes, A. M., Baldwin, R. C., & Connolly, M. J. (2006). Depression and anxiety in elderly patients with chronic obstructive pulmonary disease. *Age and Ageing*, 35(5), 457–459.

Case 2.12 What's Shaking?

By Donna Packo Diaz, MS, RN, and Cathi A. Thomas, MS, RN, CNRN

Mr. M, a 65-year-old Caucasian male, was referred to the neurological practice for evaluation of a new onset tremor of his right hand. He was accompanied by his wife of 42 years.

Mr. M reports a tremor of his right hand over the last 10 months. The tremor "comes and goes"; and, more recently, it has been "harder to hide." Mr. M notices it when he is watching television in the evening. It is clearly worse when he is nervous and disappears when he sleeps. The tremor does not bother him when he eats or writes. He is a recently retired chemical engineer who has worked for 30 years at a major pharmaceutical company and has lived in an urban setting in the northeastern United States. Mr. M is now teaching mathematics at the local community college 2 evenings per week. He states he has no significant difficulty performing his job; however, he feels anxious when his tremor is present. He also reports some problems manually adjusting transparencies on an overhead projector. Mr. M is father of 2 adult sons and 1 daughter. Mr. M and his wife also have 4 grandchildren. He enjoys spending time with the 2 grandchildren who live locally. He and his wife also like socializing; however, his wife notes that her husband's interest in these activities has significantly declined over the last year. Mr. M states that he is "just too tired" to do many of the things he once took pleasure in such as playing tennis, going out to dinner, and attending services at his synagogue. His wife shares that he has been much more sedentary the last 6 months. Mr. M has no history of smoking cigarettes and drinks an "occasional" beer (1–2 per month).

Case Studies in Gerontological Nursing for the Advanced Practice Nurse, First Edition.
Edited by Meredith Wallace Kazer, Leslie Neal-Boylan.
© 2012 John Wiley & Sons, Inc. Published 2012 by John Wiley & Sons, Inc.

Mr. M's medical history includes hypertension for a decade. He has been bothered by hay fever for several years and currently uses loratadine as needed. Mr. M had a right knee arthroscopy 15 years ago for a small meniscus tear. Eleven months ago, a precancerous polyp was removed during a routine colonoscopy. A report of his most recent visit to his PCP includes a normal physical examination except for the presence of the hand tremor. CBC and chemistry with a thyroid panel were within normal limits. An MRI of the brain was ordered by his PCP. Mr. M's mother, who lives in an assisted living facility nearby, is alive at 89 years of age and in remarkably good health. His father died of colon cancer at age 56. He has 2 younger brothers both with mild hypertension. He recalls a maternal aunt now deceased with significant head and voice tremors.

The following were noted during a review of systems: eyeglasses for both driving and reading, poor sense of smell for several years, well-controlled hypertension, constipation (3 bowel movements per week, with straining over the last 2 years), and nocturia with urination 2–3 times per night. He denies difficulty falling asleep; however, his wife reports restlessness of sleep with some thrashing of arms which has been "happening for years." Mr. M is sexually active with his wife and has occasional erectile dysfunction. He denies feeling depressed. His medications include: loratadine, 15 mg as needed; Lopressor, 50 mg every day; ASA, 81 mg every day for cardiac prophylaxis; Centrum Silver, 1 every day, and Tadalafil as needed. No history of metoclopramide, neuroleptics, or other dopamine-depleting agents. He reports seasonal allergies only.

OBJECTIVE

Mr. M arrived at the neurology clinic with his wife. He appears well nourished, slightly overweight, and neatly dressed. His vital signs are BP: 138/76; HR 60 and regular.

He is 5 ft 9 inches tall and weighs 197 lb. He exhibits a moderately decreased facial expression, a decreased blink rate, and a mildly monotonous voice. His neurological examination is as follows:

- **Cognition/mood/behavior:** Alert and oriented. Mini-Mental State Exam (MMSE): 29; 2/3 recall of objects. Moderately anxious.
- **Cranial nerves:** Decreased sense of smell. Visual fields full by confrontation. Fundi normal. Extraocular movements (EOM). Breakdown of smooth pursuit. Mild decreased up gaze. Facial sensation normal. Face symmetrical with tongue and palate midline. Gag reflex normal. Sternocleidomastoid and trapezius strength: 5/5.

- **Motor:** Mild cogwheel rigidity; right upper extremity greater than left. Tremor in right hand observed at rest. Mild action tremor on nose-to-finger test on right side. Decreased amplitude and slowing of finger tapping on right side. Small handwriting noted.
- **Gait/balance:** Up from a chair without difficulty. Slightly stooped posture. Initiates gait without difficulty. Mild dragging of right leg on ambulation. Decreased right arm swing with tremor of right hand. Runs with ease. Good balance with recovery on pull test (2–3 steps).
- **Sensory:** Exam normal to light touch, pinprick, vibration, and position sense. No extinction to double simultaneous stimulation.
- **Reflexes:** These were 2/4 and symmetrical in the upper extremities and knees and 1/4 at the ankles. Plantars are down-going. Positive Myerson sign.

ASSESSMENT

Idiopathic Parkinson Disease (PD): PD is a neurodegenerative disorder affecting 1.6% of the U.S. population over age 65 (Willis, Evanoff, Lian, Criswell, & Rachette, 2010). Men and Caucasians are more often affected. The average age of onset is 63, but risk increases with age. The cardinal motor signs are rest tremor, bradykinesia, and rigidity. Postural instability occurs later in the course of the illness. The onset is typically unilateral, and the disease progresses slowly to the contralateral side. Nonmotor symptoms may be present early on and sometimes precede the onset of motor symptoms by years. These include depression, anxiety, poor sense of smell, constipation, fatigue, REM behavior sleep disorder, urinary urgency, and pain in the shoulders and hips. Parkinson's symptoms are highly variable from person to person requiring an individualized therapeutic approach.

Essential/familial tremor: Essential tremor is a common movement disorder and is often misdiagnosed as Parkinson disease and visa versa (Ahlskog, 2010). About 2/3 of affected individuals have a positive family history. The tremor most often affects the hands, as well as the head and the voice. It is bilateral, present with posture and movement, and most noticeable when the subject writes or eats.

Other parkinsonian syndromes: This category includes several neurodegenerative disorders in which parkinsonism (tremor, rigidity, bradykinesia, and postural instability) is associated with other neurological signs such as severe autonomic dysfunction (multisystem atrophy), limitation of extraocular movements (progressive supranuclear palsy), or early dementia and hallucinations (dementia with Lewy bodies).

The diagnosis of these conditions is based on clinical examination, followup (as these other signs may not be present initially), and response to medication. In general, these syndromes are not associated with the typical PD rest tremor and do not respond well to levodopa/carbidopa preparations.

DIAGNOSTICS

The diagnosis of PD is based on the clinical history and examination performed by an experienced practitioner. If the findings fit the standard profile of PD, generally no other testing is necessary. However, additional diagnostic tests are performed when the presentation is not typical or when the diagnosis is not clear cut. An MRI of the brain may be performed to rule out normal pressure hydrocephalus or a multiinfarct state which would present primarily as a gait disorder. In this case an MRI performed 2 months ago showed no atrophy, no enlargement of ventricles, and a few small areas of increased T2 signal bilaterally in corona radiate.

A DAT (Dopamine Transporter) scan will soon be available to differentiate between essential tremor and PD in cases presenting with a complex tremor. Fluorodopa PET scanning is mostly used in research settings to follow progression of the disease. Genetic testing is not routinely done. Genetic forms of PD are rare, and the majority of individuals with PD do not carry one of the genes identified so far. Testing may be considered in the setting of a positive family history or in patients with young onset PD.

Another feature that helps support the diagnosis of PD is a clear improvement of symptoms with carbidopa/levodopa. In addition, occurrence of abnormal involuntary movements (dyskinesias) after being on this medication for several years may also be supportive of the diagnosis later in the course of the disease. Despite the numerous diagnostic limitations, studies have shown that a movement disorder specialist is 90% accurate when making a diagnosis of PD (Schrag, Ben-Shlomo, & Quinn, 2002).

CRITICAL THINKING

What is the most likely differential diagnosis and why?

What is the plan of treatment?

What are the interventions for evaluating and treating Mr. M's constipation?

RESOLUTION

What is the most likely differential diagnosis and why?
Mr. M most likely has idiopathic Parkinson disease. Upon examination, Mr. M presents with a tremor that occurs mostly at rest with slight action. He also has other motor signs typically seen in early Parkinson disease, including mild rigidity, decreased facial expression, slowness of movement, and difficulty with bimanual tasks. In addition, he has nonmotor symptoms supporting a diagnosis of idiopathic Parkinson disease including anosmia, fatigue, mild depression, constipation, and sleep disturbance. His REM behavior disorder preceded his motor signs by years.

A diagnosis of essential tremor is unlikely even with a positive family history of an aunt with head and voice tremors because of coexisting motor and nonmotor signs and symptoms. The red flags associated with other parkinsonian syndromes such as early cognitive changes, early severe autonomic dysfunction, gaze difficulty, upper motor neuron or cerebellar signs, apraxia, or early falls are not present.

What is the plan of treatment?
Because Parkinson disease is a chronic, progressive, complex disorder, it requires an interdisciplinary approach to treatment. These strategies may include both pharmacological management and nonpharmacological interventions particularly in the areas of education, psychosocial support, and rehabilitation.

In order to assess which of Mr. M's manifestations require (or will require) intervention and then to design an effective plan of care, the health care team needs to include both Mr. and Mrs. M and significant others in the decision-making process. The primary objective of medical management after establishment of a diagnosis is to identify targets of therapy (i.e., tremor, rigidity, and depression) and to select which agents will control the symptoms with the fewest side effects. Treatment goals also include slowing the disease progression, as well as reducing the risks of complications of therapy over time. Several classes of medications are available to decrease both motor and nonmotor symptoms. Levodopa remains the gold standard of therapy. Efforts are underway to identify an agent that will modify the disease process, but this has not yet been accomplished. (Dhah & Simuni, 2009).

Several orally administered drugs are approved as therapy in "early" Parkinson disease. These include rasagiline (an MAO inhibitor), ropinirole and pramipexole (dopamine agonists), levodopa/carbidopa, amantadine, and some anticholinergics. There is significant debate among prescribers on when to initiate therapy and which medications to use. Avoiding long-term motor and psychiatric complications drives this discussion. Age of diagnosis, disability including impairment of

ADL, cognitive status, employment status, lifestyle, and patient prefer-
ence are all taken into consideration.

In addition to managing the motor problems associated with PD,
more recently the nonmotor manifestations are being evaluated by
practitioners for proper and adequate treatment. The American
Academy of Neurology recognizes that without proper interventions,
these nonmotor issues can cause as much difficulty and distress as the
movement problems themselves and can greatly affect quality of life.
Some suggested interventions are isosmotic macrogol for constipation
and sildenafil citrate for erectile dysfunction. (Zesiewicz et al., 2010).

Mr. M and his family will benefit greatly from education early on
about the disease process and its uniqueness as a chronic condition. It
is important for them to understand that the presentation of Parkinson
disease, its progression, and its responsiveness to medications and
other therapies are all highly individual. Hence, significant time must
be spent on patient/family teaching. This particularly encompasses the
topics of proper timing of medications, as well as recognition of the
difference between PD symptoms and the possible adverse effects of
the drugs.

Currently, a variety of reliable community sources of education are
available for Mr. and Mrs. M and the family. For example, the American
Parkinson Disease Association, Inc. (APDA) sponsors numerous local
centers and chapters. At the grass-roots level, these are staffed by professionals and volunteers. Telephone help lines, free information about
the disease and daily living, newsletters, Web sites, resource libraries,
referrals, support groups, lectures, and community programs are provided. Patients need to be guided in use of these resources and given
the tools to discern between which are solid sources of information and
which are not (Diaz & Thomas, 2009).

Receiving the diagnosis of Parkinson disease is overwhelming
for most patients and families. Individuals who were involved in the
PD Quality of Life research study described their experience at the
time of diagnosis as "chaotic." They likened it to a bomb shattering
their lives and tearing apart their previous existence (Phillips, 2006).
There are those individuals who express some degree of relief that
their nagging and subtle symptoms now point to an actual disease
that has a name. However, the majority wrestle with fear and anxiety
about the uncertainties of their future. If and when Mr. M, his wife,
and/or family are ready in the disease coping process to reach out for
help, there are many organizations that sponsor Parkinson support
groups. The benefits of these self-help programs are invaluable in
providing camaraderie, education, and hope. Because of his anxiety,
he may also benefit from individualized care from a mental health
professional who offers counseling as well as coping and relaxation
techniques. A mild antidepressant and/or antianxiety medication
might be prescribed.

A referral to the rehabilitation team is essential in helping patients maintain and/or improve function and quality of life. Many studies support the efficacy of exercise in Parkinson disease (Goodwin, Richards, Taylor, Taylor, & Campbell, 2008). The physical therapist can assist in providing a comprehensive evaluation and initiating an effective plan of care. With regard to exercise, Mr. M may benefit from a program that includes stretching, aerobics, strengthening, and conditioning. Many individuals also benefit from other movement modalities, including yoga, tai chi, and dance.

In addition, a speech and language pathologist can assess communication patterns and provide treatment strategies to address Mr. M's soft, monotone voice. If hand tremor and rigidity interfere with his ADL, a referral to an occupational therapist may be warranted. Also, a meeting with a nutritionist to discuss dietary concerns and strategies to deal with constipation may be helpful.

What are the interventions for evaluating and treating Mr. M's constipation?

Many patients report a change in bowel habits often predating the diagnosis of PD (Zesiewicz et al., 2010). With Parkinson's, changes in the autonomic nervous system cause slowing of gastric and bowel motility. Medications used to treat PD can contribute to this problem as well. Decreased exercise and diminished fluid intake can also make the issue worse. This often results in varying degrees of constipation. In order to effectively manage Mr. M's constipation, it is best to use a stepwise approach as described in the Practice Guidelines of the American Rehabilitation Nurses (ARN) (Folden, 2002). Also, given Mr. M's family history as well as his personal history of precancerous polyp removal, periodic physical examinations as well as colorectal cancer screening are indicated.

Based on Mr. M's history, physical, and interview, he will start medication therapy with rasagiline 1 mg per day. This MAO inhibitor will provide mild symptomatic relief. He will also be referred to a physical therapist who specializes in movement disorders and is knowledgeable about resources including PD wellness and fitness programs. In addition, he will be provided with information to best manage his constipation beginning with lifestyle changes including increasing exercise levels and intake of dietary fiber and fluids.

Mr. M was given contact information for the coordinator of the local APDA Information and Referral Center. A call was made by the clinician to Mr. M's primary health care provider to discuss Mr. M's plan of care. Mr. M was encouraged to call the clinic with any questions or concerns. He will follow up with his neurological team in 1 month to be evaluated for his response to medication and therapies as well as his coping strategies. Through the delivery of this comprehensive and individualized patient/family plan of care by the health care team, Mr.

M will be in an optimal position to receive a "good start" in order to "live well" with his Parkinson disease.

REFERENCES

Ahlskog, J. E. (2010). Pearls: Parkinsonism. *Seminars in Neurology, 30*(1), 10–14.

Dhah, B., & Simuni, T. (2009). Key clinical trials in pharmacological treatment of early Parkinson's disease. *U.S. Neurology, 5*(1), 25–29.

Diaz, D. P., & Thomas, C. A. (2009). The American Parkinson Disease Association—Information and referral center coordinators—Making the connection. *U.S. Neurology, 5*(1), 22–24.

Folden, S. L. (2002). Practice guidelines for the management of constipation in adults. *Rehabilitation Nursing, 27*(5), 169–175.

Goodwin, V. A., Richards, S. H., Taylor, R. S., Taylor, A. H., & Campbell, J. L. (2008). The effectiveness of exercise intervention for people with Parkinson's disease: A systematic review. *Movement Disorders, 23*(5), 631–640.

Phillips, L. J. (2006). Dropping the bomb: The experience of being diagnosed with Parkinson's disease. *Geriatric Nursing, 27*(6), 362–369.

Schrag, A., Ben-Shlomo, Y., & Quinn, N. (2002). How valid is the clinical diagnosis of Parkinson's disease in the community? *Journal of Neurology, Neurosurgery, Psychiatry, 73,* 529–534.

Willis, A. W., Evanoff, B. A., Lian, M., Criswell, S. R., & Rachette, B. A. (2010). Geographic and ethnic variation in Parkinson's disease: A population based study of U.S. medicare beneficiaries. *Neuroepidemiology, 34*(3), 143–151.

Zesiewicz, T. A., Sullivan, K. L., Arnulf, I., Chaudhuri, K. R., Morgan, J. C., Gronseth, G. S., . . . Weiner, W. J. (2010). Practice parameter: Treatment of nonmotor symptoms of Parkinson disease. *Neurology, 74,* 924–993.

Case 2.13 Too Much to Manage

By Melanie J. Holland, BSN, MS

Mrs. D is a 72-year-old patient of an inner city primary care clinic, where she has been seen every 3–6 months for the last 8 years. She has a 10-year history of Type 2 diabetes. After her initial diagnosis, she was able to control her diabetes with diet and lifestyle changes. Seven years ago she was started on metformin, 1000 mg twice a day. She is also under treatment for hypertension and hypercholesterolemia. Mrs. D has had no surgeries or hospitalizations, other than for childbirth. She has yearly ophthalmologist appointments and sees a podiatrist regularly for foot care. Mrs. D lives in her own home with her spouse of 45 years. She has 3 grown children and 5 grandchildren, none of whom live locally. Mrs. D and her spouse own a 2-family home, where they rent the first floor and occupy the second and third floors. She has never used tobacco but admits to occasional social alcohol use. Mrs. D retired at age 60 after working as a secretary for 35 years. She and her spouse subsist on income from rent and social security, and each has a small pension. Mrs. D has been active in her church and senior citizens groups. She walks for 30 minutes 4–5 days a week in the mall with friends. Her spouse is reported to be in good health. Both parents are deceased; her mother was diabetic and died in her seventies from a heart problem. Her father died at the age of 61 from lung cancer. Mrs. D has one 65-year-old male sibling who is alive and well with "borderline diabetes" that he controls by diet. During this visit Mrs. D complains of feeling "tired and worn out". This fatigue has worsened over the past 2–3 months. She also complains of a numb, tingling sensation in both of her feet. These symptoms have caused a decline in her

Case Studies in Gerontological Nursing for the Advanced Practice Nurse, First Edition.
Edited by Meredith Wallace Kazer, Leslie Neal-Boylan.
© 2012 John Wiley & Sons, Inc. Published 2012 by John Wiley & Sons, Inc.

activity level and have made climbing the stairs in her home increasingly difficult. She denies shortness of breath, dyspnea, or chest discomfort. She has had no difficulty with constipation or diarrhea and has had no episodes of nausea or vomiting. She admits to occasional dizziness when arising from lying or sitting positions, which passes if she does not get up too quickly. Mrs. D admits to nocturia, which is not a new symptom for her. She denies urgency, pain, or burning with urination and incontinence, but admits to some recent weight gain, which she attributes to her decline in activity level. She tests her blood glucose levels sporadically and did not bring a blood glucose log or glucometer with her to the clinic.

Mrs. D states that her fasting blood glucose levels are "mostly less than 140 (mg/dl)." She states that she is careful about her diet with an occasional "cheat" on special occasions. She had dietary counseling by a registered dietician several years ago. Mrs. D continues to describe a tired and worn out feeling; she has checked finger stick glucose when the fatigue was overwhelming and found it to be within normal range. She is distressed by the numbness and tingling in her feet. These symptoms have caused a decrease in her normally busy social schedule and have limited participation with her mall-walking group. Her medications include the following: metformin, 1000 mg twice daily; atorvastatin calcium, 20 mg daily; hydrochlorothiazide, 25 mg daily; enteric-coated aspirin, 81 mg daily; and Tylenol, 650 mg as needed for headaches. She has no known allergies (NKA).

OBJECTIVE

Mrs. D appears clean, with clothing that is appropriate to the season. She is alert and oriented. Her height is 5 ft 2 inches. Her weight is 140 lb with a body mass index of 26. She is afebrile; pulse: 80 beats per minute; respirations: 18 per minute; O_2 Sat: 96%; BP lying: 130/80 mmHg: BP sitting: 128/78, BP standing: 126/75; random capillary blood glucose (3 hours post prandial): 148 mg/dl. She wears corrective lenses, pupils are equal, round, and reactive to light and accommodation (PERRLA), and her fundi are clear. Mrs. D's lungs are clear to auscultation. Her heart rate and rhythm are regular with no abnormal sounds. Her abdomen is soft and nontender; there are positive bowel sounds in all 4 quadrants. A vascular assessment indicates no carotid bruits, positive pedal pulses bilaterally and trace pedal edema, bilaterally. The neurologic assessment shows a steady, slightly broad-based gait with full range of motion of all extremities. There is a bilateral loss of vibratory sense and pinprick below the ankle. Monofilament is felt above the ankles bilaterally, and ankle reflexes are brisk bilaterally. Rectal exam shows no abnormalities and stool is guaiac negative.

ASSESSMENT

Type 2 diabetes: Mrs. D has come to the clinic for her annual exam, one year ago her hemoglobin A1c was 7.4%, and her new complaints may indicate a need for a change in her diabetic treatment plan. Poor glycemic control may be a contributing factor to her symptoms of weakness and fatigue.

Hypertension (HTN): A 40% increase in rate of HTN has been noted in the diabetic population, and it is one of the most prevalent cardiovascular diseases among older adults. Mrs. D is taking hydrochlorothiazide and lisinopril, an ACE inhibitor, for management of HTN and therapeutically for prevention of nephropathy. Some of Mrs. D's complaints may be related to adverse effects of these medications. Positional BP changes may be responsible for her complaints of dizziness; however, this was not evidenced by her positional BP assessment.

Hyperlipidemia: Mrs. D is taking a daily dose of atorvastatin (Lipitor). As she presents for her annual exam, it is reasonable to reassess cholesterol and triglyceride levels, risk factors that are modifiable by dietary changes and medication adjustment.

Neuropathy: The patient's symptoms of numbness and tingling in her lower extremities, as well as loss of vibratory sense and pinprick on exam may be attributed to neuropathy. Neuropathy is a chronic complication of diabetes mellitus that is experienced by nearly 60% of diabetics (American Diabetes Association, 2010a).

Fatigue: The patient's recent complaints of weakness and fatigue may have manifestations of different medical origins. Mrs. D is taking hydrochlorothiazide which can contribute to fluid and electrolyte imbalance. Subclinical hypothyroidism can cause fatigue, and it occurs in 15% of postmenopausal woman (Guessekloo et al., 2004). The prevalence of anemia increases with age. Adults 65 years and older are at particular risk for anemia; the estimated prevalence in this age group is 20% (Conrad, 2006). With regard to depression, according to Hu et al. (2007) and McKellar et al. (2004), older adults with diabetes have twice the likelihood of comorbid depression; it is present in about 20% of those patients.

DIAGNOSTICS

Mrs. D agreed to complete a self-administered depression assessment tool. There are several such assessment tools available. The patient completed the Geriatric Depression Scale (GDS) short form (www.

geriatricsatyourfingertips.org.). This is a 15-question, yes-or-no assessment of how the patient has been feeling over the past week. Her scored response was not suggestive of depression. A stool test for guaiac and urine for microalbumin are obtained. Mrs. agrees to return the following day for fasting lab work. Laboratory orders include hemoglobin A1c, complete metabolic panel, lipid panel, liver function tests, thyroid stimulating hormone (TSH), free T4, complete blood count (CBC), serum folate, ferritin, RBC folate, total iron binding capacity (TIBC), and a serum cobalamin. The stool test for guaiac was negative. Complete metabolic panel, lipid panel, liver function tests, TSH, T4, serum folate, ferritin, RBC folate, TIBC, and urine for microalbumin were all within normal limits. Hemoglobin A1c was 7.4% (normal range ≤7%); hemoglobin: 11.0 grams/dl (normal range 12–14 grams/dl); hematocrit: 33% (normal range 36%–43%); and serum cobalamin (B12): 106 pg/mL (normal range 190–914 pg/mL).

CRITICAL THINKING

What is the most likely etiology of the patient's symptoms of fatigue and bilateral foot numbness?

What should the target range of hemoglobin A1c be for an older adult patient with Type 2 diabetes mellitus?

Are there any guidelines that can be used in the assessment and care of older adults with diabetes? How were these guidelines used in Mrs. D's annual physical examination and plan of care?

RESOLUTION

What is the most likely etiology of this patient's symptoms of fatigue and bilateral foot numbness?
Decreased sensation and painful nerve damage in the feet is commonly experienced by older adults with diabetes. Minor foot problems can rapidly progress to major problems, including amputation (American Diabetes Association, 2010b). Physical assessment of the diabetic foot should include observation of dermatologic conditions, absence of hair, a decrease in turgor, dry or rough skin, fissures, calluses, hyperpigmentation, ulcers, and nail problems. Vascular status should be evaluated by checking peripheral pulses, temperature, edema, and color. Neurologic status should be evaluated by testing deep tendon reflexes, response to pain by touch, pin prick, and vibration sense (Jarvis, 2004). Mrs. D was seeing a podiatrist every 3 months for nail and foot care.

The lower extremity numbness, paresthesias, and impaired vibration sense experienced by Mrs. D can easily be attributed to diabetic neuropathy. However, review of her lab results revealed a serum cobalamin level of 106 pg/mL (normal range is 190–914 pg/mL). Vitamin B12 deficiency is common in older adults, but often goes unrecognized and untreated. It is often misdiagnosed in diabetics due to its resemblance to diabetic neuropathy (Pflipsen et al., 2009).

Vitamin B12 is a water soluble vitamin that is found in foods of animal origin (meat, fish, shellfish, and dairy products). The human body is able to store several years' worth of this vitamin. It is an essential micronutrient to the development of red blood cells. In synergy with folic acid, vitamin B12 plays a role essential to red blood cell DNA synthesis. Deficiencies of either of these micronutrients lead to macrocytosis and a decrease in bone marrow red blood cell production. Vitamin B12 is essential for nervous system function; deficiencies damage the myelin which can lead to mental status changes, neuropathies, balance problems and spinal cord disease and paralysis. B12 deficiency is also related to a higher risk of vascular events, such as stroke and myocardial infarction. Symptoms of deficiency are often vague and can appear as pallor, orthostatic hypotension, tachycardia, exertional dyspnea, weakness, dizziness, fatigue, syncope, and cognitive dysfunction (Spader, 2006).

During Mrs. D's visit, her dietary habits were reviewed. At a previous clinic encounter, she met with a dietician and has been adherent to the dietary and lifestyle advice she received. Dietary intake does not appear to be the source of her B12 deficiency as she eats a variety of foods, including those rich in vitamin B12. The most likely etiology of her deficiency is her long-term use of metformin. Research has shown that metformin can cause a dose-dependent vitamin B12 deficiency through interference with calcium metabolism, causing a decrease in absorption of this nutrient. Metformin induced malabsorption of vitamin B12 affects 30% of patients with diabetes. Each gram of metformin causes 3 times the risk of B12 deficiency. This risk is also increased by the length of time the patient is on metformin. The risk is doubled for those taking metformin for 3 years or more (Dharmarajan, Adiga, & Norkus, 2003). Mrs. D's reflexes remained intact, despite the sensory loss in her feet. This is a "red flag" that the etiology may be vitamin B12 deficiency (Bell, 2010). Once treatment is begun, reversal of signs and symptoms occurs rapidly, and a sense of well-being is reported within 24 hours. Neurologic changes present for less than 6 months can be reversed; however, neurologic reversal is not likely if these changes have been present for a protracted period (Fitzgerald, 2007).

Mrs. D had been taking metformin for 7 years. Clearly this puts her at risk for metformin-induced B12 deficiency. Treatment with intramuscular injection of B12, 1000 mcg, was initiated; and her fatigue and neurologic symptoms resolved. Metformin was not discontinued.

Mrs. D had achieved good glycemic control on this medication. It is a good choice for older adults because it does not produce hypoglycemia when it is used alone.

Treatment guidelines are evolving. Bell (2010) recommends that patients on long-term metformin have vitamin B12 levels monitored annually and feels that one annual 1000 mcg B12 injection may be enough for most patients as a preventive measure. Metformin use and advanced age are associated with vitamin B12 deficiency. Subtle vitamin B12 deficiency is clinically significant, and it should be detected early and aggressively treated to prevent irreversible complications.

What should the target range of hemoglobin A1c be for an older patient with diabetes mellitus?
Outcomes of the Diabetes Control and Complications Trial (DCCT) research indicate conclusively that prevention of microvascular and macrovascular complications for the diabetic patient is directly related to glycemic control. Although participants in the DCCT research were insulin-dependent diabetics, the findings have been generalized to diabetics who are not insulin dependent. A reduction in hemoglobin A1c has been associated with a 37% drop in microvascular complications and a 21% drop in other comorbid complications. The American Diabetes Association recommends a target hemoglobin A1c of 7% or less. Care of older adults with diabetes is often complicated by coexisting medical problems. It is important to consider comorbid factors when deciding if an older adult is a candidate for tight glycemic control. Many older adults with diabetes mellitus are active and have little comorbidity; others are frail with limited physical and cognitive function or underlying chronic conditions. The life expectancy and the quality of life need to be examined when setting goals for this heterogeneous population. A goal A1c of 7% or less is reasonable for healthy older adults with good functional status. The American Geriatrics Society (2007) recommends that hemoglobin A1c goals be individualized for older adults. A goal of 8% or less may be a more reasonable for frail older patients with life expectancy of 5 years and those whose risk of tight glycemic control outweigh the benefits.

Mrs. D's hemoglobin A1c is 7.4%, which is above the goal for an active older adult. The results were discussed with her, and she felt that her "numbers would drop" when she was able to resume activities. It was agreed not to make any medication adjustments at this time and reassess laboratory values after treatment for vitamin B12 deficiency and activity resumption.

Are there any guidelines that can be used in the assessment and care of older adults with diabetes? How were these guidelines used in Mrs. D's annual physical examination and plan of care?
The California Healthcare Foundation/American Geriatrics Society Panel on Improving Care of Elders with Diabetes (2003) developed

evidence-based guidelines individualized for persons aged 65 or older with diabetes mellitus and recommendations for screening and detection of geriatric syndromes.

The recommendations for the older adult with diabetes are as follows:

1. **Aspirin 81–325 mg daily,** unless contraindicated or unless the patient is on other anticoagulant therapy. The American Diabetes Association (2010a) says aspirin use has been shown to reduce cardiovascular mortality in older adults and persons with diabetes mellitus. Mrs. D is on a daily dose of aspirin, 81 mg.

2. **Smoking cessation:** Older adults who smoke should be offered counseling and pharmacological intervention to assist with smoking cessation. Smokers have a higher risk of mortality and premature death; substantial benefit may be obtained through smoking cessation. Mrs. D was not a smoker.

3. **Hypertension management:** The older adult with diabetes requires medical therapy when the BP is 140/80; lowering the BP to 130/80 produces further benefit. Older adults may have a decreased tolerance for BP reduction; therefore, hypertension should be treated gradually to avoid complications. Older adults with diabetes and hypertension should be offered dietary and behavioral interventions to lower blood pressure. Individuals whose hypertension is managed with the use of an ACE inhibitor or ARB should have renal function and serum potassium monitored within 1–2 weeks of therapy initiation, with each dose change, and annually. Those managed with thiazide or loop diuretics should have electrolytes checked within 1–2 weeks of therapy initiation, with each dose change, and annually.
   Mrs. D's hypertension was controlled with lisinopril (an ACE inhibitor) and hydrochlorothiazide (a thiazide diuretic). Renal function and electrolytes were assessed and found to be within normal limits.

4. **Glycemic control:** Individualized targets for older adults have been discussed here previously. In patients with stable hemoglobin A1c, annual measurement over several years may be appropriate. At a minimum, the older adult whose target is not being met should have hemoglobin A1c measured. Self-monitoring of blood glucose should be considered in older adults. Functional and cognitive abilities need to be taken into consideration when teaching the patient this skill. Older adults managed with insulin should have a schedule for self-monitoring of blood glucose based on the goals of care and their particular needs. Frail older adults are at an increased risk for hypoglycemia; self-monitoring reduces the risk of serious hypoglycemia and hypoglycemic coma. The American Diabetes Association and the National

Diabetes Education Program guidelines (2010) suggest that self-monitoring improves outcomes when combined with review of blood glucose levels and adjustment of therapy to attain target glycemic control. Frequency of self-monitoring should be adjusted with any changes in medication for glycemic control. Individuals with severe and frequent hypoglycemia require further evaluation. Referral to a diabetic educator or endocrinologist may be indicated, as well as more frequent contact between the patient and caregivers and the health care team. Older adults who are taking oral antidiabetic agents should not be prescribed chlorpropamide as it is associated with an increased risk for hypoglycemia (Shekelle et al., 2001). Aging is associated with a decline in renal function; older adults who take metformin should have regular monitoring of renal function. According to the American Association of Clinical Endocrinologists medical guidelines for patients with diabetes (2007), older adults with a creatinine clearance that indicates reduced renal function should not be prescribed metformin because of increased risk of lactic acidosis. Those on metformin should have serum creatinine measured at least annually; and, with any increase in dose, individuals 80 years of age or greater or those with decreased muscle mass should have a timed urine collection for creatinine clearance. Mrs. D's serum creatinine of 1.0 mg/dl was within normal limits.

5. *Dyslipidemia*: When overall health status permits, efforts should be made to correct lipid abnormalities. Low levels of high density lipoproteins (HDL), high levels of low density lipoproteins (LDL), and elevated triglycerides are more commonly found in the diabetic population and contribute to an increase in cardiovascular risk.

    According to guidelines offered by The American Association of Clinical Endocrinologists for Diagnosis and Treatment of Dyslipidemia (2000), older adults with diabetes whose LDL cholesterol levels are 100 mg/dl or less should have their lipid statuses checked every 2 years. Those with levels of 100–129 mg/dl should increase physical activity, should have dietary evaluations and education, and should have their lipid statuses checked annually. In older diabetic adults with LDL levels of 130 mg/dl or greater, pharmacologic therapy is required in addition to lifestyle modifications. The American Diabetes Association (2010b) recommends HDL greater than 40 mg/dl and triglycerides lower than 150 mg/dl. Older adults with normal or nearly normal LDL and low HDL or elevated triglycerides should be offered a fibrate in addition to nutritional therapy. Mrs. D's lipid panel results were LDL (calculated) 84 mg/dl, HDL 44 mg/dl, and triglycerides of 148 mg/dl, necessitating no change in her current dietary habits or medication.

Older adults with diabetes who have been started on a statin or niacin or those who have had a dose change should have an alanine aminotransferase level checked within 12 weeks. Those taking a fibrate should have annual liver enzyme evaluation.

Mrs. D is currently prescribed a statin (atorvastatin calcium, 20 mg, Lipitor). During her annual examination, a lipid panel and liver function tests were drawn and found to be within normal limits; no change was needed in treatment.

6. **Eye care:** Older adults newly diagnosed with diabetes should have a dilated eye exam by a specialist with funduscopy training. Incidence of retinopathy is associated with, among other things, the level of glycemic control over the prior 6 years and higher blood pressure. The progression of retinopathy is associated with older age, male sex, and hyperglycemia. Older adults with diabetes and at high risk for eye disease should have an eye exam by a specialist at least annually. Mrs. D has an ophthalmologist whom she sees annually.

7. **Foot care:** Older adults with diabetes should have annual foot examinations to note any bony deformities, check skin integrity, check for sensory loss, and check for perfusion. Regular foot exams permit identification of foot lesions and diabetic neuropathy, which could progress to ulcers and amputation. The American Diabetes Association (2010b) recommendations specify that foot examination be done at all nonurgent outpatient visits. Mrs. D goes routinely to a podiatrist for nail cutting. Foot examination at her annual visit did reveal sensory loss, initially attributed to the development of neuropathy, but later discovered to be caused by vitamin B12 deficiency. Her sensory loss and related symptoms resolved after treatment with vitamin B12.

8. **Nephropathy:** The American Diabetes Association (2010a) recommends a urine test for microalbuminuria be performed at diagnosis of Type 2 diabetes and annually. Presence of protein in the urine requires interventions to prevent a decrease in renal function. As renal function decreases, blood urea nitrogen and creatinine will increase. Interventions include tighter glycemic control, a dietary evaluation for decrease in protein and adding an ACE inhibitor. Mrs. D's urine was negative for protein; no changes in treatment were indicated.

9. **Diabetes education:** The National Diabetes Education Prog Guiding Principles for Diabetic Care (http://ndep.r media/GuidPrin_HC_Eng.pdf) provides specific gu well as educational materials and resources for d tion. Multidisciplinary interventions that prov blood glucose monitoring, medication use hypo- and hyperglycemia can improv

should be provided to older adults with diabetes, family members, and caregivers. All involved in care should be given guidelines as to when a health care provider should be contacted. Patients should be evaluated for functional and cognitive impairments that may impede their ability to learn or increase physical activity. Physical activity of older adults should be routinely evaluated. The benefits of regular exercise should be reinforced, and strategies for becoming more active should be made available. Referral to a registered dietician for assessment of dietary and nutritional status is recommended; culturally sensitive dietary plans are important considerations. Diet and goals should be reviewed at each nonurgent medical visit. Nutritional knowledge and an increase in physical activity can reduce weight and enhance glycemic, lipid, and blood pressure control. Knowledge regarding medication is of great importance to the patient, as well as any caregiver; they should be made aware of the purpose of the drug, how it is to be taken, its side effects, and any adverse effects. Education regarding foot care, risk of ulcers, and other complications should be provided. Many older adults, because of visual, physical, or cognitive impairment do not have the ability to conduct proper foot care and surveillance. In these cases, multidisciplinary intervention is important. Educational materials provided to the older adult should take into consideration health literacy, readability (large fonts), and language. There are many diabetes curricula appropriate to the needs of individuals with diabetes mellitus. Two culturally and linguistically diverse sources are www.niddk.nih.gov/health/diabetes/pubs/type1-20 and http://nedp.nih.gov/materials/2001campaign/spanishbrochure.pdf. Annual diabetes self-management training is a covered benefit under Medicare Part B (http//www.medicare.gov). Mrs. D demonstrates a solid understanding of diabetes and its treatment, is careful with her diet, and walks for exercise. She is a regular attendee of diabetic education seminars offered by the medical center.

10. **Depression:** Older adults with diabetes should be assessed for symptoms of depression at their initial evaluation and with any unexplained decline in status. Depression is common in older adults with diabetes, and it can impair self-management. The Geriatric Depression Scale is a useful tool which is available in several languages (http://www.stanford.edu/~yesavage/GDS.html). Patients who present with new onset or recurrent depression should be referred within 2 weeks or immediately if they are a danger to themselves. Patients who have received therapy should be evaluated within 6 weeks of initiation (Shekelle et al., 2001). Mrs. D was evaluated for depression because of her report

of fatigue and decrease in activity; results were previously discussed here.

11. **Polypharmacy:** Older adults with diabetes should maintain a current medication list of prescription and non-prescription drugs. In this population the risk for drug side effects and drug-to-drug interaction is high. Medication reconciliation should be done at every visit; and adverse reactions to medications should be considered as a sources for those who present with new onset of depression, cognitive impairment, or falls.

12. **Cognitive impairment:** Type 2 diabetes mellitus in older adults has been associated with a decrease in cognitive function, manifested as decrease in memory, learning, and verbal skills (Gregg et al., 2000). A standardized screening tool should be used during the initial evaluation and with any decline in clinical status. The Mini-Mental State Examination (MMSE) is a tool often used to detect impairment in older adults with diabetes (Folstein, Folstein, & McHugh, 1975). As noted previously, the medication list should undergo review. If there is evidence of cognitive impairment and delirium has been excluded, the American Academy of Neurology guidelines recommend screening for depression, vitamin B12 deficiency, hypothyroidism and structural neuroimaging to identify lesions (Knopman, DeKosky, & Cummings, 2001).

13. **Urinary incontinence:** During health care screening of older adults with diabetes, symptoms of incontinence should be evaluated. Urinary incontinence is commonly under-reported. Risk factors in diabetic older adults include polyuria, autonomic insufficiency, urinary tract infection, overflow secondary to neurogenic bladder, *candida* vaginitis, and fecal impaction due to autonomic insufficiency (Dugan et al., 2000). If there is evidence of urinary incontinence, then treatable causes should be evaluated.

14. **Falls:** Falls often go unreported; older adults with diabetes should be questioned about falls. Falls may be associated with reversible factors or may be associated with functional decline. The American Geriatric Society Guideline for the Prevention of Falls in Older Persons (2010) provides recommendations on this issue.

15. **Pain:** Older adults with diabetes are at risk for neuropathic pain and are often undertreated (Greene, Stevens, & Feldman, 1999). Many in this population are reluctant to report pain, therefore a targeted history and physical examination should be used to screen for pain; and appropriate therapy should be offered. The American Geriatrics Society has recommended Guidelines for the Management of Persistent Pain in Older Adults (http://www.americangeriatrics.org/health_care_professionals/education/persistent_pain_cme_program/).

REFERENCES

American Association of Clinical Endocrinologists (2000). AACE medical guidelines for clinical practice for the diagnosis and treatment of dyslipidemia and prevention of atherogenisis. *Endocrine Practice, 6,* 162–213.

American Association of Clinical Endocrinologists (2007). AACE medical guidelines for the management of diabetes mellitus: The AACE system of intensive diabetes self-management. *Endocrine Practice, 13*(Suppl. 1), 1–68.

American Diabetes Association (2010a). Diagnosis and classification of diabetes mellitus. *Diabetes Care, 33*(Suppl. 1), S62–S69.

American Diabetes Association (2010b). Standards of medical care in diabetes. *Diabetes Care, 33*(Suppl. 1), S11–S61.

American Geriatric Society, British Geriatric Society, & American Academy of Orthopedic Surgeons Panel on Falls Prevention (2010). Guideline for prevention of falls in older persons. *Journal of the American Geriatrics Society, 49,* 664–672.

Bell, S. H. (2010). Vitamin B12 deficiency: A chronic complication of metformin therapy that can cause irreversible neuronal damage. *Southern Medical Journal, Retrieved* February 2, 2010, from doi:10.1097.SMJ.0b013e3181ce0e4d

California Healthcare Foundation/American Geriatrics Society Panel in Improving Care for Elders with Diabetes. (2003).Guidelines for improving the care of the older person with diabetes mellitus, Article first published online: 29 May, 2003, *Journal of the American Geriatrics Society, 51*(5s), 265–280. DOI: 10.1046/j.1532-5415.51.5s.1.x

Conrad, M. (2006). Anemia E Medicine. Retrieved from http://www.emedicine.com/med/topics132,1188.htm.

Dharmarajan, T. S., Adiga, G. U., & Norkus, E. P. (2003). Vitamin B12 deficiency: Recognizing subtle symptoms in older adults. *Geriatrics, 58*(3), 30–38.

Dugan, E., Cohen, S. J., Bland, D. R., Preisser, J. S., Davis, C. C., Suggs, P. K., & McGann, P. (2000). The association of depressive symptoms and urinary incontinence among older adults. *Journal of the American Geriatrics Society, 48*(4), 413–416.

Fitzgerald, M. (2007). Drug induced vitamin B12 deficiency. *The Nurse Practitioner Journal, 32*(9), 1–6.

Folstein, M. F., Folstein, S. E., & McHugh, P. R. (1975). "Mini-Mental State". A practical method for grading the cognitive state of patients for the clinician. *Journal of Psychiatric Research, 12,* 189–198.

Greene, D. A., Stevens, M. J., & Feldman, E. L. (1999). Diabetic neuropathy. Scope of the syndrome. *The American Journal of Medicine, 107,* 2S–8S.

Gregg, E. W., Yaffe, K., Cauley, J. A., Rolka, D. B., Blackwell, T. L., Venkat Narayan, K. M., & Cummings, S. R. for the Study of Osteoporotic Fractures Research Group. (2000). Is diabetes associated with cognitive impairment and cognitive decline among older women? Study of osteoporotic fractures research group. *Archives of Internal Medicine, 160,* 174–180.

Guessekloo, J., van Exel, E., de Craen, A. J. M., Meinders, A. E., Frölich, M., & Westendorp, R. G. J. et al. (2004). Thyroid status, disability and cognitive function, and survival in old age. *The Journal of the American Medical Association, 292*(21), 2591–2613.

Hu, J., Amoako, E. P., Grubert, K., & Rossen, E. K. (2007). The Relationships among Health Functioning Indicators and Depression in Older Adults with Diabetes. *Issues in Mental Health Nursing*, *28*, 133–150.

Jarvis, C. (2004). *Physical examination and health assessment*. St. Louis, MO: Elsevier.

Knopman, D. S., DeKosky, S. T., & Cummings, J. L. (2001). Practice parameter: Diagnosis of dementia. Report of the quality standards subcommittee of the American academy of neurology. *Neurology*, *56*, 1143–1153.

McKellar, J. D., Humphreys, K. & Plette, J. (2004). Depression increases diabetes symptoms by complicating patients' self-care adherence. *The Diabetes Educator*, *30*, 485–492.

National Diabetes Education Program (2010). The power to control diabetes is in your hands [on-line]. Retrieved June, 2010, from http://ndep.nih.gov/materials/2001campaign/spanishbrochure.pdf.

The National Diabetes Education Program. Guiding Principles for Diabetic Care. http://ndep.nih.gov/media/GuidPrin_HC_Eng.pdf

Nelson, J. M., Dufraux, K., Cook, P. F. (2007). The relationship between glycemic control and falls in older adults. *J Am Geriatr Soc*, *55*(12), 2041–2044.

Pflipsen, M. C., Oh, R. C., Saguil, A., Seehusen, D. A., Seaquist, D., & Topolski, R. (2009). The prevalence of vitamin B12 deficiency in patients with Type 2 diabetes: A cross-sectional study. *The Journal of the American Board of Family Medicine*, *22*(5), 528–534.

Pharmacologic Management of Persistent Pain in Older http://www.americangeriatrics.org/health_care_professionals/education/persistent_pain_cme_program/

Pharmacologic Management of Persistent Pain in Older Persons. http://www.americangeriatrics.org/health_care_professionals/education/persistent_pain_cme_program/

Shekelle, P. G., MacLean, C. H., Morton, S. C., & Wenger, N. S. et al. (2001). ACOVE quality indicators. *Annals of Internal Medicine*, *135*, 653–667.

Spader, C. (2006). Valuable vitamin essential to good health. *Nursing Spectrum*. pp. 1–6. Retrieved from http://community.nursing spectrum.com/MagazineArticles/articles.ctm?AID=21816.

Stabler, S. P. (1995). Screening the older population for colbalamin (vitamin B12) deficiency. *Journal of the American Geriatrics Society*, *43*(11), 1290–1297.

Case 2.14 Them Bones, Them Bones

By Ivy M. Alexander, PhD, APRN, ANP-BC, FAAN

Ms. O, a 63-year-old female, presents with upper mid-back pain that began after lifting her 3-year-old granddaughter 3 days ago. The pain began right after lifting her 25-pound granddaughter up over her head and placing her into the high chair. Ms. O has done this many times without any pain in the past. The pain is sharp, originates in her back, and radiates into her lower chest and around to her abdomen. Ms. O's pain is constant and heavy but does wane with rest (5–7 on a 1–10 scale). It is unaffected by nonsteroidal antiinflammatory drugs (NSAIDs), acetaminophen, or topical rub, each of which she tried once. She feels slightly short of breath, which she describes as "hard to take a full breath in because it hurts." She found it difficult to put on a turtleneck shirt this morning.

She denies prior chest pain, palpitations, DOE, peripheral edema, or a history of blood clots. Ms. O's overall health is "good." She is enjoying retirement and caring for her granddaughter. She reports that she has good energy, that she usually sleeps well, but that she has not slept well since this pain began. Ms. O reports no specific systemic complains. She denies general fatigue and says she did not have terrible hot flashes like her sister did with the change of life. She feels well.

She has well-controlled hypertension and rheumatoid arthritis (RA) as well as fall seasonal allergies. She previously used oral steroids for her RA for about 6 years. She now takes a single DMARD. She has

Case Studies in Gerontological Nursing for the Advanced Practice Nurse, First Edition.
Edited by Meredith Wallace Kazer, Leslie Neal-Boylan.
© 2012 John Wiley & Sons, Inc. Published 2012 by John Wiley & Sons, Inc.

some morning stiffness that is relieved with a warm shower and movement. She gets regular exercise and is quite active in caring for her granddaughter with daily walks, often pushing the stroller, getting her in and out of the high chair, and playing with her on the swings at the park. Ms. O lives with her husband of 35 years and the family cat in a private home that they own. She is a retired elementary schoolteacher and currently provides daycare for her granddaughter while her daughter works. Ms. O's mother died from breast cancer. Her father had DMT2, HTN, and some dementia. Her sister is alive and well. Her medications include over-the-counter antihistamines for allergies, as needed; nasal spray for allergies, as needed; multivitamin daily; calcium (when she remembers); HCTZ, 25 mg daily; glucosamine sulfate with chondroitin, 1500 mg in a divided dose daily; omega-3 supplements (fish oil), 2 g daily; and leflunomide, 10 mg daily. She has no known drug or food allergies (NKDA, NKFA).

OBJECTIVE

Ms. O's vital signs are as follows: BP: 130/78 (L) sitting; P: 74; RR: 10; weight: 130 lb; height: 5 ft 5 inches; and BMI: 21.6. She appears uncomfortable with slow careful movements and limited use of upper extremities, is neatly dressed with appropriate affect. Her neck is supple, without lymphadenopathy. Her thyroid is nontender without palpable masses or enlargement. The carotids are without bruits. She has limited range of motion (ROM) in her neck, especially chin to chest, due to pain. Her lungs are clear to auscultation; however, she is unwilling to take a full inhalation due to pain. Her heart rate is regular with normal S1 and S2 and without murmurs, rubs, or gallops. There is pain with manual compression to anterior and posterior chest wall. Her breasts are without masses, skin changes, or discharge bilaterally. The abdomen is soft, nondistended and nontender with positive bowel sounds x4. She has good ROM in the spine at the waist and for twisting with the lower spine. Her thoracic spine has limited ROM due to pain, with tenderness over T7 and T8. Her extremities are without edema or clubbing; +2 pulses bilaterally. There is limited upper spine mobility; and the upper extremities are limited for full overhead movements. There is slight tenderness and swelling over MCP and PIP joints of both hands. Her joints are without crepitus. There are no digital ulnar deviations, swan neck, boutonniere deformities, or nodules. Her neurological exam reveals cranial nerves II–XII are grossly intact; she has 5/5 motor strength, but limited effort of bilateral upper extremities. Her gait and Romberg are normal.

ASSESSMENT

Vertebral compression fractures: Ms. O's acute upper mid-back pain after lifting her 3-year-old granddaughter may be caused by vertebral compression fractures (VCFs) related to osteoporosis (OP). This is a common presentation of OP as bone loss is painless until a fracture occurs (National Osteoporosis Foundation [NOF], 2010; North American Menopause Society [NAMS], 2010).

Back strain or costochondritis: Ms. O's acute onset of pain with activity is suggestive of back strain. Costochondritis is more often associated with overuse and develops gradually. However, as Ms. O does have a high amount of upper body activity and lifting when caring for her granddaughter, it is one of the differentials that needs to be considered.

DIAGNOSTICS

Diagnostic testing is needed to diagnose both OP and VCFs. A complete history and physical examination is needed in addition to selected laboratory testing to identify secondary OP and to provide information to support selecting various pharmacotherapeutic agents.

CBC, ESR, CRP: Ms. O's CBC showed slight anemia of chronic disease, a common finding with RA. A CBC is also useful to rule out secondary causes of OP and to determine overall health status (Alexander & Lewiecki, 2008). ESR and CRP are nonspecific markers for inflammation and are indicative of disease activity with RA; however, they are not highly specific and will be elevated with other inflammatory processes as well (Colglazier & Sutej, 2005). Ms. O's levels were both slightly elevated, as is common with RA.

LFTs, BUN/creatinine, eGFR, and phosphorous: These tests are often measured to assess general health and are appropriate tests for Ms. O to evaluate for secondary causes of OP. Knowing her liver and kidney function status may be important when determining whether to use pharmacotherapeutics to manage her OP and VCFs. Ms. O's levels were normal.

TSH: Ms. O's TSH is evaluated for secondary causes and is in the normal range.

Fasting serum calcium, 24-hour urinary calcium, and serum 25-OH-D (vitamin D): These tests are done to identify calcium and vitamin D levels and are important when OP is suspected as low calcium levels may suggest underlying pathology or secondary OP and must be rectified prior to starting any antiresorptive medication (Alexander & Lewiecki, 2008). Similarly, low vitamin D levels (below 30 ng/ml) need to be corrected (NOF, 2010). Adequate vitamin D is needed both for normal bone resorption processes and for calcium absorption. Ms. O's laboratory testing revealed normal fasting serum calcium, 24-hour urinary calcium, and a serum 25-OH-D of 20 ng/ml, suggesting nutritional insufficiency.

Spine films: Spine films can be used to diagnose VCFs. OP can be seen on x-ray examination if there is >30% bone loss. A dual-energy x-ray absorptiometry (DXA) is then ordered. Her spine films revealed stage 1 VCFs at T7 and T8 (20%–25% deformity).

DXA with FRAX®: DXA is considered the gold standard for diagnosis of OP (NAMS, 2010; NOF, 2010; U.S. Department of Health and Human Services [DHHS], 2004). Results are provided that include both T-scores and Z-scores; and since early 2009 most reports also include the 10-year risk probability for hip and major OP fractures identified by the FRAX® algorithm. T-scores identify how the patient's bone density compares to that of a normal young adult of the same gender. The Z-score identifies how the patient's bone density compares to others of the same age and gender. Both T-scores and Z-scores are reported as standard deviations, with 0 meaning it is an exact match and normal extending from −1 to +1. Low bone mass, or osteopenia, is identified with T-scores of below −1 to −2.5, and osteoporosis is identified with T-scores below −2.5. Severe OP is identified with T-scores below −2.5 in the presence of fragility or low-trauma fracture (DHHS, 2004; World Health Organization [WHO], 1994). FRAX® is an individualized algorithm that identifies the probability of fracture over the next 10 years based on the patient's height, weight, and bone density raw score, as well as the presence or absence of 11 additional risk factors such as smoking, history of RA, steroid use, and parental history of hip fracture (World Health Organization [WHO], 2007a, 2007b). FRAX® is used to assist with determining whether a specific patient would benefit from the use of pharmacotherapeutics to prevent fracture and thus is used for patients who have not previously been treated with medication. Cutoffs based on U.S. population analyses suggest that it is cost effective to treat those with a 10-year risk of hip fracture of above 3% or a 10-year risk of major OP fracture of above 20% (Dawson-Hughes et al., 2008; NOF, 2010; Tosteson et al., 2008). OP is not diagnosed based solely on DXA results. All patients, even those with a T-score of below −2.5, require a detailed history and physical exam with selected laboratory tests to evaluate for secondary causes of OP to treat and determine safety in using possible pharmacotherapeutic agents (NOF, 2010). Ms. O's DXA revealed a T-score of −2.6 at her lower spine, −2.0 at her hip, and −1.7 for her total hip. Her FRAX® 10-year fracture risk at the hip was 3.0% and for any major OP fracture was 22%.

CRITICAL THINKING

What is the most likely differential diagnosis and why?

What is the plan of treatment?

What is the plan for follow-up care?

Does Ms. O's psychosocial history affect her management plan?

What if Ms. O also had diabetes or hyperlipidemia or were male?

Are there any standardized guidelines that the clinician will use to assess or treat Ms. O?

RESOLUTION

What is the most likely differential diagnosis and why?
VCFs due to OP are the most likely diagnoses for Ms. O. She has a common presentation of VCF with acute onset of pain following minor trauma or daily activities. Her physical examination findings are consistent with thoracic VCFs, and VCFs were identified on spine films. Her DXA results support a diagnosis of OP.

VCFs commonly occur with usual activities when the spine is hyperextended or flexed, which crushes the anterior or posterior edges of the weakened vertebral bones and changes them into a wedge rather than square shape leading to the classic forward bent posture seen in patients with kyphosis of the spine. VCFs may present with height loss or kyphosis as about two-thirds of these patients do not experience significant pain. OP often presents with a fracture because there are no symptoms associated with bone loss until an actual fracture occurs, thus early screening is advocated (NAMS, 2010; NOF, 2010; DHHS, 2004).

Ms. O is at risk for secondary OP because she has a high-risk disease (RA) and has needed to take high-risk medications (oral steroids) for many years in the past (NAMS, 2010; NOF, 2010; DHHS, 2004). The rate of bone loss also normally increases significantly in women during the early postmenopausal years (bone loss of up to 5% per year can occur); thus it is likely that Ms. O's OP is partly due to her postmenopausal status and partly due to her RA and prior steroid use.

Musculoskeletal causes of back or chest wall pain that are unrelated to OP must also be considered. Such differentials would include back strain and costochondritis. Her physical examination findings of pain upon movement and tenderness with chest wall compression support each of these differentials. Back strain is the more likely of these differentials because of the history of physical activity that precipitated the onset of Ms. O's pain. Costochondritis is less likely as it tends to develop over time with overuse and inflammation as opposed to acute injury. However, neither of these differentials is supported by the physical examination finding of vertebral tenderness; this finding is more indicative of VCF.

What is the plan of treatment?

Ms. O and her clinician need to address both of her diagnoses. She has documented VCFs identified by x-ray as well as OP identified by DXA. The plan for her pain management for the VCFs will be of a short-term nature, while OP management will be long term.

Self-Management Lifestyle Changes—Ms. O needs to avoid activities that increase her pain initially. A return to activity as soon as possible is important, though it may take 3 months before she is fully healed. It will be important for her to see the physical therapist for pain modalities early on, as well as for strengthening exercises for her upper mid-back and body mechanics retraining later to prevent further injury.

For OP management she will need to adjust her activity and intake of vitamin D and calcium. Ms. O's activity needs to increase and include both resistance and weight bearing activities daily. These activities will increase osteoblast activity and thus strengthen bone. Ms. O also needs a daily intake of 800 to 1000 IU vitamin D and 1200 mg calcium (NAMS, 2010; NOF, 2010; DHHS, 2004). This level of vitamin D intake is enough to rectify her vitamin D deficiency within about a 3-month period (Dawson-Hughes, 2010). Since most people cannot achieve the recommended daily intake of vitamin D and calcium through diet alone, it is likely that Ms. O will require ongoing calcium and vitamin D supplementation. Many different supplement brands and types are available. Calcium citrate is less constipating than calcium carbonate and can be taken with or without meals. Calcium carbonate must be taken with meals, as an acid environment is needed for it to be absorbed. Calcium carbonate would not be an appropriate option for Ms. O if she used antacids of any kind. Both calcium carbonate and calcium citrate are also available as a combination tablet with vitamin D.

Ms. O needs to prevent falls that could cause fracture (NAMS, 2010; NOF, 2010; DHHS, 2004). Ms. O will need to remove any loose rugs or cords that she might fall or trip on, ensure adequate lighting in case she needs to get up at night, ensure removal of snow, ice, or wet leaves, and keep uncluttered walkways around her home to reduce the risk of a fall.

Light massage therapy or acupuncture may provide some pain relief. While neither of these therapies will necessarily increase bone strength, each may help to reduce her pain while the VCFs are healing and continuing with these therapies may increase her tolerance for exercise later as well. Other relaxation therapies that may be beneficial include yoga, aromatherapy, and meditation. Yoga should not be initiated until the VCFs have healed and will need to be modified to avoid any forward bending (flexion) of the spine.

Soy products do not appear to offer consistent benefit for bone health (Liu et al., 2009). While most soy products are available for purchase over-the-counter (OTC) Fosteum Rx® is available via prescription (see Table 2.14.1). Herbs that are marketed to increase bone strength are usually those that are thought to increase estrogen levels. These include herbs such as black cohosh, ginseng, cypress, sage, and licorice (Decker & Meyers, 2001).

Pharmacotherapeutic agents for both Ms. O's VCF pain and management of her OP are reasonable. Her pain may be adequately managed by consistent use of acetaminophen, dosed at 1000 mg orally every 6 hours, or in combination with an NSAID. If an NSAID is used, she must take it with food to reduce the likelihood of developing gastrointestinal irritation, especially if she is prescribed a bisphosphonate for her OP. If acetaminophen or acetaminophen combined with NSAIDs is ineffective, then acetaminophen combined with a narcotic analgesic, such as acetaminophen with codeine, may be tried. A return to usual activity as soon as possible is the goal.

Ms. O meets criteria established by both the NOF and NAMS for pharmacotherapeutic treatment of her OP. Both organizations recommend initiating medication therapy in individuals with documented OP, which Ms. O has. In fact, Ms. O also meets the diagnostic criteria established by the WHO for severe OP, because she has a spine T-score of −2.5 on DXA plus fragility fractures (WHO, 1994). Even if Ms. O's DXA scores had not indicated OP and she did not have VCFs, her clinician would still consider pharmacotherapeutic therapy for her as her FRAX® 10-year risk for major OP fracture was above the cut-off of 20%. This suggests that it would be cost effective to treat Ms. O with medications for OP, based on U.S. population calculations (Dawson-Hughes et al., 2008; Tosteson et al., 2008).

The goal of pharmacotherapy for OP is to reduce fracture incidence and its related sequelae. Several different effective medications for OP management are currently available in the U.S. and approved by the FDA, including bisphosphonates, calcitonin, estrogen agonist/antagonists, hormone therapy (estrogen or estrogen-progestin therapy), a RANK-ligand inhibitor, and parathyroid hormone (see Table 2.14.1). These medications can be categorized into the following two groups: antiresorptive or anabolic. Antiresorptive agents increase bone

TABLE 2.14.1. Prescription Agents for Osteoporosis Management.

Medication	FDA Approved Use and Dose	Considerations
Alendronate (Fosamax)	PMO prevention—5 mg by mouth daily or 35 mg by mouth weekly SIO—5 mg by mouth daily or 10 mg by mouth daily if postmenopausal and off estrogen PMO and MOP treatment—10 mg by mouth daily or 70 mg by mouth weekly	Take oral doses first thing in the morning on an empty stomach with 8-oz glass of plain water. Remain upright and take no other food or drink for 30–60 minutes. Take oral doses 2 hours before antacids/calcium. Caution with oral forms if upper gastrointestinal disease, clinical association with dysphagia, esophagitis, or ulceration. • Beneficial effects may last for years after medication is discontinued. • Fosamax plus D—combined bisphosphonate and vitamin D_3 in a single tablet taken weekly
alendronate + cholecalciferol (Fosamax Plus D)	PMO and MOP treatment—70 mg plus 2800 IU vit D_3 or 70 mg plus 5600 IU vit D_3 in combined tablet by mouth weekly	• Actonel with Calcium—blister pack for 28-day use, provides Actonel in 1 tablet taken on day 1 and calcium in the other 6 tablets taken on days 2–7; repeated sequence over 4 weeks. • IV ibandronate and zoledronic acid are not associated with gastrointestinal side effects or limitations on timing dose around food, water, calcium, or medication intake.
risedronate (Actonel)	PMO prevention or treatment—5 mg by mouth daily, 35 mg by mouth weekly, 75 mg by mouth 2 consecutive days each month, or 150 mg by mouth monthly SIO—5 mg by mouth daily MOP—35 mg by mouth weekly	• Hypocalcemia must be corrected prior to use. • Osteonecrosis of the jaw (ONJ), exposed bone in the mouth for >3 ms with nonhealing lesions, has been associated with high dose IV bisphosphonate therapy among individuals with cancer-related bone disease (2%–10%); cancer patients with dental problems, gum injury, oral bony abnormalities, or taking medications that interfere with healing; and, in very rare cases, healthy individuals with similar risk factors who are on bisphosphonates for osteoporosis (incidence estimated at 0.001%–0.002%). Consider stopping therapy for 2–3 months if invasive dental procedures are required and resume after healing is complete. Encourage usual dental care (e.g., cleaning, fillings, and crown work).
Risedronate plus; calcium carbonate (Actonel with Calcium)	PMO prevention or treatment—35 mg risedronate on day 1; 1250 mg (500 mg elemental) calcium carbonate on days 2–7	

ibandronate (Boniva)	PMO prevention or treatment—2.5 mg by mouth daily or 150 mg by mouth monthly PMO treatment—3 mg IV every 3 months	• Subtrochanteric fracture is an extremely rare event that has been associated with bisphosphonate use. Advise patients that the risk of this extremely rare event is far less than the risks associated with hip fracture, and encourage them to take their prescribed bisphosphonates consistently.
zoledronic acid (Reclast)	PMO prevention—5 mg IV every 2 years PMO, MOP, and SIO treatment—5 mg IV yearly	
calcitonin (Miacalcin, Fortical NS)	PMO treatment—200 IU intranasal spray daily (Miacalcin or Fortical NS) or 100 IU subcutaneously 3 times each week (Miacalcin)	• Usually administered as nasal spray • Alternate nares for nasal spray • Most often used for analgesic effect on acute pain due to vertebral compression fractures
denosumab (Prolia)	PMO treatment—60 mg injection (subcutaneous) every 6 months	• Denosumab is for those with multiple risks for fracture, those with osteoporotic fracture history, and those who have not responded to other treatments. • Requires administration by a health care professional • Individuals with latex allergy should not handle grey needle cover. • Hypocalcemia must be corrected prior to use. • Use may be associated with ONJ, over suppression of bone turnover, skin infections, and dermatologic conditions.

TABLE 2.14.1. (Continued)

Medication	FDA Approved Use and Dose	Considerations
estrogen (e.g., Alora, Climara, Estrace, Estraderm, Menest, Menostar, Premarin, Vivelle, Vivelle Dot)	PMO prevention—doses and routes vary.	• Also effective in alleviating most symptoms related to menopause (even Menostar, which has a very low dose and was shown to effectively reduce severity and frequency of hot flashes in a 2007 study) • Available in several forms (e.g., pills, patch, ring, cream, and gel)
estrogen-progestin combination products (e.g., Activella, Climara Pro, Femhrt, Prefest, Premphase, Prempro)	PMO prevention—doses and routes vary.	• Use for 2–3 years immediately following menopause may provide some beneficial effects on bone health after discontinuation.
genistein + citrated zinc + cholecalciferol (Fosteum Rx®)	Prevention—1 capsule twice daily (Each capsule contains 27 mg genistein, 20 mg citrated zinc, 200 IU cholecalciferol.)	• Medical food • Meets FDA standards for GRAS (generally recognized as safe) • Not recommended if taking HT, estrogen agonist-antagonists
raloxifene (Evista)	PMO prevention or treatment—60 mg by mouth daily	• May cause hot flashes • Not recommended if taking ET or EPT • Also approved for prevention of breast cancer in women at high risk for invasive breast cancer
teriparatide [recombinant human PTH 1-34] (Forteo)	PMO, MOP, and SIO treatment (high fracture risk)—20 mcg subcutaneously daily (A teriparatide patch for osteoporosis is under investigation.)	• Reserved for use after failure of first-line agents • Most effective when used sequentially following bisphosphonate

Source information on following page.

Adapted from: Alexander, I. M., & Andrist, L. A. (2005). Menopause (Chapter 11, pp 249–289). In F. Likis & K. Shuiling (Eds.), *Women's Gynecologic Health*. Sudbury, MA: Jones and Bartlett.

Sources: U.S. Department of Health and Human Services. *Bone health and osteoporosis: A report of the Surgeon General*. Rockville, MD: U.S. Department of Health and Human Services, Office of the Surgeon General; 2004; Dawson-Hughes B. A revised clinician's guide to the prevention and treatment of osteoporosis. *J Clin Endocrinol Metab.* Jul 2008; 93(7):2463–2465; Micromedex. Available to subscribers at: http://www.thomsonhc.com/hcs/librarian and accessed January 27, 2010; ePocrates. Computerized pharmacology and prescribing reference. Updated daily. Available at: www.epocrates.com. Accessed January 27, 2010; North American Menopause Society. Management of osteoporosis in postmenopausal women: 2010 position statement of The North American Menopause Society. *Menopause.* Jan–Feb 2010; 17(1):25–54; Fosteum Prescribing Information. Available at: www.fosteum.com. Accessed February 27, 2008; North American Menopause Society. Government-Approved Postmenopausal Osteoporosis Drugs in the United States and Canada. *North American Menopause Society.* June 2009. Available for members at: http://www.menopause.org/otcharts.pdf. Accessed February 2, 2010; Novartis Pharmaceuticals. Reclast Prescribing Information. *Novartis Pharmaceuticals* [pdf]. August, 2007. Accessed October 26, 2007; Roche Laboratories. Boniva Tablet Prescribing Information. *Roche Laboratories.* August, 2006. Available at: http://www.rocheusa.com/products/Boniva/PI.pdf. Accessed October 26, 2007; Roche Laboratories. Boniva Injectable Prescribing Information. *Roche Laboratories.* February, 2007. Accessed October 26, 2007. Available at: http://www.rocheusa.com/products/Boniva/Injection_PI.pdf; Bachmann GA, Schaefers M, Uddin A, Utian WH. Lowest effective transdermal 17beta-estradiol dose for relief of hot flushes in postmenopausal women: A randomized controlled trial. *Obstet Gynecol.* Oct 2007; 110(4):771–779; Maggon, L. Denosumab (Prolia, Amgen) FDA review and approval. Available at: http://knol.google.com/k/denosumab-prolia-amgen-fda-review-approval#. Accessed January 27, 2010; Cosman F, Lane NE, Bolognese MA, et al. Effect of transdermal teriparatide administration on bone mineral density in postmenopausal women. *J Clin Endocrinol Metab.* Jan 2010;95(1):151–158; Rizzoli R, Burlet N, Cahall D, Delmas PD, Eriksen EF, Felsenberg D, et al. Osteonecrosis of the jaw and bisphosphonate treatment for osteoporosis. Bone 2008; 42(5):841–7; McClung MR. Osteonecrosis of the Jaw. Menopause e-Consult 2007; 3(2); American Association of Oral and Maxillofacial Surgeons. AAOMS position paper on bisphosphonate related osteonecrosis of the jaw. In: American Association of Oral and Maxillofacial Surgeons; 2006; Shane E, Goldring S, Christakos S, Drezner M, Eisman J, Silverman S, et al. Osteonecrosis of the jaw: More research needed. J Bone Miner Res 2006;21(10):1503–5; Bilezikian JP. Osteonecrosis of the jaw—Do bisphosphonates pose a risk? N Engl J Med 2006;355(22):2278–81; Bolland M, Hay D, Grey A, Reid I, Cundy T. Osteonecrosis of the jaw and bisphosphonates—Putting the risk in perspective. N Z Med J 2006;119(1246):U2339; Bagger YZ, Tanko LB, Alexandersen P, Hansen HB, Mollgaard A, Ravn P, et al. Two to three years of hormone replacement treatment in healthy women have long-term preventive effects on bone mass and osteoporotic fractures: The PERF study. Bone 2004; 34(4):728–35; Black DM, Kelly MP, Genant HK, et al. Bisphosphonates and Fractures of the Subtrochanteric or Diaphyseal Femur. N Engl J Med 2010; 10.1056/NEJMoa1001086, nejm.org, accessed November 2, 2010; Prolia Prescribing Information, available at: http://pi.amgen.com/united_states/prolia/prolia_pi.pdf, accessed March 8, 2011.

PMO = Postmenopausal Osteoporosis; SIO = Steroid Induced Osteoporosis; MOP = Male Osteoporosis.

strength by inhibiting the function of the osteoclasts and include bisphosphonates, calcitonin, estrogen agonist/antagonists (which were previously known as selective estrogen receptor modulators [SERMs]), and hormone therapy (HT, estrogen or estrogen-progestin therapy). Denosumab is also in this category and increases bone density by binding with RANK-ligand, which ultimately inhibits osteoclast formation and function. Anabolic agents stimulate bone formation by increasing osteoblast activity and include one agent, teriparatide. The prescription medical food Fosteum Rx® meets FDA GRAS criteria for "generally regarded as safe" and is also available by prescription.

For Ms. O, selecting an agent will focus on identifying an effective therapy that is acceptable to her, does not interfere with her current medications, and has a reasonable side-effect profile. Because she has established OP, she needs a medication that is approved for OP treatment, this means that hormone therapy is not an appropriate option. If Ms. O had osteopenia and was also experiencing significant menopause-related symptoms, then HT might be a good option (NAMS, 2010). Bisphosphonates are frequently identified as first line options for OP. Several different medications are now available in this class with varied frequency of dosing and also varied routes of administration. Some are also available in generic formulation, which can significantly reduce their cost. A precise procedure for taking oral bisphosphonates must be followed to reduce the risk of esophageal irritation. Other rare side effects are also possible (see Table 2.14.1). If Ms. O starts with a bisphosphonate and is unable to follow the oral medication regimen or has a low bone density response, she might have better adherence with an injectable bisphosphonate or denosumab. If Ms. O was at high risk for breast cancer, raloxifene might be a better option for her. Calcitonin is sometimes used for the pain associated with VCFs and might be considered for Ms. O. However, other OP medications have better fracture prevention data and Ms. O's pain will likely be well managed with analgesics instead. Teriparatide is an unlikely option for Ms. O as it is generally reserved for use in patients who do not respond to first line medication options. Poor adherence to OP medication is well documented (Gold, Alexander, & Ettinger, 2006). Therefore, it is important that Ms. O is an active participant in deciding which medication to use. She is much more likely to continue with the medication if it is taken on a schedule that works for her.

What is the plan for follow-up care?
In addition to re-evaluating Ms. O's ability to follow the management plan, including both medications and self-management strategies at every visit, a follow-up DXA scan will be ordered in about 1–2 years to evaluate the efficacy of Ms. O's management strategies (NOF, 2010). It is repeated every 1–2 years until her results are stable. If her T-scores

do not improve after a few years, her clinician might consider changing the pharmacotherapeutic agent to an alternate class or consider referral to an OP specialist.

Does Ms. O's psychosocial history affect her management plan?
Consideration of Ms. O's psychosocial history is important when developing a management plan with her. Consideration of her health care insurance coverage of medications, physical therapy, and DXA evaluations is important. Many insurance companies dictate which pharmacotherapeutic agents are covered and have rules governing the frequency of covered DXA testing and length of physical therapy treatments. These issues are taken into account when deciding on a management plan with Ms. O so that financial barriers to the cost of medications, follow-up DXA testing, or PT do not become barriers to her ability to follow the plan.

What if Ms. O also had diabetes or hyperlipidemia or were male?
Several of the medications available for OP treatment and prevention do not carry FDA approval for use in men, so agent selection options would be narrowed if Ms. O were male (see Table 2.14.1). Conversely, the disease processes of hyperlipidemia and diabetes themselves would not alter Ms. O's plan of care. However, pharmacotherapeutic agent selection for managing diabetes and hyperlipidemia would potentially be altered. Statins (e.g., Lipitor and Mevacor) have been demonstrated to improve bone health, though not enough to be used as OP agents, and they might be a preferred class of agent for Ms. O if she also had hyperlipidemia (DHHS, 2004). Thiazolidinediones (TZDs; e.g., Actos and Avandia) have been identified as potentially increasing risk for bone loss and may need to be avoided if Ms. O also had diabetes (NOF, 2010). Incidentally, hydrochlorothiazide diuretics have been identified as bone preserving medications (DHHS, 2004); thus the fact that Ms. O's hypertension is treated with HCTZ is optimal with regard to her OP.

Are there any standardized guidelines that the clinician will use to assess or treat Ms. O?
The U.S. Surgeon General's 2004 Report *Bone Health and Osteoporosis* helped to raise awareness about the importance of bone loss and its consequences (DHHS, 2004). Since that report, the NOF has published at least 2 sets of guidelines for clinicians about managing OP and osteopenia, the most recent of which was updated in 2010 (NOF, 2010). In 2010, the NAMS also published guidelines for OP and osteopenia management in their updated position statement; these are specifically geared to the postmenopausal woman (NAMS, 2010).

*This case is reprinted in part in *Clinical Case Studies for the Family Nurse Practitioner.* (Neal-Boylan, L., Ed.). Ames: Wiley-Blackwell.

REFERENCES

Alexander, I. M., & Lewiecki, E. M. (2008). Prevention, identification and treatment of postmenopausal osteoporosis (online CME/CE program). *Medscape.* Retrieved from http://www.medscape.com/viewprogram/17528

Colglazier, C. L., & Sutej, P. G. (2005). Laboratory testing in the rheumatic diseases: A practical review. *Southern Medical Journal, 98*(2), 185–191.

Dawson-Hughes, B. (2010). Treatment of vitamin D deficient states. Up-To-Date, Retrieved November 1, 2010, from http://www.uptodate.com/online/content/topic.do?topicKey=bone_dis/11247&selectedTitle=1%7E139&source=search_result/

Dawson-Hughes, B., Tosteson, A. N., Melton, L. J., 3rd, Baim, S., Favus, M. J., Khosla, S., et al. (2008). Implications of absolute fracture risk assessment for osteoporosis practice guidelines in the USA. *Osteoporosis International, 19*(4), 449–458.

Decker, G. M., & Meyers, J. (2001). Commonly used herbs: Implications for clinical practice. *Clinical Journal of Oncology Nursing, 15*(2), 13, pullout insert.

Gold, D. T., Alexander, I. M., & Ettinger, M. P. (2006). How can osteoporosis patients benefit more from their therapy? Adherence issues with bisphosphonate therapy. *The Annals of Pharmacotherapy, 40*(6), 1143–1150.

Liu, J., Ho, S. C., Su, Y. X., Chen, W. Q., Zhang, C. X., & Chen, Y. M. (2009). Effect of long-term intervention of soy isoflavones on bone mineral density in women: A meta-analysis of randomized controlled trials. *Bone, 44*(5), 948–953.

National Osteoporosis Foundation (NOF) (2010). *Clinician's guide to prevention and treatment of osteoporosis.* Washington, DC: National Osteoporosis Foundation.

North American Menopause Society (NAMS) (2010). Management of osteoporosis in postmenopausal women: 2010 position statement of The North American Menopause Society. *Menopause, 17*(1), 25–54. quiz 55–26.

Tosteson, A. N., Melton, L. J., 3rd, Dawson-Hughes, B., Baim, S., Favus, M. J., Khosla, S., et al. (2008). Cost-effective osteoporosis treatment thresholds: The United States perspective. *Osteoporosis International, 19*(4), 437–447.

U.S. Department of Health & Human Services (DHHS) (2004). *Bone health and osteoporosis: A report of the Surgeon General.* Rockville, MD: U.S. Department of Health and Human Services, Office of the Surgeon General.

World Health Organization (WHO) (1994). *Assessment of fracture risk and its application to screening for postmenopausal osteoporosis. Technical report series.* Geneva: WHO.

World Health Organization (WHO) (2007a). *WHO FRAX Technical Report.* Retrieved June 6, 2008, from http://www.shef.ac.uk/FRAX/

World Health Organization (WHO) (2007b). *WHO scientific group on the assessment of osteoporosis at primary health care level: Summary meeting report.* Brussels, Belgium: WHO Press. Geneva, Switzerland.

Section 3

Health Promotion

Case 3.1 Never Too Old to Quit

By Geraldine Marrocco, EdD, APRN, CNS, ANP-BC
and Amanda LaManna, MSN, RN, NP-C

Mrs. K is a 76-year-old female who presents to the clinician with chronic fatigue, leg pain, and weakness. She describes weakness associated with increasing difficulty in sustaining any lengthy walking. She describes that walking even in her neighborhood grocery store is difficult and that she often needs to stop and rest. She denies leg pain, but reports weakness. Mrs. K wants to know why she is so tired all of the time. She denies chest pain. She reports no joint pain, no shortness of breath, an occasional nonproductive cough, no abdominal pain, no paresthesia of the extremities, and no dizziness or headache.

Mrs. K's past medical history includes diverticulitis, colectomy in 2003, peripheral vascular disease (PVD), chronic obstructive pulmonary disease (COPD), dyslipidemia, osteoporosis, and cataract surgery in 2008. She does not drink alcohol; however, she has smoked 1 pack per day (PPD) for the last 50 years. She reports no illegal substance abuse. She has a high-school education, is of Italian American heritage, and was a former beauty pageant award winner. She reports that she does not engage in senior events or activities. She exercises little and does not drive anymore.

Her father died at age 82 of a stroke; he was a smoker. Her mother died at age 58 of a brain tumor; she also was a smoker. Her brother is alive at age 72 with coronary artery disease (CAD) and dyslipidemia; he is a smoker. Her husband died at age 58 (ETOH abuse, smoker). She has 3 children. One son has ETOH abuse and is a smoker. Her daughter

Case Studies in Gerontological Nursing for the Advanced Practice Nurse, First Edition.
Edited by Meredith Wallace Kazer, Leslie Neal-Boylan.
© 2012 John Wiley & Sons, Inc. Published 2012 by John Wiley & Sons, Inc.

has illegal substance abuse and is a previous smoker, and another son is estranged from the family.

Her medications include Spiriva, 1 puff daily; ASA, 81 mg daily; Fosamax, 70 mg weekly; fish oil from the health food store; calcium with D, 600 mg twice a day. She refuses statins because they cause her "severe muscle pain". She is on a fixed income and is noncompliant with medications when money is tight and samples are unavailable. She is up to date with influenza and Pneumovax vaccinations.

OBJECTIVE

Mrs. K is a well-developed, well-nourished female who looks her stated age. Vitals: BP: 130/70; pulse: 86 and regular; temperature: 97.6; RR: 16; pulse ox: 92 at rest. Her skin is clear with some periorbital edema. She has a pleasant, talkative, husky voice. HEENT: Normocephalic, atraumatic, and wears glasses for near and far. Throat: Erythematous, chronic post nasal drip, and wears upper and lower dentures. She shows no evidence of oral pathology and has no palpable lymph nodes. Chest: Distant breath sounds, clear to auscultation. Her most recent chest x-ray demonstrates emphysema. A CT scan of the chest reveals a tortuous aorta. Heart: RRR, murmur unchanged. Pulses positive in all extremities; no edema. Abdomen: Well-healed incision, BS+, symmetrical, nontender, no organomegaly. Recent relevant labs: H/H: 17.1/38; metabolic panel: normal; renal function: normal; total cholesterol: 251; HDL: 42; LDL: 140. TSH: normal; urinalysis: negative.

ASSESSMENT

Smoking cessation Mrs. K is 76-year-old patient with a long history of smoking and denial of consequences of smoking. She refuses most medications because she thinks her body is too sensitive to them. She refuses statins, antidepressants, nicotine patch, and Nicorette gum. Smoking cessation is addressed at every visit to the primary care office. Her daughter, who successfully quit smoking 15 months ago, is supportive of her mother's quitting.

CRITICAL THINKING

What are the considerations in revisiting smoking cessation strategies for this patient?

What is the next plan of treatment and followup?

Is she a candidate for alternative nonpharmacological treatments?

RESOLUTION

What are the considerations in revisiting smoking cessation strategies for this patient?

It is reported that over 4.5 million Americans age 65 and older are smokers (PHS Guideline Update Panel, Liaisons, and Staff, 2008). The habit doubles the mortality rate of those older than 65. In addition, smoking can complicate common diseases of older adults, including heart disease, hypertension, circulatory insufficiency, ulcers, osteoporosis, and diabetes. Also, as older adults tend to take more medications than younger adults, smoking can interfere with the efficacy of pharmacotherapy (Morgan et al., 1996). Men and women smokers lose, on average, 13.2 and 14.5 years of life, respectively, due to smoking (Doolan & Froelicher, 2008). It is overwhelmingly clear that this is a problem that needs increasing attention by primary care providers.

It is no surprise that smoking is common among older adults, as many of them grew up in a time when smoking was glorified and even endorsed by physicians. Through years of research and rising trends in smoking-related disease and death, we now know that there appears to be little or no benefit of smoking and that the risks are too numerous to list.

Despite public health campaigns and numerous efforts to bring about smoking cessation in the primary care setting, older adult smokers seem to be slipping through the cracks. As with any treatment, smoking cessation must be tailored to the individual, taking into account the most effective modalities for the specific population. The average smoker sees an outpatient provider more than 4 times annually, which gives many opportunities for intervention (Morgan et al., 1996).

There are several common misconceptions about smoking cessation in the older adult. First, it is thought that there is little benefit to smoking cessation at an older age; this assumes the damage is done. Another thought is that simply decreasing the number of cigarettes daily can be effective. A third mindset is that one cannot teach an old dog new tricks, implying that the older adult is too set in his or her ways to be able to quit smoking. All of these suggestions are false.

Even older smokers like Mrs. K can benefit from quitting smoking. Benefits include a decrease in the risk of death from heart disease, COPD, and lung cancer. In addition, there is a decrease in the risk of osteoporosis. Quitting smoking also results in a quicker recovery from smoking-exacerbated diseases, along with an improvement in cerebral blood flow (PHS Guideline Update Panel, Liaisons, and Staff, 2008).

There have been many recent efforts in harm reduction, including decreasing the number of cigarettes smoked daily or using filters. However, these methods do not reduce exposure to nicotine, tar, or carcinogens. While reducing the number of cigarettes smoked daily may reduce the long-term risk of lung cancer, it does not reduce the risk for other smoking-related diseases such as heart disease or COPD (Cataldo, 2007).

It is a misconception that the desire to smoke declines with age, yet it has been found that older adults may be less likely to receive smoking cessation medication and treatment due to this common misconception (PHS Guideline Update Panel, Liaisons, and Staff, 2008). Nevertheless, according to the literature, older age has been consistently found to be associated with successful smoking cessation. Success rates continue to increase after 65 years old. The older old are more likely to quit and less likely to relapse than those age 65–69. After age 84, the prevalence of success drops, though this is due to mortality, as smokers rarely live past age 84 (Cataldo, 2007).

What is the next plan of treatment and followup?

There has been limited research looking at the success rates of different treatment modalities on smoking cessation in the older adult, though the research that has been done is promising. Older studies focused mainly on different styles of counseling and self-help that were tailored to the older adult, but results were not incredibly consistent or specific. Group oriented smoking cessation treatment for older adults like Mrs. K were found to offer benefits through the "same as me" atmosphere and bonding (Morgan et al., 1996). Using the 4 A's assessment model (which has now been expanded to the 5 A's model), Morgan et al. (1996) combined older adult-specific literature with phone call followup to achieve a 17.8% six-month abstinence rate, versus a 9.3% rate in the control group. The literature used was *Clear Horizons* which is a guide tailored to adults older than 50 years. It is written at an eighth grade reading level and outlines strategies for cessation per decade. The strategies are broken down per stages of change, including deciding to quit, preparing to quit, initial cessation, and maintenance. *Clear Horizons* is still available today through the National Cancer Institute's public health campaign, at http://www.myclearhorizons.com/. According to Rimer et al. (1994), tailoring information to a specific age group is, in fact, effective and should be utilized whenever possible.

Doolan and Froelicher (2008) found that pharmacotherapy was more effective in older adults than advice and counseling alone. Specific treatment, whether through nicotine replacement therapies (NRT) or other pharmacologic agents, doubles the odds for lasting cessation over going "cold turkey" alone (Cataldo, 2007). It is important to begin with an assessment of whether or not Mrs. K is ready and willing to quit. A reputable approach for someone who is not willing to quit is the 5 R's motivational intervention: Relevance, risk, reward, road block, and repetition. For someone who is willing to quit, the 5 A's model is a gold standard for beginning treatment: Ask, advise, assess, assist, and arrange (for followup) (Cataldo, 2007). The current approved therapies for smoking cessation are as follows:

- Bupropion (Wellbutrin SR)
- Varenicline (Chantix)
- Nicotine gum
- Nicotine inhaler
- Nicotine nasal spray
- Nicotine patch

During the assess aspect of the 5 A's method, it is important to decipher which treatment method will be most appropriate for a specific individual.

Is she a candidate for alternative nonpharmacological treatments?
It has been shown that the most effective method is through multiple modalities, meaning that combining counseling and followup with one of the above therapies is imperative (Cataldo, 2007).

Barriers to counseling for Mrs. K may be mobility and transportation with the older adult, so consider telephone counseling and/or group therapy options as they may be most likely for her successful adherence. For those who have tried to quit multiple times using NRT, it would be appropriate to consider first bupropion or varenicline as initial pharmacotherapy. The cost of therapy may be a concern, but the good news is that smoking cessation treatment is covered by Medicare Part D for older adults (PHS Guideline Update Panel, Liaisons, and Staff, 2008).

It is unfair and untrue to assume that it is too late to begin smoking cessation with the older adult. There are still benefits to quitting at an older age, and there is no decrease in the desire to quit. Cessation rates are quite successful in older adults when treatment is approached correctly. Pharmacotherapy may be crucial in the older adult, so the clinician should consider bupropion, varenicline, or a form of NRT in addition to individualized counseling. The results will be beneficial to the health, finances, and overall well-being of the older adult who is willing to quit.

REFERENCES

Cataldo, J. K. (2007). Clinical implications of smoking and aging: Breaking through the barriers. *Journal of Gerontological Nursing*, *33*(8), 32–41. Retrieved from http://ovidsp.ovid.com/ovidweb.cgi?T=JS&NEWS=N&PAGE=fulltext&D=medl&AN=17718376

Clear Horizons. Retrieved at http://www.myclearhorizons.com/

Doolan, D., & Froelicher, E. S. (2008). Smoking cessation interventions and older adults. *Progress in Cardiovascular Nursing, 23*(3), 119–127. doi:10.1111/j.1751-7117.2008.00001.x

Morgan, G. D., Noll, E. L., Orleans, C. T., Rimer, B. K., Amfoh, K., & Bonney, G. (1996). Reaching midlife and older smokers: Tailored interventions for routine medical care. *Preventive Medicine, 25*(3), 346–354. doi:10.1006/pmed.1996.0065

PHS Guideline Update Panel, Liaisons, & Staff. (2008). Treating tobacco use and dependence: 2008 update U.S. Public Health Service clinical practice guideline executive summary. *Respiratory Care, 53*(9), 1217–1222. Retrieved from http://ovidsp.ovid.com/ovidweb.cgi?T=JS&NEWS=N&PAGE=fulltext&D=medl&AN=18807274

Rimer, B. K., Orleans, C. T., Fleisher, L., Cristinzio, S., Resch, N., Telepchak, J., & Keintz, M. K. (1994). Does tailoring matter? The impact of a tailored guide on ratings and short-term smoking-related outcomes for older smokers. *Health Education Research, 9*(1), 69–84. Retrieved from http://ovidsp.ovid.com/ovidweb.cgi?T=JS&NEWS=N&PAGE=fulltext&D=med3&AN=10146734

Case 3.2 Protection by Prevention

By Kimberlee-Ann Bridges, MSN, RN-BC, CNL

Mr. W is an 88-year-old male who is being seen today in the primary care practice. He is accompanied today by his daughter. She made the appointment for him yesterday after she visited him at his apartment. She noticed during the visit that he did not seem to be able to follow the conversation and was forgetting things. He seemed tired and somewhat weak. He also had not been participating in his usual activities for the past several days. He was last seen at the practice for his annual physical 7 months ago. At that time, he was in generally good health and his chronic conditions were well managed. He declined the flu and pneumonia vaccines. His past medical history includes mild BPH, coronary artery disease, hypertension, internal hemorrhoids, arthritis, and cataracts. His past surgical history includes an appendectomy 30 years ago, coronary artery stenting 5 years ago, and cataract surgery 11 years ago. Mr. W is a retired postal worker. He resides in an assisted living facility. He was married for 52 years and lost his wife 6 months ago. He has 1 daughter who lives nearby and visits him regularly. He has 1 son who lives out of state and visits about twice a year. He has 5 grandchildren. He goes in annually for a complete physical exam by his primary care physician. He also sees a cardiologist annually. He has a colonoscopy every 10 years. Both parents are deceased. His father died at the age of 74 of respiratory failure due to COPD. His mother died of colon cancer at the age of 92. He walks 2 miles daily with one of his friends at the assisted living facility, but he has not walked in the last 3 days due to his current illness. He has no history of smoking. He drinks occasionally in social situations. He participates in many of the

Case Studies in Gerontological Nursing for the Advanced Practice Nurse, First Edition.
Edited by Meredith Wallace Kazer, Leslie Neal-Boylan.
© 2012 John Wiley & Sons, Inc. Published 2012 by John Wiley & Sons, Inc.

activities offered at the assisted living facility. He goes to his daughter's house once a week to have dinner with her family. He does not drive. He is not currently sexually active, but he states that he and his wife had a satisfactory sex life up until her death. He states that he has some stiffness and discomfort in his fingers a few times a week for which he takes ibuprofen with good effect. He does state that he has noticed that he has trouble concentrating on things the last several days. He does not complain of headaches or any episodes of syncope. He has some shortness of breath with exertion. He denies chest pain, shortness of breath, palpitations, abdominal pain, diarrhea, nausea, or vomiting. He complains of occasional difficulty initiating urination, but he has no issues with incontinence or retention. He states that his last bowel movement was this morning. He does occasionally notice bright, red blood in his stools; but he does not recall seeing any today. His current medications include lisinopril, 10 mg once daily; Zocor, 40 mg once daily; aspirin, 81 mg once daily; multivitamin, once daily; and ibuprofen, 600 mg, as needed for arthritis pain. He is allergic to penicillin.

OBJECTIVE

Mr. W is a well-groomed, well-nourished adult male in no apparent distress. He is 6 ft 1 inch and weighs 190 lb. BP: 124/72; P: 74; RR: 22; T: 98.9 oral; O$_2$ Sat 90% RA. Currently Mr. W is alert, but is slow to answer questions and seems unsure of some of his answers. He knows who he is, where he is, and what year it is. He recognizes his daughter. His gait is WNL with FROM of his extremities; no balance or coordination deficits. He has 2+ deep tendon reflexes and equal strength bilaterally. Cranial nerves II–XII grossly intact. He has a moist, nonproductive cough. His respirations appeared somewhat labored while walking to the exam room, but they are unlabored while he is at rest. His lung sounds are clear, but diminished bilaterally. Cardiac exam reveals a regular rate and rhythm, with no murmurs rubs or gallops; normal S1 and S2. His abdomen is soft, nontender, nondistended with +bowel sounds in all 4 quadrants. He has a faded scar in the right lower quadrant. His skin is warm, dry, and intact. He has no pedal edema and positive pedal pulses. His sclerae are clear with PERRLA. His ears are clear with normal tympanic membranes bilaterally. Oral mucosa is pink and moist; teeth are intact. Digital rectal exam reveals no abnormalities. Stool is guaiac negative.

ASSESSMENT

Depression: Mr. W lost his wife recently and may be having difficulty dealing with her death. He has withdrawn from social activities recently and has been tired and forgetful, which can be symptoms of depression in older adults.

Anemia: Mr. W has a history of rectal bleeding. He has been tired and forgetful lately, and he is now short of breath on exertion. These are all symptoms of anemia.

Pneumonia: Mr. W is at higher risk for developing pneumonia due to his advanced age (Middleton et al., 2008). He is afebrile, but the elderly often do not experience fever as symptom of pneumonia. He has a cough, his pulse ox is low, and he is short of breath on exertion. All of these symptoms can be signs of pneumonia in older adults.

DIAGNOSTICS

A chest x-ray is ordered to determine if there are lung infiltrates, which would indicate pneumonia. A CBC is ordered to check Mr. W's white blood cell count, and an H&H is ordered to check for an infection or anemia. A UA is ordered and found to be negative for UTI. An EKG is ordered as a precautionary measure, to ensure that there is no cardiac component to his symptoms. The chest x-ray reveals bilateral infiltrates. The CBC reveals a WBC of 16.8; H&H: 12 & 38.2; EKG reveals sinus rhythm with a rate in the 70s, no ST changes.

CRITICAL THINKING

What is the most likely differential diagnosis and why?

What is the plan of treatment?

What is the plan for follow-up care?

Does the patient's psychosocial history impact how the clinician might treat this patient?

What if the patient lived in a rural or isolated setting?

What if this patient also had diabetes? Would that affect the treatment plan? If so, how?

Are any referrals needed?

Are there any potential complications from the illness or treatment about which the clinician should educate Mr. W and his daughter at his follow-up appointment?

Are there any standardized guidelines the clinician should use to assess or treat this patient?

RESOLUTION

What is the most likely differential diagnosis and why?

Depression is a likely diagnosis given the recent death of Mr. W's wife. He has withdrawn from activities and is tired and forgetful, which can all be symptoms of depression. Depression in older adults can be underdiagnosed and undertreated. However, Mr. W has an elevated WBC and a positive chest x-ray, which rule out the diagnosis of depression as an immediate problem. The next differential would be anemia. Mr. W is exhibiting symptoms of anemia, such as lethargy and forgetfulness. His H&H comes back normal, so anemia is ruled out as a diagnosis.

The final differential is pneumonia. This is Mr. W's diagnosis. He has a cough, low pulse ox, lethargy, and confusion, which are all symptoms of pneumonia. His WBC is elevated, and the chest x-ray shows bilateral infiltrates. Older adults generally do not have a fever with pneumonia, as their fever response is slower than that of younger people. Confusion is frequently a sign of infection in older adults, and Mr. W is showing signs of new onset confusion. Also of note is that Mr. W refused the pneumonia vaccine during his last physical. Older adults are at far greater risk for developing pneumonia than younger people (Fisman, Abrutyn, Spaude, Kim, Kirchner, & Daley, 2006).

What is the plan of treatment?

Mr. W probably should be hospitalized at this point due to his combination of symptoms and advanced age. He should be started on intravenous antibiotics, O₂ and monitored closely for any changes in his condition. Older adults are at increased risks of developing complications related to pneumonia and of dying as a result (Centers for Disease Control [CDC], 2009). Pneumonia is the fourth leading causes of death in the United States (Maggi, 2010). He should receive the pneumococcal vaccination during his hospitalization according to CDC guidelines (CDC, 2009). The pneumonia vaccination has shown to be effective in preventing pneumococcal pneumonia and its complications in older adults (Middleton et al., 2008). Current Medicare guidelines require vaccination of patients who are hospitalized with a diagnosis of community-acquired pneumonia (Shorr & Owens, 2009). Vaccination is the only effective measure in the prevention of pneumococcal pneumonia (Martin, 2008). Complications and mortality rates are significantly reduced in patients who have been vaccinated but who still get a pneumococcal infection, (Fisamn et al., 2006).

What is the plan for follow-up care?

Mr. W should be seen back in the office within 3 or 4 days of his discharge from the hospital. He should be reassessed to ensure that his pneumonia has improved and his symptoms have resolved. He should also be reassessed for possible depression at that time. His symptoms of depression could have been overlooked while he was being treated for his more immediate medical problem.

Does the patient's psychosocial history impact how the clinician might treat this patient?

Mr. W seems to be able to manage his health care needs and has a supportive social network. His daughter is nearby and able to drive him to his doctors' appointments. It should be stressed upon Mr. W that he should call the office and make an appointment when he first starts to have symptoms of an illness. A seemingly mild problem can progress rapidly in older adults, and he should not delay treatment.

What if the patient lived in a rural or isolated setting?

Mr. W would likely need to be monitored more closely if he lived in an isolated setting. If that were the situation, he might need to stay with his daughter for a week or 2 after his hospitalization, until he makes a full recovery. His daughter would be able to make sure he got to his medical appointments and would monitor his symptoms to make sure they were improving. If Mr. W were to stay by himself in an isolated setting after his hospitalization, he might not be able to get to his follow-up appointments. He may have a reduced capacity for self-care after his hospitalization and would likely need someone close by to ensure that his needs are being met.

What if this patient also had diabetes? Would that affect the treatment plan? If so, how?

If Mr. W were diabetic, his blood glucose would need to be monitored closely and kept within tight control during and immediately after the infection. The infection would likely affect his blood sugar levels. The clinician would need to ensure that Mr. W was checking his blood sugar regularly and was knowledgeable about his diabetes medications.

Are any referrals needed?

Mr. W should not need any further referral once his pneumonia resolves. If he seems to be exhibiting symptoms of depression at his follow-up appointment, he should be referred for further evaluation.

Are there any potential complications from the illness or treatment about which the clinician should educate Mr. W and his daughter at his follow-up appointment?

Mr. W should be encouraged to receive the pneumonia vaccine at his follow-up appointment if he did not receive it in the hospital. The risks and benefits of vaccination should be discussed with him. He would only need to be vaccinated one time in order to have long-term protection against pneumococcal pneumonia and its complications (CDC, 2009). He should be vaccinated against pneumonia even though he was just hospitalized for the illness, because he is still at risk for developing pneumonia. He should not experience any complications related to the treatment of his pneumonia.

Are there any standardized guidelines the clinician should use to assess or treat this patient?
The CDC has published a full set of guidelines regarding the treatment of pneumonia. These guidelines include information regarding antibiotic and vaccination administration, among other treatments. In order for CMS providers to get reimbursed fully for their services, they must follow these guidelines.

REFERENCES

Centers for Disease Control (CDC). (2009). (n.d.). Pneumococcal disease. Retrieved March 26, 2010, from http://www.cdc.gov/vaccines/pubs/pinkbook/downloads/pneumo.pdf

Fisman, D. N., Abrutyn, E., Spaude, K. A., Kim, A., Kirchner, C., & Daley, J. (2006). Prior pneumococcal vaccination is associated with reduced death, complications and length of stay among hospitalized adults with community acquired pneumonia. *Clinical Infectious Diseases, 42,* 1093–1101.

Maggi, S. (2010). Vaccination and healthy aging. *Expert Reviews, 9*(3), 3–6.

Martin, J. (2008). Pneumococcal disease. *Practice Nursing, 19*(11), 566–568.

Middleton, D. B., Jin, C. J., Smith, K. J., Zimmerman, R. K., Nowalk, M. P., Roberts, M. S., . . . Fox, D. E. (2008). Economic Evaluation of Standing Order Programs for Pneumococcal Vaccination of Hospitalized Elderly Patients. *Infection Control and Hospital Epidemiology, 29*(5), 385–394.

Shorr, A. F., & Owens, R. C. (2009). Guidelines and quality for community-acquired pneumonia: Measures from the joint commission and the centers for medicare and medicaid services. *American Journal of Health-System Pharmacy, 66*(4), 52–57.

ADDITIONAL RESOURCES

Andrews, J., Nadjm, B., Grant, V., & Shetty, N. (2003). Community-acquired pneumonia. *Current Opinion in Pulmonary Medicine, 9,* 175–180.

Brenner, Z. R., & Salathiel, M. (2009). The nurse's role in CMS quality indicators. *Medsurg Nursing, 18*(4), 242–246.

Centers for Disease Control http://cdc.gov/features/pneumonia

Cleveland Clinic Center for Continuing Education http://www.clevelandclinicmeded.com/medicalpubs/diseasemanagement/infectious-disease/community-acquired-pneumonia

Niederman, M. S. (2002). Community-acquired pneumonia: Management controversies, Part 1; Practical recommendations from the latest guidelines. *Journal of Respiratory Diseases, 23,* 7–10.

Case 3.3 Is Being Careful Enough?

By Bonnie Cashin Farmer, PhD, RN

Ms. I, a 76-year-old retired school cafeteria worker presents to the community health clinic for a post fall exam. Four weeks ago, she fell from a small step stool while washing her apartment windows. She sustained some moderate facial bruising and a laceration to her left leg that required 4 sutures. Ms. I lives alone in a partially subsidized 2-bedroom apartment in a small urban area of a rural state. Her husband of 47 years died 3 years ago at the age of 79. Her only sister is deceased, and her sister's adult children live several states away. She continues to maintain contact with her many friends who were "like family" to her and her husband. Prior to this fall, Ms. I had essentially been an independent and healthy individual. She confirms some complaints of arthritis in her knees, feet, and hands; mild hypertension; and an early cataract in her right eye. She expresses discouragement with her weight gain despite her attempts at "healthy eating". During her post-fall examination, her clinician discusses with her the importance of regular exercise in preventing further falls, as well as the promotion and maintenance of her health. She states that she has never really liked to exercise and has preferred baking and homemaking types of activities. She has always liked to knit and do crossword puzzles. She also enjoys watching television, especially *Judge Judy* and cooking shows. Ms. I expresses concern that she might fall if she did try to "exercise". "I am fine. I just need to be more careful." Her medications include HCTZ, 25 mg; Lipitor, 10 mg; ibuprofen, 400 mg; calcium with vitamin D, 600 mg; and a multivitamin for seniors every day. She has no known allergies (NKA).

Case Studies in Gerontological Nursing for the Advanced Practice Nurse, First Edition.
Edited by Meredith Wallace Kazer, Leslie Neal-Boylan.
© 2012 John Wiley & Sons, Inc. Published 2012 by John Wiley & Sons, Inc.

OBJECTIVE

Ms. I is 5ft 5 inches and weighs 177 lb; a recent weight gain of 4 lb is noted. Results of prior bone density tests are considered to be within normal limits. Since Ms. I had a fall requiring medical attention, a multifactorial fall risk assessment (i.e., focused history, physical examination, functional assessment, and environmental assessment) is conducted (American Geriatric Society/British Geriatric Society [AGS/BGS], 2010). A focused history of falls reveals a previous "stumble about 6 months ago" with no injury. Medications are reviewed and considered appropriate at this time. Other risk factors (e.g., acute or chronic medical problems) are negative. Physical examination of gait, balance, mobility levels, and lower extremity joint function reveals moderate bilateral supination, slow-to-moderate pace, slightly rounded shoulders with some leaning, satisfactory balance, minimal unsteadiness, and some limited bilateral range of motion in knees and hips. Neurological functions are all within normal limits. Some weakness in lower extremity muscle strength is noted. Cardiovascular status is within a normal range, with a BP 136/74. Visual acuity has improved since the change in her eyeglass prescription 4 months ago. Feet appear normal with no significant calluses or bunions. Her footwear consists of white, flat, tie sneakers. The outer edges of both shoes, including the outer heels, are worn down. Functional disability is not evident, and no assistive device is being used. Activities of daily living (ADL) are intact. Perceived functional ability and fear related to falling are noted as minimally compromised. Although Ms. I denies a fear of falling, she states that she needs to "be more careful".

ASSESSMENT

Risk for falls: Ms. I demonstrates increased susceptibility for future falls related to her identified risk factors: a fall with injury, prior fall within the last 6 months, advancing age, altered gait, poor footwear, and cataracts, combined with a sedentary lifestyle. In the United States, more than one-third of adults ≥65 years of age fall each year. Falls are the leading causes of death from injury among older adults (Center for Disease Control [CDC], 2010).

Fear of falling: Ms. I demonstrates potential for compromised activity related to fear of falling. The symptom, fear of falling, is known to contribute to the limitation of physical activity, loss of self-confidence, and functional decline of older adults (CDC, 2010; Dukyoo, Juhee, & Sun-Mi 2009).

Sedentary lifestyle/sedentarism: Ms. I's physical inactivity and lack of exercise pose significant risk factors for additional falls, morbidity, and premature mortality. Also, risks for chronic disease, related disabilities, and increasing dependency are exacerbated by a sedentary lifestyle (Agency for Health care Research and Quality [AHRQ], 2010). Regular physical activity is essential for healthy aging (National Guideline Clearinghouse [NGC], 2007).

CRITICAL THINKING

What is the most modifiable risk factor that could prevent Ms. I from future falls?

What is the plan of treatment?

What is the plan for follow-up care?

Does the patient's psychosocial history impact how the clinician might treat this patient?

What if the patient also had one or more of the following: Type I diabetes, peripheral vascular disease, or impaired mobility with the use of an assistive device?

Are there any standardized guidelines that the clinician should use to treat this case?

RESOLUTION

What is the most modifiable risk factor that could prevent Ms. I from future falls?

Ms. I is representative of the older adult population who does not exercise or has not exercised for many years, if ever. By age 75, 1 in 3 men and 1 in 2 women do not engage in regular physical activity (U.S. Department of Health and Human Services [USHHS], 2010). Ms. I's controlled hypertension, which is considered a clinically significant chronic condition (NGC, 2007), does not affect her ability to be active. Physical activity and exercise are sometimes used interchangeably, yet each term suggests specific criteria for implementation and evaluation. Physical activity is considered to be an activity that includes voluntary bodily movement that burns calories (National Institute on Aging [NIA], 2010). Physical activity may be considered incidental, such as activities of daily living (ADL) and instrumental activities of daily living (IADL), or intentional, such as walking the dog, gardening, or raking leaves. Exercise, as a form of physical activity, is a specifically planned, structured, and repetitive activity for the purpose of improving one or more aspects of aerobic activity (NIA, 2010). Examples of exercise include tai chi, strength or weight training, and aerobics class. For clarity of purpose and content, exercise and physical activity are deliberately delineated within the literature and in practice. Exercise and physical activity are complex processes that are often oversimplified by common and generic advice from the health care provider (Handcock & Jenkins, 2003).

Although the differentials of risk for falls and fear of falling are present, a sedentary lifestyle presents the most comprehensive focus for intervention. Among the most evidence-supported components of an intervention program for fall prevention, in addition to an adaptation or modification of the home environment, is the recommendation for an exercise program that incorporates balance, strength, and gait training, combined with flexibility and endurance training (AGS/BGS, 2010). Even when assessment scores may be satisfactory, regular physical activity can improve an older adult's level of fitness and wellness and reduce the risk for falls, serving as an intervention for addressing the potential fear of falling.

What is the plan of treatment?

Many choices for exercise and physical activity are available for a patient like Ms. I, for whom physical activity is at a reasonably low risk level. Health care providers need to regard the recommendations of exercise and physical activity as specific treatment interventions, just as writing a prescription/treatment plan for bladder training or medication management. A successful example is the Green Prescription program, a New Zealand public health initiative first introduced in 1998 for the purpose of increasing physical activity levels (Handcock & Jenkins, 2003). The Green Prescription is written physical activity advice from the health care provider and then facilitated by a government-supported network. Making physical activity and exercise a priority intervention/treatment by the health care provider continues to gain popularity, as evidenced by the Healthy People 2020 proposed objectives of prescriptions for exercise (USHHS, 2010). However, since "there is 'no one size fits all' approach" (AHRQ, 2010), the many options for exercise and physical activity interventions can be overwhelming for both the patient and the health care provider.

One recommendation is for the organization, facility, practice, or service to establish a protocol for the effective delivery of exercise and physical activity recommendations. Such protocol may include, for example, direct patient education and intervention based upon specific activity needs (AGS/BGS, 2010; Dukyoo et al., 2009). The health care provider or team "conducting the fall risk assessment should directly implement the interventions or should assure that the interventions are carried out by other qualified health care professionals" (AGS/BGS,

2010). Exercise recommendations related to fall prevention may vary according to source; and most include multifactorial interventions combining balance, endurance, flexibility, and gait training (AGS/BGS, 2010; NGC, 2007). Given Ms. I's prior sedentary lifestyle, an initial gradual approach that incorporates less-than-recommended levels to increase physical activity is called for (NGC, 2007).

One of the most effective strategies for becoming more active is incorporating incidental and intentional activity into normal daily routines (AHRQ, 2010). Given Ms. I's homemaking interests, emphasis on the inclusion of lifestyle physical activities may be warranted. Following an assessment of individual needs, two of the most important first steps for older adults in beginning an exercise and physical activity program are getting ready and getting started by reviewing current activity and setting short- and long-term goals (National Institute on Aging [NIA], 2009a). Educational material indicating specific local resources with varying foci (e.g., individual, group), activities (e.g., tai chi, walking/pedometer), and formats (e.g., electronic, online, meetings) can be useful. For example, A Matter of Balance program sponsored by an area agency on aging, a senior center walking program, or tai chi might be very appropriate for Ms. I if such programs are available, accessible, affordable, convenient, and of interest. Assessment of actual resources is an integral step in developing a sustainable and effective exercise and physical activity plan. Even when community resources are available, in addition to referrals to community resources, an individual review and physical activity handout for older adults (e.g., NIA, 2009a) offered at the time of assessment are still recommended.

Simple generic physical activity and exercise recommendations have rarely been found to be effective (Handcock & Jenkins, 2003). The following treatment/intervention plans are illustrative of the recommended content.

Best:

- Explore reasons with the patient as to why she is not more active.
- Give need-specific handouts/references with guidelines for goal setting, strategies, specific exercises, examples, and motivational advice (NIA, 2009a, 2009b).
- Direct intervention—For example, an intervention including the components of patient goal setting; written exercise prescriptions; individually tailored physical activity programs; and electronic, mailed, or telephone followup to name a few (AHRQ, 2010).
- Refer the patient to community resources, per the established practice protocol (AHRQ, 2010).

Good:

- Explore reasons with the patient as to why they are not more active.

- Give need-specific handouts/references with guidelines for goal setting, strategies, specific exercises, examples, motivational advice (NIA, 2009a, 2009b).
- Refer the patient to community resources, per the established practice protocol (AHRQ, 2010).

Poor:

- Advise the patient to get more exercise and be more physically active.

What is the plan for follow-up care?

Realistically the health care provider may not be in a position to follow up. Although followup with the health care provider may be recommended, self-monitoring is the goal for most physical activity plans. At the time of assessment or immediate follow-up care, the distributions of resources that can enable the patient to establish a sustainable physical activity plan are essential.

Does the patient's psychosocial history impact how the clinician might treat this patient?

Current evidence underscores the importance of assessment for classification of the patient' physical abilities and specific needs (AGS/BGS, 2010). For example, Ms. I identifies the importance of her friends, which suggests that group activities may be appropriate.

What if the patient also had one or more of the following: Type I diabetes, peripheral vascular disease, or impaired mobility with the use of an assistive device?

As risk increases, options need to become even more specific. The fundamental structure and content of the assessment would remain essentially the same. The assessment results would indicate the specific needs of the patient who is beginning an exercise and physical activity program. For example if the patient had impaired mobility and used a walker, beginning with sitting/chair-based exercises might be appropriate.

Are there any standardized guidelines that the clinician should use to treat this case?

Yes. Recommended guidelines are available from:

Agency for Healthcare Research and Quality (2010). Physical activity and older Americans. Retrieved from http://www.ahrq.gov/ppip/activity.htm

NGC (2007). Physical activity and public health in older adults: Recommendation from the American College of Sports Medicine and the American Heart Association. Retrieved from http://www.ngc.gov/summary/summary.aspx?doc_id=11691&nbr=006038&string=fall s+A

REFERENCES

Agency for Healthcare Research & Quality. (2010). Physical activity and older Americans. Retrieved from http://www.ahrq.gov/ppip/activity.htm

American Geriatric Society/British Geriatric Society. (2010). Clinical practice guidelines: Prevention of falls in older persons. Retrieved from http://www.americangeriatrics.org/health_care_professionals/clinical_practice/clinical_guidelines_recommendations/2010/

Center for Disease Control. Falls—Older adults. Retrieved in 2010 from http://www.cdc.gov/HomeandRecreationalSafety/Falls/index-fs.html

Dukyoo, J., Juhee, L., & Sun-Mi, L. (2009). A meta-analysis of fear of falling treatment programs for the elderly. *Western Journal of Nursing Research, 31*(1), 6–16. doi:10.1177/0193945908320466

Handcock, P., & Jenkins, C. (2003). The green prescription: A field of dreams? *The New Zealand Medical Journal, 116*(11870). Retrieved from http://www.nzma.org.nz/journal/116-1187/713/

National Guideline Clearinghouse. (2007). Physical activity and public health in older adults: Recommendation from the American College of Sports Medicine and the American Heart Association. Retrieved from http://www.ngc.gov/summary/summary.aspx?doc_id=11691&nbr=006038&string=falls+A

National Institute on Aging. (2009a). Exercise and physical activity: Your everyday guide from the National Institute on Aging. Retrieved from http://www.nia.nih.gov/HealthInformation/Publications/ExerciseGuide/

National Institute on Aging. (2009b). Exercise and physical activity: Getting fit for life. Retrieved from http://www.nia.nih.gov/HealthInformation/Publications/exercise.htm

U.S. Department of Health & Human Services. (2010). Healthy people 2020. Retrieved from http://www.healthypeople.gov/hp2020/Objectives/TopicArea.aspx?id=39&TopicArea=Physical+Activity+and+Fitness

ADDITIONAL RESOURCES

American College of Sports Medicine. http://www.acsm.org/AM/Template.cfm?Section=Home_Page&TEMPLATE=CM/HTMLDisplay.cfm&CONTENTID=7764#Over_65_or_50_64

American Society on Aging. http://www.asaging.org/cdc/module6/home.cfm

Center for Disease Control and Prevention. http://www.cdc.gov/physicalactivity/everyone/guidelines/olderadults.html

National Institute on Aging. http://www.nia.nih.gov/healthinformation/publications/exercise.htm

NIH Senior Health. http://nihseniorhealth.gov/exerciseforolderadults/toc.htmlc

Case 3.4 Sick and Tired of Being Sick and Tired

By Kathleen Lovanio, MSN, APRN, F/ANP-BC,
Patricia C. Gantert, MSN, RN-BC,
and Susan A. Goncalves, DNP(c), MS, RN-BC

Mr. D is a 78-year-old obese retired pharmacist who lives alone in an assisted living facility. His wife of 52 years died last year of heart failure. Mr. D has 2 grown sons and 5 grandchildren who live in a neighboring state. When his wife was alive, they would drive to visit their sons and grandchildren 2–3 times a year; but since her death, Mr. D no longer wishes to make the trip alone. He states that he misses his wife dearly but "she is in a better place." He continues to stay in touch with his sons weekly by phone.

Mr. D's oldest son is his durable power of attorney, and his living will has been prepared. His close friends at the assisted living facility have tried encouraging him to participate in card games and other activities that he once enjoyed when his wife was alive; but he refuses their invitations and replies, "I'm too tired, maybe tomorrow." He has been found numerous times napping in a chair in the lounge, and he fell asleep twice in conversation with other residents while eating dinner in the dining room. His friends are concerned about his excessive daytime sleepiness (EDS) and have urged him to talk to his health care provider (HCP) about it. Knowing they were probably right, he made an appointment for a physical examination.

On the way to his medical appointment, he fell asleep at the wheel of his car while stopped at a red light; and a passerby had to knock on his car window to awaken him. Mr. D was clearly shaken over this incident, and he asked his HCP to prescribe something that will help him sleep at night and stay awake during the day. Mr. D reports that his EDS started about 10 months ago, and he attributed it to his 20

Case Studies in Gerontological Nursing for the Advanced Practice Nurse, First Edition.
Edited by Meredith Wallace Kazer, Leslie Neal-Boylan.
© 2012 John Wiley & Sons, Inc. Published 2012 by John Wiley & Sons, Inc.

pound weight gain since his wife died. During that same time, he stopped his 2 mile morning walks. He drinks 4–5 cups of coffee a day and 2–3 glasses of wine at night; he denies tobacco use. On a typical night, he falls asleep on his reclining chair watching TV and goes to bed when he wakes to go to the bathroom. He reports watching TV some nights until 2–3 in the morning. He wakes frequently at night and experiences 2–3 episodes of nocturia with difficulty falling back to sleep. When he wakes in the morning, he feels tired and drowsy for the rest of the day, thus needing frequent naps.

When asked if he snores, Mr. D states, "Oh, yes. In fact, when my wife was alive, we slept in separate bedrooms because of my snoring." He complains of frequent morning headaches but denies dizziness. He wears glasses for reading and states that his last eye examination was over a year ago. He notices no changes in hearing. Mr. D denies chest pain, discomfort, or palpitations. However, he reports shortness of breath (SOB) when walking up one flight of stairs. He complains of moderate lower back and knee pain, which are aggravated by activity and are relieved by rest; extra strength acetaminophen provides little relief.

Mr. D's appetite is good, and he eats most of his meals in the dining room of the assisted living facility. He often orders out for a late-night pizza. He experiences heartburn often, and some nights he wakes up because of burning in his throat. His bowel movements are regular with no complaints of pain or straining. There is no frequency or urgency with urination. He reports having problems with concentration and memory, but no change in mood. In case of an emergency, Mr. D states that he can call a good friend who lives next door.

Mr. D's present medical history includes hypertension (HTN), hyperlipidemia, gastroesophageal reflux disease (GERD), and osteoarthritis (OA). His medications include hydrochlorothiazide (HCTZ), 25 mg; lisinopril, 20 mg, Lipitor, 40 mg; Nexium, 20 mg; Extra Strength Tylenol, 500 mg as needed. He is allergic to penicillin and codeine.

OBJECTIVE

Mr. D is sitting quietly and is hunched over. His hands are over his eyes, and his voice sounds tired when he begins to speak. He appears unshaven, with messy hair. There is no unpleasant odor; his clothes are appropriate, but wrinkled. His vital signs reveal that he is afebrile, 97.8 oral; BP: 156/78; P: 96, regular rhythm; RR: 22, nonlabored; O_2 Sat: 96% on room air; BMI: 34. His eye exam reveals PERRLA, arcus senilis, with lower lids slightly ectopic. His vision and hearing are grossly intact. His oral mucosa is pink, and dentition is good. Further examination reveals negative; carotid pulse without bruits; neck circumference of 18.5 inches; thyroid thin and smooth, no adenopathy; cranial nerves (CN) II–XII are intact. Lungs are clear to auscultation (CTA); no adventitious breath sounds are auscultated. S1 and S2 are heard with no extra heart sounds. There is an early systole grade 2 murmur at the midclavicular line (MCL) 5th intercostal space (ICS) with no radiation.

The upper extremities reveal no obvious deformity, tenderness, or swelling, with the exception of a Heberden node on the distal interphalangeal joint of the left index finger. There is full range of motion in all extremities, and hand-grip strength is equal. His abdomen is protuberant and nontender. There are no masses. Bowels sounds are positive, and digital rectal examination (DRE) is negative. Lower extremities reveal superficial varicosities. His knees are enlarged; and crepitis is noted with flexion and extension, with atrophy of the quadriceps muscle bilaterally. His gait is steady; a timed get-up-and-go test was 18 seconds.

ASSESSMENT

Insomnia: "Insomnia is a common sleep complaint in the older adult and is characterized by difficulty falling asleep, staying asleep, or having nonrestorative sleep, resulting in negative daytime function" (APA, 2000, p. 267).

Obstructive Sleep Apnea (OSA): This case is suggestive of OSA, which is the most common type of sleep-related breathing disorder in older adults. Older age, male gender, family history, neck circumference greater that 17 inches, and obesity are risk factors associated with OSA. OSA is characterized by partial cessation of breathing (hypopnea) and/or complete cessation of breathing (apnea) lasting at least 10 seconds. The number of apneas and hypopnea per hour of sleep is called the "apnea-hypopnea index" (AHI). Events are clinically significant when they last at least 10 seconds and occur 15 or more times per hour of sleep. The cessation of breathing during sleep results in repeated arousals from sleep and reductions in oxygen levels over the course of the night. The two hallmark symptoms of OSA are loud snoring and EDS.

Restless Leg Syndrome (RLS)/Periodic Limb Movements in Sleep (PLMS): RLS is a common neurological movement disorder associated with a sleep complaint, and its prevalence increases with age. Patients with RLS can suffer an irresistible urge to move their legs, which is worse during inactivity and results in discomfort, sleep disturbances, and fatigue. It has been estimated that 90% of individuals with RLS have PLMS. PLMS is characterized by clusters of leg jerks, causing brief arousal or awakening that occurs approximately every 20–40 seconds over the course of a night.

DIAGNOSTICS

Since EDS is associated with significant morbidity and mortality, identification of the cause and management are paramount (Dew et al., 2003). The Epworth Sleepiness Scale (ESS) is a self-administered questionnaire with 8 questions and is one of the most valid and reliable instruments used to assess the severity of EDS (Johns, 1991). On a 4-point scale (0–3), the individual rates their usual chances of dozing off or falling asleep in 8 different situations or activities in which most people engage as part of their daily lives. Each question is answered with a number from 0 (not at all likely to fall asleep) to 3 (very likely to fall asleep). This yields a total score of 0 (minimum) to 24 (maximum). The Pittsburgh Sleep Quality Index (PSQI) is a self-rating scale that measures sleep quality, sleep patterns, and general sleep disturbances; information regarding use of sleep aids; and daytime function over the past month. The PSQI global score has a possible range of 0–24 points. A global score of 5 or more indicates poor sleep quality. The higher the score, the worse the quality (Buysse, Reynolds, Monk, Berman, & Kupfer, 1989). The ESS and PSQI can each be used for an initial assessment and ongoing comparative measurements.

Diagnostic criteria for OSA are based on clinical signs and symptoms and findings identified by polysomnography (PSG). PSG or a sleep study is the "gold standard" for confirmation of the diagnosis and the severity of OSA (Figure 3.4.1) (Epstein et al., 2009). A comprehensive PSG includes measurements to document the following:

- Sleep-disordered breathing (oxygen saturation, rib cage and abdominal movement, nasal and oral airflow, and snoring sounds
- Data regarding sleep and stages of sleep (electroencephalography (EEG), electrical activity of the brain, electrooculography (EOG), recording of eye movements
- Electromyogram (EMG) to evaluate and record the electrical activity produced by skeletal muscles) and electrocardiogram and leg electromyogram to document the presence of periodic leg movements.

Because EDS can also result from hypothyroidism, anemia, cognitive impairment, and depression, the following laboratory work and screening tests will be performed:

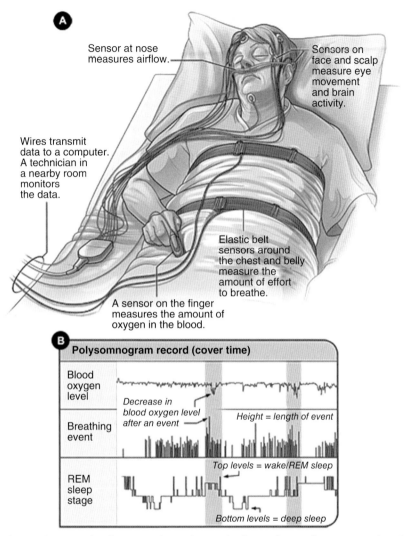

Figure 3.4.1. This illustration shows the standard setup for a polysomnogram (PSG). In Figure 3.4.1A, the patient lies in a bed with sensors attached to his body. In Figure 3.4.1B, the PSG recording shows the blood oxygen level, breathing event, and rapid eye movement (REM) sleep stage over time. (Provided by the National Heart, Lung, and Blood Institute as a part of the National Institutes of Health and the U.S. Department of Health and Human Services.)

- Complete blood count (CBC)
- Thyroid stimulating hormone (TSH)
- Geriatric Depression Scale (GDS)
- Mini Mental State Examination (MMSE).

His CBC and TSH were within normal limits. Geriatric Depression Scale (GDS): 3; Mini Mental State Examination (MMSE): 27; PSQI: 19;

Epworth Sleepiness Scale: 19 (normal is <10/24). PSG results indicated that during the first 75 minutes of sleep Mr. D experienced 83 apneas and 28 hypopneas for an elevated AHI of 97 events per hour. His lowest SaO_2 during the pre-CPAP period was 73%. CPAP was applied at 5 cm H_2O and sequentially titrated to a final pressure of 11 cm H_2O. At this pressure his AHI was 4 events per hour and the low SaO_2 increased to 90%. No evidence of RLS/PLMS noted.

CRITICAL THINKING

What is the most likely differential diagnosis and why?

Are any referrals needed?

What is the plan of treatment?

What is the plan for follow-up care?

Does the patient's psychosocial history impact how the clinician might treat this patient?

What if this patient lived in a long-term care setting?

What if the patient had dementia?

Are there any standardized guidelines that the clinician should use to assess or treat this case?

RESOLUTION

What is the most likely differential diagnosis and why?
Difficulty falling asleep or staying asleep for at least 1 month and impairment in daytime functioning, resulting from difficulty sleeping, are required for a diagnosis of insomnia.

Mr. D definitely meets these criteria; however, at this point it is important to determine if the insomnia is caused by a primary or comorbid condition. Poor sleep hygiene, lifestyle choices, pain of osteo-arthritis, nocturia, medications, and multiple chronic conditions can all be contributing to Mr. D's insomnia.

The prevalence of OSA in older adults has been reported to be as high as 70% in men and 56% in women (Ancoli-Isreal, Kripke, & Klauber, 1991). Mr. D's gender, age, obesity (BMI of 34), neck circumference greater than 17 inches, and hypertension put him at high risk for the development of OSA. Moreover, Mr. D presented with the two cardinal symptoms of OSA—EDS and snoring. These findings make this case highly suspect for the OSA. Results of the PSG confirmed the diagnosis of OSA and ruled out RLS/PLMS.

Are any referrals needed?
In this case, due to Mr. D's dangerously high EDS and hypertension, a referral to a sleep specialist for a sleep study is mandatory.

What is the plan of treatment?
While medications are traditionally used to treat insomnia, recent studies have shown that cognitive behavioral therapy (CBT) is more effective and is recommended as the first line of treatment of insomnia (Bloom et al., 2009). The cognitive portion of CBT deals with misconceptions or unrealistic expectations about sleep (e.g., the requirement of 8 hours or more of sleep), while the behavioral component involves a combination of sleep restriction therapy, stimulus control, and teaching sleep hygiene techniques. Sleep restriction consists of curtailing the amount of time spent in bed to increase the percentage of time asleep. This improves the patients sleep efficiency (time asleep/time in bed). For example, a person who reports staying in bed for 8 hours but sleeping an average of 5 hours per night would initially be told to decrease sleep time in bed to 5 hours. The allowable time in bed per night is increased 15–30 minutes as sleep efficiency improves. Stimulus control treatment consists of the behavioral instructions of going to bed only when sleepy; using the bed and bedroom only for sleep and sex; getting out of bed if unable to fall asleep after 15–20 minutes and going into another room, returning only when sleepy; having a regular time to get out of bed in the morning, even if one only had a little sleep the night(s) before; and not taking naps during the day. Sleep hygiene includes a variety of behavioral changes such as avoiding caffeine, nicotine, alcohol, exercise, and heavy meals at bedtime; reducing light, noise, and extreme temperatures in the sleep environment; limiting bedtime fluid intake; avoiding daytime naps; limiting time in bed; and maintaining a regular sleep schedule.

Continuous positive airway pressure (CPAP) is the first line of treatment for OSA. CPAP involves wearing a mask that is placed over the nose and is connected to a machine that generates positive air pressure. The CPAP machine blows air at a prescribed pressure (titrated pressure) at which most apneas and hypopneas will be prevented.

What is the plan for follow-up care?
OSA is a chronic illness and requires long-term care management. Patients come in frequently for followup, especially during the first 6 months after the start of treatment, to assess their response to treatment and to monitor their adherence to CPAP. A weight loss program should be part of the treatment plan in overweight patients. Patients with OSA require followup for their comorbidities, especially patients with hypertension. Patients treated with CPAP may have a change in their

requirements for antihypertensive medications (Bloom, et al., 2009). Improvements in both the ESS and PSQI can be used for ongoing comparative measurements.

Does the patient's psychosocial history impact how the clinician might treat this patient?

Social isolation and bereavement can lead to sleep complaints. Mr. D's dangerously high EDS is preventing him from taking part in activities with residents of the assisted living facility. While he misses his wife, he accepted her death and proceeded through the grieving process appropriately. Mr. D should be encouraged to stay socially and physically active.

What if this patient lived in a long-term care setting?

It has been estimated that 50%–75% of long-term care residents have at least mild OSA. OSA is associated with cognitive impairment, falls, agitated behaviors, and increased mortality (Martin & Fung, 2007). Studies have not been conducted on CPAP use in long term care, but recent findings in community-dwelling older adults with dementia have the same level of compliance with CPAP as other patients without dementia. Martin and Fung (2007) report that some nursing home residents who used CPAP prior to institutionalization continued to use CPAP while in the nursing home. CPAP should be considered the treatment of choice among individuals in the long-term care setting with OSA.

What if the patient had dementia?

There is considerable evidence that dementia affects sleep, and the severity of the sleep disturbance increases with the severity of the dementia (Ancoli-Israel et al., 2008). Individuals with dementia may experience EDS, nighttime wandering, confusion, and agitation (sundowning). In community-dwelling older adults with dementia, it is important to address and manage sleep disturbances to postpone institutionalization due to caregiver burden and distress. With sleep disturbances, these individuals should be assessed for primary sleep disorders and screened for depression. Their medications should be reviewed, and a thorough assessment of pain from medical illnesses should be done. Depending on the severity of the dementia, an overnight sleep study may not always be appropriate. In this case, actigraphy (a non-invasive method of monitoring sleep patterns and circadian rhythms) may be useful. Treatment should be guided by the specific disorder identified, and maintenance of regular physical activity and social interaction should be encouraged.

Are there any standardized guidelines that the clinician should use to assess or treat this case?

The adult OSA task force of the American Academy of Sleep Medicine developed evidenced based guidelines to assist health care providers in the evaluation, management, and long-term care of OSA found at http://www.aasmnet.org/Resources/ClinicalGuidelines/OSA_ Adults.pdf.

Evidence-based recommendations for the assessment and management of sleep disorders in older adults have been developed by an expert panel of professionals with expertise in sleep disorders and in the clinical care of older adults. These can be found at http://www. uw-crmsd.org/handouts/GR_Vitiello_handout.pdf.

With regard to excessive sleepiness, evidence-based geriatric nursing protocols for best practice can be accessed at http://www.guideline. gov/summary/summary.aspx?ss=15&doc_id=12263&string=; http:// www.guideline.gov/Compare/comparison.aspx?file=OSAPNEA4.inc.

REFERENCES

American Psychiatric Association. Diagnostic and Statistical Manual of Mental Disorders, 4th Ed. Text Revision. DSM-IV-TR. Washington, D.C.: APA, 2000: 267.

Ancoli-Isreal, S., Kripke, D. F., & Klauber, M. R. (1991). Sleep disordered breathing in community dwelling elderly. *Sleep, 14*, 486–495.

Ancoli-Israel, S., Palmer, B. W., Cooke, J. R., Corey-Bloom, J., Fiorentino, L., Natarajan, L., . . . Loredo, J. S. (2008). Cognitive effects of treating obstructive sleep apnea in Alzheimer's disease: A randomized controlled study. *Journal of the American Geriatrics Society, 56*(11), 2076–2071.

Ayalon, L., Ancoli-Israel, S., & Drummond, SP. (2009). Altered brain activation during response inhibition in obstructive sleep apnea. *Journal of Sleep Research, 18*(2), 204–208.

Bloom, H. G., Ahmed, I., Alessi, C. A., Ancoli-Israel, S., Buysse, D., Kryger, M. H., . . . Zee, P. C. (2009). Evidence-based recommendations for the assessment and management of sleep disorders in older persons. *Journal of the American Geriatrics Society, 57*(5), 761–789. doi:10.1111/j.1532-5415.2009. 02220.x

Buysse, D. J., Reynolds, C. F., Monk, T. H., Berman, S. R., & Kupfer, D. J. (1989). The Pittsburgh Sleep Quality Index: A new instrument for psychiatric practice and research. *Journal of Psychiatric Research, 28*(2), 193–213.

Dew, M. A., Hoch, C. C., Buysse, D. J., Monk, T. H., Begley, A. E.., Houck, P. R., . . . Reynolds, C. F. (2003). Healthly older adults' sleep predicts all-cause mortality at 4 to 19 years of follow-up. *Psychosomatic Medicine, 65*, 63–73.

Epstein, L. J., Kristo, D., Strollo, P. J., Friedman, N., Malhotra, A., Patil, S. P., . . . Weinstein, M. D. (2009). Clinical guideline for the evaluation and long-term care of obstructive sleep apnea in adults. *Journal of Clinical Sleep Medicine, 5*(3), 263–276.

Johns, M. W. (1991). A new method for measuring daytime sleepiness: The Epworth Sleepiness Scale. *Sleep, 14*, 540–545.

Martin, J. L., & Fung, C. H. (2007). Quality indicators for the care of sleep disorders in vulnerable elders. *Journal of the American Geriatrics Society*, 55(52), S424–S430. doi:10.1111/j1532-5415.2007.01351.x

ADDITIONAL RESOURCES

Medline Plus National Library of Medicine. http://www.nlm.nih.gov/medlineplus/tutorials/sleepdisorders/htm/index.htm

My Healthy Vet—United States Department of Veteran Affairs. http://www.myhealth.va.gov

National Center on Sleep Disorders Research National Institutes of Health (NCSDR). http://www.nhlbi.nih.gov/about/ncsdr

Case 3.5 To Screen or Not to Screen

By Meredith Wallace Kazer, PhD, APRN, A/GNP-BC, FAAN

Mr. C, a 75-year-old man, presents to the primary care practice for his 6-month checkup. He has visited every 3–6 months over the past 6 years. Mr. C is generally healthy, with well-managed hypertension and coronary artery disease. In addition to his semiannual visits to our practice, he also sees a cardiologist annually. He has no surgical history. He lives at home with his wife and works part-time at a local grocery store. He has a son and a daughter, who are both married professionals and live close by. He has 4 grandchildren. He has an occasional social drink, but does not smoke. His income comes primarily from social security and a small pension from his previous career as a banker. He also supplements his income with his part-time job. He is very involved with his family and attends Catholic services weekly. Mr. C is generally in good health and visits his primary care provider every 6 months for followup of his chronic medical illnesses. His family is healthy. Both parents are deceased. His father died in his "fifties" of a heart attack. His mother recently died at age 92.

During this visit, Mr. C's review of systems is negative. He denies shortness of breath (SOB), dyspnea on exertion (DOE), chest pain, palpitations, headaches, dizziness, nausea, vomiting, or diarrhea. He complains of a little urinary hesitancy and difficulty starting his stream. This has been going on for "some time now". He says it does not bother him much and he is getting used to it. He denies pain and burning on urination. He denies a history of urinary tract infection or problems with his prostate gland. His bowels are regular with an occasional need

Case Studies in Gerontological Nursing for the Advanced Practice Nurse, First Edition.
Edited by Meredith Wallace Kazer, Leslie Neal-Boylan.
© 2012 John Wiley & Sons, Inc. Published 2012 by John Wiley & Sons, Inc.

for prune juice or Metamucil. He is sexually active with his wife, and sexual function is adequate with the assistance of oral erectile agents. His medications include HCTZ, 25 mg; lisinopril, 20 mg; Lipitor, 20 mg every day; and Metamucil and Cialis as needed. He has no known allergies (NKA).

OBJECTIVE

Mr. C is awake, alert, and oriented with an erect posture. He appears clean and well kept. His clothes are appropriate. His vitals are height: 5 ft 9 inches; weight: 180 lb; BP: 164/92; P: 110; 02 sat: 99%. He is afebrile with a temperature of 97.8. His lungs are clear. Cardiac exam reveals a regular heart rate, S1, S2; and no adventitious sounds. His abdomen is soft and nontender, and his bowel sounds are present in all 4 quadrants. He has no scars or lesions on his abdomen, and his umbilicus is midline. His skin is dry and intact. He has no pedal edema and has positive pedal pulses. His eyes reveal clear normal sclerae with PERRLA. His ears reveal mild wax buildup and normal tympanic membranes bilaterally. His mouth indicates normal oral mucosa. Neurological exam reveals 2+ deep tendon reflexes bilaterally and equal strength. His gait is normal, and he has full range of motion of all extremities. His digital rectal examination (DRE) reveals no abnormalities.

ASSESSMENT

Urinary tract infection: Mr. C's urinary hesitancy and difficulty starting stream may be related to an infectious process. It is important to note in older adults that the fever response to infection is variable. Thus, the absence of a fever does not rule out infection in this case.

Benign Prostatic Hypertrophy (BPH): BPH is very common among older men and provides a good rationale for his symptoms. The disease entails a benign enlargement of the prostate gland, which anatomically surrounds the urethra. Inflammation of the gland puts pressure on the urethra and manifests in the types of symptoms Mr. C describes.

Prostate cancer: In the United States, prostate cancer is the most commonly diagnosed cancer in men (American Cancer Society [ACS], 2008), and 64% of all prostate cancers are diagnosed in men older than 65 years (ACS, 2008). A tumor growing in the prostate gland will produce pressure on the urethra and manifest in the symptoms described.

DIAGNOSTICS

An important point to consider is whether or not this patient should have had a PSA test at all. Controversy exists as to whether the PSA test should be used to screen men for the presence of disease as the goal of screening is to decrease mortality and improve quality of life. The U.S. Preventive Services Task force has recently recommended that men over 75 years of age forego PSA screening due to limited benefit and increased risk for physical and psychological harm (2008). During this routine visit, the patient agrees to have a complete metabolic panel drawn, complete blood count (CBC), and prostate specific antigen (PSA). Because of the urinary symptoms, the clinician also orders a urinalysis, culture and sensitivity. Diagnosis of prostate cancer may be confirmed following biopsy guided by transrectal ultrasound. The ultrasound is used in order to direct the placement of the needle to extract the specimens. The urologist may opt for a transperineal or transrectal approach to perform the biopsy (ACS, 2008). A summary of the USPSTF recommendations is shown below:

> The USPSTF concludes that the current evidence is insufficient to assess the balance of benefits and harms of prostate cancer screening in men younger than age 75 years. Thus, the USPSTF recommends against screening for prostate cancer in men age 75 years or older. This recommendation is a level D. This means that the USPSTF recommends against it because there is moderate or high certainty that the screening has no net benefit or that the harms outweigh the benefits.
>   Accessed from http://www.uspreventiveservicestaskforce.org/uspstf/uspsprca.htm

The CBC and metabolic panel are within normal limits. The urinalysis is negative; the PSA reading is 6.2ng/dL. His readings over the past 4 years are shown in the Figure 3.5.1.

CRITICAL THINKING

What is the most likely differential diagnosis and why?

What is the plan of treatment?

What is the plan for follow-up care?

Does the patient's psychosocial history impact how the clinician might treat this patient?

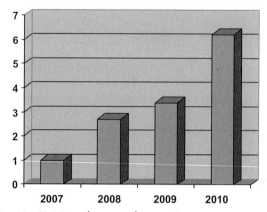

Figure 3.5.1. Mr. C's PSA values over the past 4 years.

What if the patient also had kidney failure?

What are the best treatment options for this patient with each of the differentials listed?

Are there any standardized guidelines that the clinician should use to assess or treat this case?

RESOLUTION

What is the most likely differential diagnosis and why?
Urinary tract infection (UTI) is an obvious differential given the symptoms that Mr. C presented with. UTIs are relatively rare in adult males, but they increase dramatically after the age of 60 related to conditions of the prostate (Howes & Pillow, 2009). A UTI could be confirmed or ruled out with a simple in-office normal urinalysis. In this case, Mr. C did not have a UTI. If he had had a urinary tract infection, the urinalysis would have revealed white blood cells. If this had been the case, culture and sensitivity testing of the urine sample would have revealed an antibiotic that would have been appropriate to treat him.

The next differential would be benign prostatic hyperplasia. Gerber (2009) states that BPH is a condition resulting from benign enlargement of the prostate gland. This is very common in adult males over the age of 50. Urinary symptoms result from increased pressure on the urethra from the surrounding enlarged prostate. An enlarged prostate can easily be determined through the use of a digital rectal examination (DRE) in the office or upon referral to a urologist. BPH may also be accompanied by an elevated PSA value. BPH is effectively treated with alpha-1-adrenergic antagonists to relax prostate and bladder muscle contractility—tamsulosin (Flomax); terazosin (Hytrin). Men should be cautioned about the hypotensive effects of these medications. Alternative medications in the form of 5-alpha-reductase inhibitors to reduce the size of the prostate gland (finasteride [Proscar]; dutasteride [Avodart]) may be prescribed but could have a side effect of erectile dysfunction. In the case of Mr. C, a digital rectal exam revealed a normal size prostate. However, he was referred to a urologist for further evaluation.

What is most curious in the case of Mr. C is his rapidly rising PSA value over the past year. Normal PSA values are between 0- and 4.0 ng/mL; values greater than 4.0 may warrant additional followup, depending on a number of patient characteristics including but not limited to age, ethnicity, body mass index, height, and a family history of prostate cancer. The PSA levels revealed in the graph are very suspicious for prostate cancer. Most telling is the doubling of the PSA values over the past year. However, elevated PSA levels may also be the result of benign prostatic hypertrophy, older age, inflammation, or ejaculation within 2 days of testing (ACS, 2008). Values lower than 4.0 in African American men and those who are obese also call for additional followup by a health care provider, as research has shown that these factors may result in high risk for prostate cancer. (Freedland et al., 2008; Sanchez-Ortiz et al., 2006).

What is the plan of treatment?
In the case of Mr. C, symptoms have been present for some time; and his PSA values have been gradually increasing over the past several years. However, over the past year, the PSA has doubled, which is cause for concern and referral. The next steps for Mr. C would be referral to a urologist. The diagnostic testing would likely entail a digital rectal exam (DRE). DRE is helpful in finding abnormities in the prostate; but the exam covers only the small, palpable portion of the gland. Thus, if a tumor is in an area of the prostate gland that is not palpable, it may not be detected. Transrectal ultrasound (TRUS) guided biopsy of the prostate gland would likely be the next step in the diagnosis of this patient. The biopsy results are categorized using a grading system, referred to as the Gleason Grading system. This system assigns a grade to each of the two largest areas of cancer in the biopsy samples. Grades range from 1 to 5, with 1 being the least aggressive and 5 the most aggressive. The two grades are then added together to produce a Gleason score. A score of 2 through 4 is considered low grade; 5 through 7, intermediate grade; and 8 through 10, high grade. A high Gleason score indicates that the cancer is more likely to grow quickly (ACS, 2008). Mr. C had a positive biopsy for Gleason stage 6 prostate cancer.

Treatment options for Mr. C include radical prostatectomy, external beam radiotherapy, brachytherapy, cryotherapy, and active surveillance (AS). The treatment decision will be made by Mr. C in discussion with his family and health care provider. However, given his age and the modest survival benefits of treatment, as well as the fact that all available therapeutic modalities for localized prostate cancer result in significant risk of adverse effects such as sexual dysfunction, urethral strictures, urinary incontinence, and bowel problems, active surveillance may be a good option. Active surveillance is becoming a more accepted prostate cancer management option. For men like Mr. C, with early-stage, low-risk prostate cancer, AS provides an alternative to surgery or radiation therapy. With AS, men make the decision to actively monitor their disease with the knowledge that treatment remains an option.

What is the plan for follow-up care?
Regardless of the treatment choice, Mr. C will continue followup with a urologist. However, he will continue to visit primary care for followup of other medical problems. During these visits, he should be questioned to ensure that he visits the urologist every 6 months at a minimum. PSA values can be drawn with annual blood work and sent to the urologist for followup. Of course, changes in PSAs should be reported to the patient and urologist immediately, as rising PSAs after treatment are problematic in the prostate population. PSAs should still be monitored after treatment completion.

Does the patient's psychosocial history impact how the clinician might treat this patient?
The fact that Mr. C is married underscores the need to determine the impact of treatment on his sexual relationship. Thus, the adverse effects of treatment should be discussed with this patient prior to decision making. While the patient's urologist or medical oncologist will discuss this, the patient may still have questions regarding the impact of treatment on urinary and sexual structures and the subsequent impact on his quality of life. These impacts must be considered carefully.

What if the patient also had kidney failure?
As kidney failure has a potential to shorten life span and would prevent radical treatments, the presence of this disease would greatly impact treatment options. In conjunction with the patient's age, a chronic illness such as kidney failure may make this patient a good candidate for active surveillance above other treatment options.

What are the best treatment options for this patient with each of the differentials listed?
Given the patient's age at diagnosis and cancer characteristics, active surveillance is a good prostate cancer management option. In this case, Mr. C will actively monitor his disease by visits to the urologist every 3 or 6 months with the knowledge that treatment remains an option if the cancer progresses.

Are there any standardized guidelines that the clinician should use to assess or treat this case?
The American Urological Association has published guidelines on the treatment of localized prostate cancer. This is available at http://www. auanet.org/content/guidelines-and-quality-care/clinical-guidelines. cfm.

REFERENCES

American Cancer Society. (2008). *American cancer society. Cancer facts & figures 2008*. Atlanta, GA: American Cancer Society.

Freedland, S. J., Wen, J., Wuerstle, M., Shah, A., Lai, D., & Moalej, B. (2008). Obesity is a significant risk factor for prostate cancer at the time of biopsy. *Urology, 72*(5), 1102–1105.

Gerber, G. (2009). Benign prostatic hyperplasia (BPH, enlarged prostate). Retrieved from http://www.medicinenet.com/benign_prostatic_hyperplasia/article.htm

Howes, D. S., & Pillow, M. T. (2009). Urinary tract infection. Male. EMedicine. Retrieved from http://emedicine.medscape.com/article/778578-overview

Sanchez-Ortiz, R. F., Troncoso, P., Babaian, R. J., Lloreta, J., Johnston, D. A., & Pettaway, C. A. (2006). African-American men with nonpalpable prostate cancer exhibit greater tumor volume than matched white men. *Cancer, 107*(1), 75–82.

ADDITIONAL RESOURCES

American Cancer Society. http://www.cancer.org/docroot/lrn/lrn_0.asp

American Urological Association treatment guidelines and resources. http:// www.auanet.org/content/guidelines-and-quality-care/clinical-guidelines. cfm

John Hopkins Prostate Health Alerts. http://www.johnshopkinshealthalerts. com/alerts_index/prostate_disorders/25-1.html

National Cancer Institute. http://www.cancer.gov/cancertopics/types/ prostate

Us TOO. http://www.ustoo.org/

*This case is reprinted in part in *Clinical Case Studies for the Family Nurse Practitioner*. (Neal-Boylan, L., Ed.). Ames: Wiley-Blackwell.

Section 4

Environments of Care

Case 4.1 Who Says I Can't Go Home

By Antoinette Larkin, RGN, H. Dip. Gerontology, and
Claire Welford, RGN, DipNS, BNS–Hons., MSc, PGC–TLHE

Mr. J was admitted to a medical unit from the emergency department following a fall at home. He was found by his visiting clinician and was confused and disorientated. Mr. J is an 86-year-old man and lives alone. His home conditions are considered substandard despite support from his neighbors and from community health services. The clinician had previously referred Mr. J to a community social worker due to her concerns for his safety as a result of decreasing mobility and sight. Community professionals had highlighted the need to declutter and clean Mr. J's house, but the services to facilitate this did not follow. Mr. J is currently only receiving "meals-on-wheels", which are being delivered to his home. In early 2009, he was offered a room in a residential home for the winter months; but after considering this option, he chose to stay at home.

In recent months, Mr. J had notable deterioration in his mobility; and there was increasing evidence that he was having difficulty managing himself at home. He had not attended any of his outpatient appointments, even though both his hearing and eyesight were becoming severely impaired and he had begun to have memory problems. Again the clinician offered residential care options, but Mr. J declined all offers and insisted he wanted to remain at home for the time being.

A month or so after the initial fall, Mr. J fell again and was found by his neighbors on the side of a main road close to his home. Mr. J's clinician again offered the option of residential care, but to no avail;

Case Studies in Gerontological Nursing for the Advanced Practice Nurse, First Edition.
Edited by Meredith Wallace Kazer, Leslie Neal-Boylan.
© 2012 John Wiley & Sons, Inc. Published 2012 by John Wiley & Sons, Inc.

and Mr. J requested that he wanted to continue living at home. A neighbor contacted the clinician informing her that large amounts of money were missing from Mr J's home. This highlighted his vulnerability to theft. As a result of the concerns raised, a case conference was organized. The following weekend, Mr. J fell at home, appeared disorientated, and was found by neighbors to be confused. He was brought in by ambulance to the emergency department, where he denied any collapse or episodes of chest pain or dizziness. He was orientated to time, place, and person but not to year. He had an injury to his left ankle; and, on further questioning, he admitted that he had fallen and hurt his knee the previous week. He stated that he slipped when walking and had no loss of consciousness. He presented with a cough, which he stated had been present for a week. Mr. J's past medical history includes osteoarthritis and osteopenia. His medications include calcium; iron; omeprazole, 20 mg OD; and paracetomol, 1 g as needed. He has no known allergies (NKA).

OBJECTIVE

Mr. J presented as a clinically stable, unkempt older man in no apparent distress. His temperature is 96.2; pulse: 85 bpm; BP: 160/78; O_2 sat: 97% on room air; weight: 156 lb; height: 5 ft 7 inches; BMI: 23.8kg/m^2. His MMSE score was 9/30. He has a cough that is productive of white sputum. On examination, his chest clear. This patient is hard of hearing and is disoriented to place and time. His motor exam reveals an unsteady gait. His lungs fields are clear, and his heart sounds and borders are within normal limits. His ECG reveals a rate of 69 and normal sinus rhythm.

ASSESSMENT

Neurocognitive changes and ataxia: Mr. J's recent falls may be related to a number of factors. The cause of the falls needs to be established.

Hypertension: Blood pressure on admission is in the high category. This may also contribute to falls or vascular dementia.

Residential care or discharge back home: Mr. J's recent self-neglect suggests that he is finding it difficult to care for himself at home. His current cognitive ability for making decisions needs to be determined.

DIAGNOSTICS

A full laboratory panel, including complete blood count and electrolytes is needed. Dehydration and/or alterations in electrolyte levels may indicate heart disease, which may have led to the falls. A sputum sample is needed for culture and sensitivity due to Mr. J's cough. A routine urinalysis to rule out a UTI—often a factor in increased confusion in older people—should be ordered, as well as BP monitoring due to the raised high blood pressure recording in the emergency room. A CT scan of the brain was ordered to establish if there are any abnormalities or infarcts either causing, or as a result of, numerous falls. He should have telemetry for 24 hours to out rule cardiac arrhythmias which may also cause falls.

CRITICAL THINKING

What is the most likely differential diagnosis?

What other factors may be contributing?

What is the plan of treatment?

How can the interaction between geriatric syndromes prove to be life threatening?

What is the significance the blood test results?

What medications is the patient taking? Could there be possible side effects impacting on the patient?

How can a health care professional help an older person make autonomous decisions when there are signs of neurocognitive changes in their health status?

RESOLUTION

What is the most likely differential diagnosis?
The most obvious differential may be neurocognitive changes and possible vascular dementia related to hypertension and/or CVA. Dementia is a condition in which there is a gradual loss of brain function; it is a decline in cognitive/intellectual functioning. The main symptoms are usually loss of memory, confusion, problems with speech and understanding, changes in personality and behavior and an increased reliance on others for the activities of daily living (Alzheimer's

Association, 2011). The CT of the brain reported a small lacunar infarct and CVA. The small lacunar infarct reported from the CT brain scan may be classed as small vessel disease or microangiopathic dementia, which predominantly involves central white matter and subcortical structures (Jellinger, 2008).

Given the case history and list of presenting symptoms, the next possible differential is physical self-neglect (including decreasing vision, hearing, and mobility as a result of nonattendance at outpatient appointments). According to Pavlou and Lachs (2006), self-neglect in older adults is a complex phenomenon characterized by inattention to health and hygiene, typically stemming from an inability or unwillingness to access potentially remediating services. Some aspects of self-neglect resemble common geriatric syndromes (e.g., falling, incontinence).

What other factors may be contributing?
Increased confusion may be contributing to some, if not all, of his falls. Also, Mr. J's home environment was described as being in a state of disrepair. It is most likely damp, unclean, and cold. The clutter and general poor environment in his home may be additional risk factors for falls.

What is the plan of treatment?
In the case of Mr. J, full interdisciplinary care is indicated. Physical therapy reported that minimal assistance of 1 person was required to transfer Mr. J. Nursing staff reported to the dieticians that Mr. J was tolerating a full diet with little assistance, but was observed coughing when drinking fluids; so they suggested a speech and language therapist evaluation. The dieticians also advised nursing staff to monitor Mr. J's intake and weight weekly. They advised that there was no need for nutritional supplements at present. The speech and language therapist reported that Mr. J was very communicative with a history of a cough for several years, even without oral intake. Mr. J was started on normal fluids from a glass and was well controlled; oral phase timely swallow triggered with adequate laryngeal movement, no evidence of post swallow pooling, and no wet voice. Mr. J expressed concerns that he would not be allowed to return home.

The CT brain scan showed a CVA and also a small lacunar infarct; thus Mr. J was commenced on an angiotensin II antagonist, olmesartan, 15 mg for lowering the BP, and meloxicam for chronic pain in his left knee. It is planned for him to continue physiotherapy for vascular gait. A request for a psychiatric consultation was made in order to ascertain his capacity. The psychiatric clinician evaluated Mr. J and found no evidence of agitation. Mr. J was mildly depressed, but was not psychotic; however, Mr. J was unable to give names of supportive friends or family on whom he could count for help at home. Furthermore, Mr. J showed no insight into his cognitive and functional deficits and had no appreciation of the possible risks associated with living alone. Thus it was determined that Mr. J lacked the capacity to make an informed decision in relation to his ongoing care in view of his cognitive deficits and decreased functional status. The psychiatric clinician also advised commencing an antidepressant without anticholinergic effects, such as a serotonin reuptake inhibitor. He was started on an NMDA—receptor antagonist memantine, 5 mg, and this was to be titrated up slowly to a maximum dose of 20 mg.

The psychiatric clinician further reported that the patient had limited insight and that he believed that if he were able to walk on his own he would be able to go home. He was informed that community services and neighbors were concerned for his well-being and that all involved in his care now felt that he needed full-time care in a nursing home setting. He informed the team that he had previously spent time in a nursing home close to home and that he did not like it there. The desire to go home continued. Mr. J again expressed his unhappiness about the suggestion that he go to a nursing home and again expressed that he wanted to return home. The risks were explained again to Mr. J; however, he was anxious about his house and his dog and about looking after his personal belongings. He expressed that he would not be happy to have anyone else touch his personal items. The health care team attempted to contact a cousin of Mr. J's to no avail; a neighbor was the only person visiting, washing, and providing clean laundry to Mr. J prior to his admission to hospital. This neighbor expressed concerns for Mr. J's safety and informed the team that the conditions at his home were not good and that Mr. J had had a large sum of money taken from his house on one occasion.

How can the interaction between geriatric syndromes prove to be life threatening?

According to Musso and Nunez (2006) geriatrics has described three entities—confusional syndrome, incontinence, and gait disorders—calling them geriatric giants. These geriatric giants can appear as an acute event or as an exacerbation of an already-existing state, often being the only clinical expression of various diseases such as pneumonia, urinary infection, and cardiac infarction. Possession of a combination of any two of these can be life threatening for the older person as one illness can impact or exacerbate the other. In Mr. J's case, he was experiencing confusional syndrome and gait disorders.

What is the significance of the blood test results?

The lab values were primarily within normal limits (HB :10.7; MCV: 99.2; Plt: 201; WBC: 5.9; neut: 4.0; urea: 5.2; creat: 85; free T4: 13.1; TSH: 3.15; and K+: 3.6). However, mild anemia was present. Anemia can contribute to falls in older people (Penninx et al., 2005; Dharmarajan &

Norkus, 2004). Raised potassium levels may indicate heart disease. Urea and electrolyte levels can indicate altered physiological functioning.

What medications is the patient taking? Could there be possible side effects impacting on the patient?

The most common drug-related side effects for older people are from anticholinergics (Mintzer & Burns, 2000). Side effects include insecure movements, falls without obvious reasons, and blurred vision. Anticholinergics can affect memory and cause confusion and disorientation. Reasons older people may be particularly susceptible to these side effects may be due to reduced metabolism and elimination and also age-related deficits in cholinergic neurotransmission.

How can a health care professional help an older person make autonomous decisions when there are signs of neurocognitive changes in their health status?

Mr. J's home circumstances impact his discharge plan. Concerns had been expressed about his safety if he continues to live at home. However, it is Mr. J's expressed wish to return home. This raises an ethical dilemma for the interdisciplinary care team—should Mr. J be assisted with making an autonomous decision or should the care team exercise their duty of care to the patient and thus ensure his safety? Mr. J has no family members involved in his care and has only one neighbor keeping an eye on him. Agich (2004, p. 6) defines autonomy as "equivalent to liberty, self-rule, self-determination, freedom of will, dignity, integrity, individuality, independence, responsibility, and self-knowledge", whilst containing the qualities of self-assertion, critical reflection, freedom from obligation, absence of external causation, and knowledge of one's own interest (Agich, 2004). Beauchamp and Childress (1994) refer to what makes life one's own and how personal preferences and choices shape it. The following 4 integral ingredients help to define personal autonomy: 1) being free from the controlling influence of others, 2) being free from limitations that prevent meaningful choice, 3) being free from inadequate understanding, and 4) being able to freely act in accordance with a self-chosen plan. Burkhardt and Nathaniel (2002) believe that in order to achieve the balance between personal autonomy and restrictive health care institutions the following fundamental elements are necessary: 1) respect, 2) the ability to direct and determine personal goals, c) the capacity to be involved in a decision-making process, and d) the freedom to act on any choices made. Most importantly, personal autonomy for the older person is not diminished by their inability to independently perform self-care; instead, they can still exercise the ability to delegate their care requirements to others.

Assessment of capacity is often facilitated through use of the Mini-Mental State Examination (MMSE). Folstein, Folstein, and McHugh

(1975) developed the Mini-Mental State Examination (MMSE) and stated that it is a brief neuropsychological test for evaluating cognitive status. MMSE scores are affected by age and education level, with lower scores being associated with increasing age and lower educational level. According to Dufouil et al. (2000) the norm for an 85-year-old man is 26/30. Mr. J's scores varied from 9/30 to 3/30 to 14/30. Some of these fluctuating readings may be attributed to the hospital environment as well as his decreased vision and hearing.

A meeting to discuss Mr. J's discharge plan was subsequently arranged. Mr. J and community health care professionals were present. Some issues were readdressed, for example, Mr. J's safety. Prior to admission, Mr. J had a small dog living with him in his house and would let him out during the day. Since Mr. J's admission to the hospital, the small dog has been locked in the house. The neighbor has been feeding the dog and noticed that there is now excrement everywhere and that the house has deteriorated more significantly. Mr. J was well aware of all of this, but he still insisted on going home. With much encouragement, his good neighbors agreed to clean his house prior to his discharge; and Mr. J gave permission for them to do so. Home care services were ordered and day care was also offered, but Mr. J declined these.

Capacity was still a concern; however, it was felt that his impaired vision and hearing were also likely contributing to the poor MMSE scores, rather than any significant neurocognitive changes. Nursing staff from the unit confirmed that Mr. J was now walking out to the toilet unaided and was placing a newspaper outside his door so that he could find his way back to his room.

On review, Mr. J continued to have an unsteady gait, was continent, eating a good diet, washing his face and hands in the sink, and dressing himself; but he would need a fully assisted shower weekly. Prior to discharge, the clinician reassessed Mr. J, and his MMSE Score was now 19/30. It was deemed that he had sufficient clear insight to go home, despite the risks. The psychiatric clinician consultant was also asked to reassess Mr. J's capacity to validate the decision to safely discharge him to home. The pyschiatric NP stated that Mr. J had essential improvement in his cognitive MMSE and also scored him at 19/30. It was suggested that a trial discharge home would be appropriate. He was also started on a new medication for his memory, Rivastigime 4.6 mg patch (an acetycholinesterase inhibitor that is used for symptomatic treatment for mild-to-moderate dementia), and this was to be titrated up as prescribed.

Mr. J was finally discharged home to a caring community supported by his neighbors and the dedication of his visiting nursing team and home care services. He is also supported by the clinician and a community social worker. His dog still lives with him but sleeps in an unused old car outside the house.

REFERENCES

Agich, G. (2004). *Dependence and autonomy in old age*. Cambridge: Cambridge University Press.

Alzheimer's Association. (2011). Dementia. Retrieved June 10, 2011, from http://www.alz.org.alzheimers_disease_dementia.asp

Beauchamp, T. L., & Childress, J. F. (1994). *Principles of biomedical ethics*. Oxford: Oxford University Press.

Burkhardt, M., & Nathaniel, A. (2002). *Ethics and issues in contemporary nursing* (2nd ed.). Albany, Australia: Delmar/Thomson Learning.

Dharmarajan, T. S., & Norkus, E. P. (2004). Mild anemia and the risk of falls in older adults from nursing homes and the community. *Journal of American Medical Directors Association*, 5(6), 395–400.

Dufouil, C., Clayton, D., Brayne, C., Chi, L. Y., Dening, T. R., Paykel, E. S., O'Connor, D. W., Ahmed, A., McGee, M. A., & Huppert, F. D. (2000). Population norms for the MMSE in the very old. Estimates based on longitudinal data. *Neurology*, 55(1 of 2), 1609–1613.

Folstein, M. F., Folstein, S. E., & McHugh, P. R. (1975). "Mini-Mental State": A practical method for grading the cognitive state of patients for the clinician. *Journal of Psychiatric Research*, 12, 189–198.

Jellinger, K. A. (2008). The pathology of "vascular dementia": A critical update. *Journal of Alzheimer's Disease*, 14, 107–123.

Mintzer, J., & Burns, A. (2000). Anticholinergic side-effects of drugs in elderly people. *Journal of the Royal Society of Medicine*, 93, 457–462.

Musso, C. J., & Nunez, J. F. M. (2006). Feed-back between geriatric syndromes: General system theory in geriatrics. *International Urology and Nephrology*, 38(3–4), 785–786.

Pavlou, M. P., & Lachs, M. S. (2006). Could self-neglect in older adults be a geriatric syndrome? *Journal of the American Geriatrics Society*, 54(5), 831–842.

Penninx, B., Pluijm, S., Lips, P., Woodman, R., Miedema, K., Guralnik, J., & Deeg, D. (2005). Late-life anemia is associated with increased risk of recurrent falls. *Journal of the American Geriatrics Society*, 53(12), 2106–2111.

Case 4.2 Regressing in Rehab

By Kendra M. Grimes, MSN, APRN, GNP-BC

Mrs. D is an 86-year-old woman who was admitted to rehab after a fall with a hip fracture 3 weeks ago. Until that time, Mrs. D had lived independently in the community. The nurse explains that Mrs. D had been making good progress in therapy but that the therapist reported that Mrs. D has been much less engaged the last 2 days and is regressing in her abilities. This morning she refused AM care and declined to go to therapy. The nurse states that Mrs. D had been occasionally forgetful at baseline, but that she has seems more "out of it" today and that her oxygen saturation has dropped to 90% from her baseline of 93–94%; so the nurse has administered oxygen at 2L via nasal cannula.

Another provider admitted her to the facility; but, upon reviewing her chart, the clinician notices that she has a history of hypertension, hypothyroidism, cholecystectomy, osteoporosis, and osteoarthritis. She is currently an assist of 1 with activities of daily living (ADL) and is toe-touch weight-bearing on her right lower extremity.

Mrs. D is a widow; her husband died 5 years ago of a heart attack. She has 2 daughters in another state who are hoping she will be able to relocate after she is fully recovered. She was a church organist and a piano teacher. She smoked briefly as a teenager. She does not drink any alcohol. She received the flu vaccine this year and got the pneumonia vaccine at age 65.

Upon meeting Mrs. D, she complains of feeling very tired and not "up for" therapy today. When asked about therapy, she said it has been "very difficult" and that she had to quit yesterday because she felt

Case Studies in Gerontological Nursing for the Advanced Practice Nurse, First Edition.
Edited by Meredith Wallace Kazer, Leslie Neal-Boylan.
© 2012 John Wiley & Sons, Inc. Published 2012 by John Wiley & Sons, Inc.

exhausted and had a hard time "getting my breath." She says she has a little cough, but denies coughing up any phlegm. She denies chest pain, palpitations, headaches, dizziness, nausea, or vomiting. She denies any pain in her hip or at her incision. She has had no problems passing urine, denies any burning, pain, or frequency. Her bowels have been regular.

Her medications include lisinopril, 10 mg daily; levothyroxine, 112 mcg daily; colace, 1 capsule 2 times daily; APAP, 650 mg 4 times daily; simvastatin; 40 mg daily; alendronate, sodium 70 mg weekly; and enoxaparin, 40 mg subcutaneous injection daily. She has made no requests for as-needed pain medication in 7 days. She has no known allergies (NKA).

OBJECTIVE

Mrs. D is awake, lethargic, and oriented to person only. She reports the name of the previous hospital as her location rather than the rehab facility. She is unable to name the correct year or month. She is wearing a nightgown and appears pale but without obvious distress. She is 5 ft 3 inches; weight:136 lb; temp: 98.7; BP: 114/62; P: 110, reg; RR: 28; O_2 sat: 92% on 2 L. Lung sounds are slightly diminished with some crackles noted on the right. Cardiac exam reveals a regular heart rate, S1, S2, and no murmurs or adventitious sounds. Abdomen is soft, nontender, and nondistended with normoactive bowel sounds and a faint scar from the open cholecystectomy. Her skin is dry. Her surgical wound is healing well, with Steri-Strips in place, open to air, and no evidence of local infection. Her extremities are without edema, and her pulses are 2+ palpable.

ASSESSMENT

Coronary heart disease: Unstable angina or myocardial infarctions often do not present with chest pain in an older woman. An acute coronary syndrome could be causing Mrs. D's dyspnea, weakness, and fatigue.

Health Care–Associated Pneumonia (HCAP): Pneumonia is a very common cause of morbidity and mortality in older adults who frequent the health care system. Older adults with pneumonia may not present typical symptoms of fever, purulent cough, and pleuritic pain; but it may be causing Mrs. D's decreased therapy tolerance, decrease in oxygen saturation, and confusion.

Heart failure: Mrs. D's activity intolerance, shortness of breath, tachycardia, and confusion could be due to worsening cardiac output and pulmonary congestion.

DIAGNOSTICS

EKG, CBC, UA, BMP, CXR. EKG showed sinus tachycardia with no evidence of ischemia. A CBC with differential reveals a white blood cell count of 14,500 per mm^3, with 10% bands. Urinalysis was negative. Metabolic panel values were within normal ranges with a BUN of 15 mg/dL. PA and lateral chest x-ray findings describe "patchy opacities in the right lower lobe suggestive of pneumonia."

CRITICAL THINKING

What is the most likely differential diagnosis and why?

Does this patient need to be hospitalized?

What is the plan of treatment?

What is the plan for follow-up care?

What if this patient were living in the community?

What if this patient had advanced dementia?

What are some evidence-based interventions for prevention of pneumonia?

Are there any standardized guidelines that the clinician should use to assess or treat this case?

RESOLUTION

What is the most likely differential diagnosis and why?
Health care–associated pneumonia (HCAP) is defined by the Infectious Diseases Society of America (IDSA) and by the American Thoracic Society (ATS) as a pneumonia that develops in a patient who:

- had an acute hospitalization lasting at least 2 days in the last 90 days;
- received IV antibiotic therapy, wound care, chemotherapy in the last 30 days;

- attends a hospital or hemodialysis clinic, or
- resides in a long-term or nursing home facility (American Thoracic Society & Infectious Diseases Society of America [ATS & IDSA], 2005).

HCAP is a common illness in older adults, especially those who are exposed to pathogens in the health care setting while postoperative or medically compromised. A patient with limited mobility, uncontrolled pain, or rib fractures may be restricting her inspiratory effort; and the resulting atelectasis may predispose her to pneumonia. Unfortunately, the pathogens present in health care settings are generally different, and have developed more antibiotic resistance, than those present in the community. Common bacterial causes of HCAP in nursing homes include *Pseudomonas aeruginosa,* gram negative enterics such as *E. coli, Klebsiella,* and *Acinetobacter,* as well as *S. aureus* (including MRSA).

Pneumonia may not present in older adults as it might in younger adults, with the classic symptoms of fever, cough with sputum, shortness of breath, or pleuritic chest pain. Instead, older people may present with subtle changes in level of function, decreased appetite, worsening of mental status, or altered vital signs, especially tachypnea. Mrs. D does not have a fever, which is common in older adults; but it should be noted that she has been taking scheduled acetaminophen around the clock. In this case, the patient's change in functional and mental status suggest a possible acute illness; her vital signs and physical exam imply a possible respiratory infection, a diagnosis supported by her elevated white cell count and confirmed as pneumonia via chest x-ray.

Does this patient need to be hospitalized?
Whatever the setting, this question should be foremost when evaluating an older adult for suspected pneumonia: Does this patient need to be hospitalized?

In a skilled nursing setting, numerous factors should be weighed. Will a transfer and acute hospitalization best serve the needs of the patient and their goals of care? Can the illness be managed with the staff and resources available at the current facility? If the rehabilitation facility is able to treat appropriately and to monitor this illness to the extent desired by the patient and provider, including IV therapy, chest x-rays, and laboratory services, then sending the patient out is not necessary. A discussion with the patient and/or their chosen family members can clarify needs and wishes.

For patients in the community, the decision to admit may be more complex; and a few different tools have been developed to help guide clinicians. One validated measure is the Pneumonia Severity Index (PSI), a 19-item index that groups patients into prognostic risk categories, with categories I–III indicating lower risk and possibly appropriateness for outpatient treatment and categories IV–V suggesting higher risk and necessary hospital or ICU admission (Fine et al., 1997). Although useful, the PSI can be cumbersome to calculate, and some online calculators have been created to assist providers. A quicker measure is the CURB-65 tool, which, instead of predicting mortality risk, is an illness severity index based on 5 measures: **C**onfusion (the presence of mental status changes), **U**remia (BUN > 17), **R**espiratory rate (>30/min), **B**lood pressure (<90 mmHg systolic or <60 diastolic) and age > **65** (Lim et al., 2003). Patients with CURB scores ≥ 2 are likely candidates for hospitalization.

What is the plan of treatment?
In this case, the patient can be treated in the subacute rehab setting. Patients with HCAP should be treated empirically with antibiotics specific to the likely infectious flora until a particular organism is identified. Likely organisms are determined by any recent antibiotic use, common pathogens in the facility, and any known exposure or history to resistant organisms. Commonly used antibiotics that are used to treat HCAP and recommended by IDSA and ATS for patients without known multidrug resistant (MDR) infections include intravenous ceftriaxone, ampicillin-sulbactam, levofloxacin, moxifloxacin, or ertapenem. For patients with known past MDR infections, recent antibiotic use, concerns for resistant species of *Pseudomonas*, *Serratia*, or *Enterobacter*, as well as MRSA and *Legionella*, combination antibiotic therapy will be required (ATS & IDSA, 2005). In the case of Mrs. D, who has no known history of MDR infections, the facility's protocol calls for levofloxacin as first line, due to the known flora of their facility and the local health care community. Prior to administration of empiric antibiotics, a sputum sample is obtained for stain and culture, as are blood cultures.

What is the plan for follow-up care?
Effectiveness of the treatment regimen needs to be evaluated within 72 hours. Blood and sputum sample cultures (if obtained) should be reviewed and antibiotic therapy tailored to the specific organisms identified and their susceptibilities, if possible. The course of therapy should be determined by the patient's clinical response. Seven days may be all that are necessary, and providers should be careful to not prolong treatment once it has proven effective. Mrs. D's mental status, respiratory status, vital signs, and lab results should be closely monitored; and if she does not show improvement at 72 hours or if the cultures indicate inappropriate management, a reassessment of the both the diagnosis and the treatment must be performed.

What if this patient were living in the community?
Community-acquired pneumonia (CAP) is any pneumonia developed by an individual who obtained the illness from outside the health care setting and does not meet any of the HCAP criteria listed above. The

pathogens associated with CAP are generally different from those associated with health care–associated infections, with the most common organisms being *S. pneumoniae, Mycoplasma, Chlamydophilia, Legionella,* and *H. influenza,* as well as influenza virus and other respiratory viruses such as RSV (Mandell et al., 2007).

Older patients who live in the community may seek care in primary care centers, urgent care centers, or emergency departments with a variety of clinical presentations. Chest x-rays, CBCs, and serum chemistries are helpful in aiding diagnoses. The ATS considers sputum cultures and blood cultures to be unnecessary for CAP patients who will be treated as outpatients, unless there is clinical suspicion for legionella, influenza, community-acquired MRSA, or an agent of bioterrorism (Mandell et al., 2007).

Again, the decision on whether to admit a patient with CAP is foremost. Using the PSI or CURB tools and assessing the patient's continued ability to care for themselves (or presence and competence of caregivers) and to participate in outpatient treatment is crucial. If Mrs. D were community-dwelling, her CURB-65 score would be 2 (age > 65 and confusion); but the presence of confusion and the absence of local caregivers might require either intensive home care or hospitalization to assure her safety and clinical improvement.

IDSA and ATS also provide suggested treatment guidelines for empiric antibiotic therapy for CAP. Generally, patients who are low risk and are treated as outpatients for CAP should receive either a macrolide (azithromycin, erythromycin, clarithromycin) or, if they have comorbidities (e.g., diabetes or chronic lung, kidney, or liver disease), a respiratory fluoroquinolone (levofloxacin, moxifloxacin) or a beta-lactam (amoxicillin-clavulanate) **and** a macrolide (Mandell et al., 2007). Prompt followup and assessment within 48 to 72 hours is needed for these patients. Patients who do not improve with outpatient treatment should be admitted for cultures and further assessment.

What are some evidence-based interventions for prevention of pneumonia?
Prevention of pneumonia in older adults should be a primary nursing goal in all settings of care. The Centers for Disease Control (CDC) have provided guidance regarding prevention of health care–associated infections. (Tablan, Anderson, Besser, Bridges, Hajjeh, & CDC & Healthcare Infection Control Practices Advisory Committee, 2004). Infection control and surveillance is of foremost importance. Status of influenza and pneumonia vaccines should be determined for every patient and administered if appropriate, and health care workers should also receive annual influenza vaccines. Older adults in nursing facilities should be routinely assessed for their risk of aspiration, and those receiving enteral feedings should have the head of the bed elevated between 30 and 45 degrees. Postoperative patients should be

encouraged to move, deep breathe, and ambulate as soon as medically possible; and incentive spirometry should be ordered and routinely observed.

What if this patient had advanced dementia?
Of particular interest in the institutional setting is the use of antibiotics in patients with advanced disease, particularly dementia. Decision making is very complex in these patients, who may develop recurrent pneumonias that may be caused by aspiration or complicated by drug-resistant organisms. A recent study suggests that while treating pneumonia with antibiotics may prolong survival of patients with dementia, they do not improve the patient's comfort, especially if IV treatment is necessary or the patient is hospitalized (Givens, Jones, Shaffer, Kiely, & Mitchell, 2010). Intravenous (IV) therapy may not improve survival over oral or intramuscular (IM) antibiotics in the institutionalized patient with dementia. Goals of care should be clarified with patients and family members before any decision is made to treat pneumonia.

Are there any standardized guidelines that the clinician should use to assess or treat this case?
Guidelines for the diagnosis and treatment of both CAP and HCAP are published by the American Thoracic Society in conjunction with the Infectious Disease Society of America. These guidelines are available for download at http://www.thoracic.org/statements/.

REFERENCES

American Thoracic Society & Infectious Diseases Society of America (2005). Guidelines for the management of adults with hospital-acquired, ventilator-associated, and healthcare-associated pneumonia. *American Journal of Respiratory & Critical Care Medicine*, 171(4), 388–416.

Fine, M. J., Auble, T. E., Yealy, D. M., Hanusa, B. H., Weissfeld, L. A., Singer, D. E., Coley, C. M., Marrie, T. J., & Kapoor, W. N. (1997). A prediction rule to identify low-risk patients with community-acquired pneumonia. *The New England Journal of Medicine*, 336(4), 243–250.

Givens, J. L., Jones, R. N., Shaffer, M. L., Kiely, D. K., & Mitchell, S. L. (2010). Survival and comfort after treatment of pneumonia in advanced dementia. *Archives of Internal Medicine*, 170(13), 1102–1107.

Lim, W. S., van der Eerden, M. M., Laing, R., Boersma, W. G., Karalus, N., Town, G. I., Lewis, S. A., & Macfarlane, J. T. (2003). Defining community acquired pneumonia severity on presentation to hospital: An international derivation and validation study. *Thorax, 58*, 377–382.

Mandell, L. A., Wunderink, R. G., Anzueto, A., Bartlett, J. G., Campbell, G. D., Dean, N. C., Dowell, S. F., File, T. M., Jr, Musher, D. M., Niederman, M. S., Torres, A., Whitney, C. G., & Infectious Diseases Society of America &

American Thoracic Society (2007). Infectious Diseases Society of America/American Thoracic Society consensus guidelines on the management of community-acquired pneumonia in adults. *Clinical Infectious Diseases,* *44*(Suppl. 2), S27–S72.

Tablan, O. C., Anderson, L. J., Besser, R., Bridges, C., Hajjeh, R., & CDC & Healthcare Infection Control Practices Advisory Committee (2004). Guidelines for preventing health-care–associated pneumonia, 2003: Recommendations of CDC and the Healthcare Infection Control Practices Advisory Committee. *Morbidity & Mortality Weekly Report. Recommendations & Reports, 53*(RR-3), 1–36.

ADDITIONAL RESOURCES

CDC Guidelines on prevention of HCAP. http://www.cdc.gov/mmwr/preview/mmwrhtml/rr5303a1.htm

Community-Acquired Pneumonia Severity Index (PSI) Calculator. http://pda.ahrq.gov/clinic/psi/psicalc.asp

Case 4.3 There's No Place Like Home

By Nicholas R. Nicholson, Jr., PhD, MPH, RN, PHCNS-BC

Recently Mr. R, an 86-year-old man, had a bout of acute delirium that required hospitalization. He was unable to create coherent thoughts and exhibited signs of severe anxiety and irritability. His family called the provider's office and described the symptoms, which resulted in Mr. R going to hospital to rule out a stroke. Initial labs drawn at the hospital revealed that the delirium was most likely due to hyponatremia (sodium level of 115 mEq/L). Mr. R was diagnosed with SIADH (syndrome of inappropriate antidiuretic hormone hyper-secretion) and was treated with hypertonic saline (5%) 150 mL per hour gradually over the course of 2–3 days to safely increase sodium levels. When Mr. R's sodium level increased to 128 mEq/L and his mental status improved to the point where he was alert and oriented, he was discharged from the hospital. Mr. R manages his health primarily on his own along with some help from his wife (70 years old); they live together in a Cape Cod style home. His daughter, 46, lives nearby but is more of a strain than a help. Mr. R is socially isolated with no close living friends, minimal social interaction from neighbors, and limited family nearby.

Upon admission to home care services, Mr. R is ordered to receive follow-up care and monitoring regarding his electrolytes, resolving delirium, and ongoing congestive heart failure (CHF). Additionally, Mr. R needs to be evaluated for physical therapy needs following his prolonged hospitalization. He is experiencing frequent shortness of breath (SOB) secondary to emphysema (50-year smoking pack history; 1 pack per day). Home care orders also include oxygen at 2 L via nasal

Case Studies in Gerontological Nursing for the Advanced Practice Nurse, First Edition.
Edited by Meredith Wallace Kazer, Leslie Neal-Boylan.
© 2012 John Wiley & Sons, Inc. Published 2012 by John Wiley & Sons, Inc.

cannula. There are many health factors that are directly and negatively impacting Mr. R's health. These include a history of an anterior myocardial infarction (AMI) with significant arterial disease, congestive obstructive pulmonary disease (COPD), CHF, hypertension (HTN), and high cholesterol. Mr. R is a veteran of World War II. Therefore, he gets the majority of his primary care from the local Veteran's Administration (VA). He receives a pension from his former employer, the state police. His wife states that he is normally much more "energetic" and talkative. Today he is answering all questions appropriately after a small delay. Mr. R denies headaches, syncope, paresthesia, or pain. Basic activities of daily living result in loud, labored breathing and coughing. Mr. R also complains of significant shortness of breath after walking the short distance up his driveway (on a hill) and climbing one set of stairs into the main floor of house. His medications include Cardizem, 60 mg every 8 hours; Prevacid, 30 mg daily; Coreg CR, 12.5 mg daily; aspirin, 81 mg daily; HCTZ, 25 mg daily; allopurinol, 100 mg daily; Ativan, 0.25 mg as needed; nitroglycerin, 0.2 mg as needed; and buspirone (BuSpar), 5 mg twice daily (taken for smoking cessation). He has no known allergies (NKA).

OBJECTIVE

Mr. R is alert and oriented, but appears tired. He is wearing pajamas and has neglected certain aspects of personal grooming, such as shaving and combing hair. His weight is 175 lb with a height of 5 ft 6 inches. His blood pressure is 100/60; pulse: 55; O_2 saturation: 91% on ambient air; and he is afebrile at 98.2 Fahrenheit. Upon auscultation of his lungs, wheezing is heard throughout all lung fields with fine crackles bilaterally in both bases. S1 and S2 are auscultated. No abnormal heart sounds are found upon auscultation. His jugular vein distention is 2 cm, and there are no bruits. There is +1 pitting pedal edema bilaterally. There are positive bowel sounds in all 4 quadrants. The eye examination reveals PERRLA. Neurological exam reveals 2+ deep tendon reflexes bilaterally with equal strength. When assessing cranial nerve VII, there is no paralysis or drooping of the face; and all expressions (frown, raising of eyebrows, wrinkle forehead, smile, whistle, puff out cheeks, and tight closing of eyes) are normal.

ASSESSMENT

Delirium: Mr. R's resolving delirium is directly impacted by low sodium levels and needs to be monitored through frequent blood draws examining electrolytes. Moving forward, a history of coronary heart disease (transischemic attacks) needs to be considered as a possible contributing factor to his change in cognition. Input and output need to be watched closely as Mr. R begins on a 1000 mL fluid restriction.

Functional dependence and need for physical therapy: Mr. R's hospitalization resulted in significant weakness, requiring the evaluation by a physical therapist to assist with building baseline endurance.

CHF: Due to the history of CHF, emphysema, and his weakened state, it is important to continue to monitor signs and symptoms of CHF exacerbation. Mr. R and his wife will need educational reminders on how to continue monitoring the CHF.

Safety of home living situation: It will be important to determine if Mr. R and his wife can manage his daily routine, including medications. Mr. R needs to be able to get up and down stairs and to complete basic activities of daily living in various parts and levels of the home. There is a 50-ft length of oxygen tubing and several throw rugs that could be fall hazards.

DIAGNOSTICS

Every 5–7 days, there will be an at-home blood draw to determine Mr. R's sodium level. Additionally, he and his wife will need to be educated regarding the early warning signs of delirium. The root cause of the SIADH was not determined in the hospital, but will need to be followed up by his primary care clinician with assistance from visiting nurses. With encouragement and additional arrangements made for a ride through the senior transportation service by his visiting nurse, Mr. R undergoes an outpatient chest x-ray. The chest x-ray showed a small mass in his right lower lobe. Mr. R's sodium level is now 137 mEq/L.

CRITICAL THINKING

What type of further diagnostic testing would the clinician order?

What can the clinician do to increase his safety in his home?

What resources may it be necessary to activate for Mr. R?

What can the clinician do to assist Mr. R and his family through the emotional distress of a potential cancer diagnosis?

If Mr. R's sodium began trending downward, what would the clinician do? What might be causing this?

How might social isolation impact the treatment plan for Mr. R?

RESOLUTION

What type of further diagnostic testing would the clinician order?

The chest x-ray showed a small mass in the lower right lobe of his lung. However, the chest x-ray alone will not distinguish between a benign or cancerous tumor. A spiral computer tomography (CT) scan may yield additional information regarding the tumor size and shape (Manser et al., 2005). A biopsy and sputum cytology will assist in determining whether the tumor is benign or cancerous, as well as whether there are any cancer cells outside of the lungs. Given the long history of smoking and the recent hospital admission for hyponatremia (which can be caused by lung cancer), these tests are warranted. Smoking is the most important risk factor for lung cancer and is the most common nonskin cancer in men and women combined in the US (US Department of Health and Human Services, 2004). Upon further testing a CT-guided biopsy combined with a sputum cytology confirmed small cell carcinoma, which is the likely cause of the SIADH and the severely decreased sodium level.

What can the clinician do to increase his safety in his home?

Now that Mr. R is home, it is important for the clinician to order a thorough home safety assessment for potential issues such as loose electrical cords, throw rugs, furniture, and other fall hazards. Additionally, it is important to take into account the steadiness of the patient's gait and whether or not handrails may be needed. This will help determine if the patient is safe to be in the home alone and whether he and his wife can move around their living space to meet their basic needs. It is very important that the patient have a way to call for help, as well as access to emergency medicines, such as nitroglycerin and inhalers. It is also necessary to assess the patient's ability to perform activities of daily living, such as toileting, bathing, transferring from bed to chair, and walking.

What resources may it be necessary to activate for Mr. R?

Since he is in a weakened state from his extended stay in the hospital, it is crucially important to call in a physical therapy consultation. He was not weak enough to require inpatient rehabilitation, but he is not likely to be strong enough to take care of all his needs alone in his living space. This is especially true due to his Cape Cod style house, which has the only bathroom on the second floor. In addition, a consultation from an occupational therapist might be warranted. The occupational therapist can provide a temporary commode chair as well as other items such as a device to assist him with putting on his shoes until he regains his strength. An in-home patient care assistant can assist with daily care, such as bathing and cleaning the commode chair until Mr. R can recover strength and his ability to perform these activities independently. Because his wife is significantly younger and must work every weekday, she cannot be around every day to assist with activities of daily living. Since Mr. R learned of a tumor in his lungs, he has acted despondent while he awaits more information about the staging of his tumor and treatment recommendations for small cell carcinoma. It will be necessary for the visiting nurse to assess Mr. R for depression and ability to cope with the new diagnosis. It will be very difficult for Mr. R to obtain his treatment and meet rehabilitation goals if he is depressed and unwilling to fully participate in his care. He should be referred to a local oncologist, and the clinician can assist with helping him make the necessary appointments with him during his office visits. Finally, a smoking cessation consult might also be appropriate so that Mr. R can receive the help he needs to quit should he choose to do so. Quitting smoking has the potential to save his lungs from any further insult. Depending on the staging and severity of the tumor and overall prognosis for Mr. R, the clinician may consider introducing the idea of hospice care, dispelling any myth or misconceptions he and his wife may have about it, so that if it becomes necessary he will have access to information required to make appropriate decisions.

What can the clinician do to assist Mr. R and his family through the emotional distress of a potential cancer diagnosis?

It is important to help Mr. R and his wife to understand the staging of the tumor and the treatment options. The clinician and visiting nurses may be helpful in providing information and resources about diagnosis and treatment of lung cancer from reliable sources such as the National Cancer Institute or the American Cancer Society. They should be prepared to discuss the goals of treatment and be sure Mr. R is comfortable with his plan of care. This may be an emotional realization for Mr. R, and it will be important to schedule extra time to discuss matters with him and his wife.

If Mr. R's sodium began trending downward, what would the clinician do? What might be causing this?

If his sodium began trending downward, it would be important to assess his cognition first. After cognition was assessed and found to be unchanged, the next steps would be to assess overall fluid balance, review the fluid restrictions, and remind Mr. R why it is important to continue to monitor fluid intake and output closely.

How might social isolation impact the treatment plan for Mr. R?
Social isolation is defined as "a state in which the individual lacks a sense of belonging socially, lacks engagement with others, has a minimal number of social contacts and they are deficient in fulfilling and quality relationships" (Nicholson, 2009, 1346). As Mr. R continues to improve physically, it is important for him to start readjusting to the routine of his life including shopping, driving, and walking. Extra coordination by the clinician and visiting nurses will be essential when Mr. R begins treatment for the small cell carcinoma, particularly because his wife has limited availability to provide rides to necessary appointments due to her work schedule. Mr. R does not have a large social network around to provide social support placing him at an increased risk of social isolation. There are numerous instruments to test for social isolation, one of which is the Lubben Social Network Scale (Lubben & Gironda, 2003). Being socially isolated may impact Mr. R's physical and emotional health.

REFERENCES

Lubben, J., & Gironda, M. (2003). Centrality of social ties to the health and well-being of older adults. In B. Berkman, L. Harootyan (Eds.), *Social work and health care in an aging society* (pp. 319–350). New York: Springer.

Manser, R. L., Irving, L. B., de Campo, M. P., Abramson, M. J., Stone, C. A., Pedersen, K. E., Elwood, M., & Campbell, D. A. (2005). Overview of observational studies of low-dose helical computed tomography screening for lung cancer. *Respirology, 10*(1), 97–104.

Nicholson, N. Jr. (2009). Social isolation in older adults: An evolutionary concept analysis. *Journal of Advanced Nursing, 65*(6), 1342–1352. doi: 10.1111/j.1365-2648.2008.04959.x.

US Department of Health and Human Services (2004). *The health consequences of smoking: A report of the surgeon general.* Atlanta, Ga: U.S. Department of Health and Human Services, CDC, National Center for Chronic Disease Prevention and Health Promotion, Office on Smoking and Health. Accessed at http://www.cdc.gov/tobacco/data_statistics/sgr/2004/index.htm

Case 4.4 Caring for the Caregiver

By Evanne Juratovac, PhD, RN (GCNS-BC)

Mrs. J is a 74-year-old, widowed, retired, African American female. She lives on the second story of a home with her 79-year-old sister, who has recurrent exacerbations of heart failure and moderate dementia. She is English speaking and a high school graduate. Though the clinician typically sees Mrs. J in the primary care older adult clinic for routine follow-up care every 3–6 months, it has been 10 months since her last exam.

Mrs. J's chief concern is that she is tired all the time but does not sleep well and has "trouble getting going" in the morning. She exhibits poor energy and exercise tolerance, experiencing dyspnea after ascending one flight of steps. Her appetite is fair, preparing and eating meals that typically consist of frozen or canned foods. The clinician notes a 5-lb weight loss since her last visit. Her sleep difficulty is positive for middle and late insomnia, and her explanation is that her sleep is often interrupted by her elder sister's needs. She feels "stressed" and "on edge" and is "lately more impatient" with her sister's repeated questions. Her mental status exam is remarkable for irritable and slightly anxious mood, with poor concentration. She attempts to abort the interview, asking how much longer the appointment will last because she "has to get going". She has stopped volunteering at her church and has not been attending services, saying she is "too busy to socialize".

Mrs. J has a documented history of hypertension (HTN) for which she is prescribed generic hydrochlorothiazide (HCTZ), 15 mg, and captopril, 25 mg daily. She has no other prescription medications listed

Case Studies in Gerontological Nursing for the Advanced Practice Nurse, First Edition. Edited by Meredith Wallace Kazer, Leslie Neal-Boylan.

in her chart and no documented allergies. She uses 2 Tylenol PM®️ over-the-counter (OTC) pills for sleep, since she regards it as safe according to the commercials on television and according to her minister. She uses no alcohol or tobacco.

OBJECTIVE

Today, Mrs. J's exam is normal except for a sitting blood pressure of 182/102 and mild (1+, nonpitting, dependent) pedal edema. Blood chemistries analyzed from earlier today are all within normal ranges for older adults. The clinician learns that her antihypertensive prescriptions have lapsed. She explains she has not called for refills since it would be hard to get to the pharmacy or the clinic. She is concerned about both money and neighborhood safety.

CRITICAL THINKING

What is the primary diagnosis for Mrs. J?

What stressors in Mrs. J's life might be related to being responsible for the care and supervision of a family member?

Is Mrs. J at high risk for depression?

What should be done for Mrs. J's sleep complaints?

What other issues should the clinician address to maintain Mrs. J's health and well-being?

What other resources should the clinician recommend to Mrs. J?

RESOLUTION

What is the primary diagnosis for Mrs. J?
The obvious challenge with this patient is poorly controlled HTN and a self-reported lapse in medication. Overtly, this case study reveals problems with adherence and self-management of a chronic health condition. A lapse in HTN therapy puts Mrs. J. at risk for more serious health complications, so reevaluating and resuming therapy is an immediate protective strategy. Additionally, Mrs. J's captopril might be more affordable in a generic equivalent, or her two medications could be offered in a combined formulation (e.g., Capozide®️). Some neighborhood pharmacies may even deliver prescriptions for her and her sister directly to their door. Some recent evidence suggests that ACE

inhibitors that cross the blood-brain barrier may be protective against dementia in addition to HTN control (Sink et al., 2009), which is an interesting health promotion consideration for this patient, given that she has a sister with dementia.

What stressors in Mrs. J's life might be related to being responsible for the care and supervision of a family member?

Mrs. J's caregiving of a family member at home requires a balance between competing responsibilities of caring for her sister while trying to maintain her own health. Dementia caregiving might pose particularly stressful challenges in striving for this balance (Farran, Loukissa, Lindeman, McCann, & Bienias, 2004), though caregivers of older adults with heart failure may have similar stressors (Saunders, 2008). As an older caregiver, Mrs. J may have additional hidden vulnerabilities. Many caregivers are dealing with their own advancing age in addition to caring for another elderly person (Johnson & Schaner, 2005), and it is more likely that older adults who reside with the care receiver are doing this work without the help of other family or formal caregivers, according to a recent survey (National Alliance for Caregiving [NAC] & American Association of Retired Persons [AARP], 2009).

Caregivers' physical health (Vitaliano, Zhang, & Scanlan, 2003) or a combination of physical and psychological health (Pinquart & Sörensen, 2003) may be in jeopardy. A disproportionate prevalence of depressive symptoms among caregivers is well documented (Gray, 2003) with a notable emphasis on dementia caregivers (Covinsky et al., 2003). Further, some clinicians may be uninformed about ethnic and age-related differences in how distress and depressive symptoms in elderly caregivers may be experienced and expressed (Sörensen & Pinquart, 2005). The odds of a caregiver having a distinct mortality risk associated with caregiving itself (Schulz & Beach, 1999) may be most alarming.

Both the caregiver and the care receiver in this dyad have potential unmet needs and risks. An inherent risk to the sister is neglect if Mrs. J is unwell and less capable of doing caregiving work; yet a distinct risk of abusive behavior toward the older adult care receiver has been identified in distressed caregivers (Beach et al., 2005). While giving this patient advice about the care of her sister may seem peripheral to her care, it is arguably this caregiving situation that has potentiated the symptoms reported in this clinic visit.

Addressing Mrs. J's health and function promotes her ability to do her caregiving work. Nursing strategies have been developed to examine the exertional aspects of family caregiving, including effort (Juratovac, 2009) and overall impact (Given et al., 1992). Evaluating her self-reported effort—that is, the energy exerted to do the workload of caregiving—may reveal how she is managing her workload as well as her self-care. Recommending caregiving resources in her community is appropriate nursing care, though it would be up to Mrs. J to determine the acceptability of services and whether they would lighten her load.

Screening Mrs. J for symptoms of caregiver strain would likely reveal affirmative responses of at least "sometimes" on all items, from the physiological perceptions to psychological upset to social consequences of caring. (See a brief/modified version of the scale at http://consultgerirn.org/uploads/File/trythis/try_this_14.pdf for further information on caregiver strain.)

Is Mrs. J at high risk for depression?

Caregivers need to be screened for depression. Because symptoms may be intermittent or suggestive of several chronic health conditions, this can confound the assessment. Positive findings in Mrs. J's depression screening include mood (irritability), energy, sleep, cognitive, appetite, self-neglect, and interpersonal symptoms of depression. She would probably not meet the frequency and persistence criteria required for a diagnosis of major depressive disorder, yet she has significant depressive symptoms (refer to DSM-IV-TR for detailed diagnostic criteria) that should be reassessed regularly. Resuming physical and social activity could be encouraged, in spite of (and because of) her caregiving responsibilities.

Not all caregivers will express the same stress and depression symptoms (Sörensen & Pinquart, 2005), further obscuring clinical discovery. Mrs. J's age and ethnic origin may influence the presentation of symptoms. For example, some older adults may not experience a sad mood as a hallmark depressive symptom (Gallo & Rabins, 1999), while the DSM-IV-TR requires sad mood as one of the two symptoms that persist and interfere with function for a diagnosis of major depression (2000). If sadness is regarded as a *sine qua non* of depression, then the absence of sad mood may lead a clinician to discount Mrs. J's other disabling depressive symptoms. Reliability of an established scale for screening depressive symptoms in older adults has been successfully demonstrated in older adults who have chronic health conditions (Zauszniewski, Morris, Preechawong, & Chang, 2004).

What should be done for Mrs. J's sleep complaints?

While Mrs. J has symptoms suggestive of a primary sleep disorder, the symptoms need to be examined in the context of her situation. Problems with sleep disruption can adversely affect the caregiver's health and interactions with the care receiver as well (Carter, 2002). Mrs. J's sleep symptoms may be due in large part to caregiving-related interruptions, rather than some more endogenous cause. If so, then problem solving about her caregiving workload may help her to develop strategies, including a reexamination of the sister's symptoms and nighttime behavior. The clinician may conduct a brief sleep assessment (http://consultgerirn.org/uploads/File/trythis/try_this_6_1.pdf) and explore whether a sleep diary would benefit this patient. It is important to educate Mrs. J about the side effects of her self-prescribed sleep aid, as this may contribute to her energy and cognitive difficulties that are conceivably bad enough with her subjectively poor sleep.

Older adults may be unaware that when they self-treat sleep problems with OTC preparations containing dipenhydramine there are real safety concerns beyond those that are advertised. Adverse effects associated with the anticholinergic effects of medications in older adults are discussed in detail in Fick et al., 2003.

What other issues should the clinician address to maintain Mrs. J's health and well-being?

Finances and access to healthy foods in her neighborhood may contribute to the nutrition choices that Mrs. J makes; these are choices that ultimately affect the health of both herself and her sister. For example, the sodium content of prepared foods is not ideal for her sister's CHF or her own HTN. Teaching this patient to read food labels with attention to serving sizes and exploring affordable ways to get fresh foods into the home promotes both sisters' nutrition. If access and safety are barriers to better nutrition, explore the availability of home-delivered meals and local senior transportation for grocery shopping. Perform a nutrition assessment (http://consultgerirn.org/uploads/File/trythis/try_this_9.pdf), and consider whether her 5-lb weight loss is clinically significant.

What other resources should the clinician recommend to Mrs. J?

The clinician should inform Mrs. J about caregiving support services so that she can make an informed choice about formal and informal supports. Some programs and Web sites are listed here to support informal caregivers:

- **Administration on Aging (U.S. Department of Health and Human Services):** An "elder care locator" is available to learn about and locate services in this patient's community at http://www.eldercare.gov/Eldercare.NET/Public/Home.aspx. Additionally, the AoA's National Family Caregiver Support Program provides information about practical support (e.g., counseling and respite services) in several languages at http://www.aoa.gov/AoARoot/AoA_Programs/HCLTC/Caregiver/index.aspx#resources
- **Alzheimer's Association:** Services for the patient and her sister may include in-home respite care, which may facilitate this patient's involvement in her faith community. See their Web site at http://www.alz.org/index.asp. Also, since she is concerned about safety, the association's Safety Center offers advice and programs such as Safe Return (e.g., in case her sister inadvertently walks away from their home) at http://www.alz.org/safetycenter/we_can_help_safety_center.asp.

- **Area Agency on Aging** (AAA): Funding for services is passed through the states to local agencies. Services for this patient may include home-delivered meals and transportation to stores and appointments.
- Additionally, with her permission, explore whether informal supports, such as her church community, have a visiting ministry or a volunteer chore service.
- Finally, some communities have a community response telephone number that is accessed by dialing 211, where a person helps the older adult or family member match their needs to local availability of and eligibility for social services to support her in her caregiving role.

Education and advocacy organizations for caregivers include the following:

- Family Caregiver Alliance: http://www.caregiver.org/caregiver/jsp/home.jsp. Full citations for this agency's reports are listed in the references section.
- National Family Caregivers Association: http://www.thefamily-caregiver.org/
- National Alliance for Caregiving: http://www.caregiving.org/. Full citations for this agency's reports are listed in the references section.
- National Alliance for Mental Illness: This site is for families dealing with neuropsychiatric and behavioral difficulties at http://www.nami.org/.

REFERENCES

Beach, S., Schulz, R., Williamson, G., Miller, L., Weiner, M., & Lance, C. (2005). Risk factors for potentially harmful informal caregiver behavior. *Journal of the American Geriatrics Society, 53*(2), 255–261.

Carter, P. A. (2002). Caregivers' descriptions of sleep changes and depressive symptoms. *Oncology Nursing Forum, 29*(9), 1277–1283.

Covinsky, K. E., Newcomer, R., Fox, P., Wood, J., Sands, L., Dane, K., . . . Yaffe, K. (2003). Patient and caregiver characteristics associated with depression in caregivers of patients with dementia. *Journal of General Internal Medicine, 18*(12), 1006–1014.

Farran, C., Loukissa, D., Lindeman, D., McCann, J., & Bienias, J. (2004). Caring for self while caring for others: The two-track life of coping with Alzheimer's disease. *Journal of Gerontological Nursing, 30*(5), 38–46.

Fick, D., Cooper, J., Wade, W., Waller, J., Maclean, J., & Beers, M. (2003). Updating the Beers criteria for potentially inappropriate medication use in older adults: Results of a US consensus panel of experts. *Archives of Internal Medicine, 163*(22), 2716–2724.

Gallo, J. J., & Rabins, P. V. (1999). Depression without sadness: Alternative presentations of depression in late life. *American Family Physician, 60,* 820-826.

Given, C., Given, B., Stommel, M., Collins, C., King, S., & Franklin, S. (1992). The caregiver reaction assessment (CRA) for caregivers to persons with chronic physical and mental impairments. *Research in Nursing and Health, 15*(4), 271–283.

Gray, L. (2003). *Caregiver depression: A growing mental health concern.* San Francisco, CA: Family Caregiver Alliance/National Center on Caregiving.

Johnson, R. W., & Schaner, S. G. (2005). *Many older Americans engage in caregiving activities. Perspectives on productive aging. (3rd issue).* Washington, DC: Urban Institute.

Juratovac, E. (2009). *Effort in caregiving and its relationship to caregiver depressive symptoms.* (Doctoral dissertation). Available from ProQuest Dissertations & Theses database. (CMI# AAT 3368061).

National Alliance for Caregiving [NAC] & American Association of Retired Persons [AARP] (2009). *Caregiving in the U. S.* Washington, DC: NAC.

Pinquart, M., & Sörensen, S. (2003). Differences between caregivers and non-caregivers in psychological health and physical health: A meta-analysis. *Psychology and Aging, 18*(2), 250–267.

Saunders, M. M. (2008). Factors associated with caregiver burden in heart failure family caregivers. *Western Journal of Nursing Research, 30*(8), 943–959.

Schulz, R., & Beach, S. R. (1999). Caregiving as a risk factor for mortality: The caregiver health effects study. *Journal of the American Medical Association, 282,* 2215–2219.

Sink, K., Leng, X., Williamson, J., Kritchevsky, S., Yaffe, K., Kuller, L., Yasar, S., . . . Goff, D. C. (2009). Angiotensin-converting enzyme inhibitors and cognitive decline in older adults with hypertension: Results from the Cardiovascular Health Study. *Archives of Internal Medicine, 169*(13), 1195–1202.

Sörensen, S., & Pinquart, M. (2005). Racial and ethnic differences in the relationship of caregiving stressors, resources, and sociodemographic variables to caregiver depression and perceived physical health. *Journal of Aging and Mental Health, 9*(5), 1–14.

Vitaliano, P. P., Zhang, J., & Scanlan, J. M. (2003). Is caregiving hazardous to one's physical health? A meta-analysis. *Psychological Bulletin, 129*(6), 946–972.

Zauszniewski, J., Morris, D., Preechawong, S., & Chang, H. (2004). Reports on depressive symptoms in older adults with chronic conditions. *Research & Theory for Nursing Practice, 18*(2–3), 185–196.

Case 4.5 Transitions

By Elizabeth McGann, DNSc, RN, and Lynn Price, JD, MSN, MPH, FNP-BC

Mr. O is a 73-year-old, cognitively intact Hispanic male discharged today from the hospital. He is transitioning to a short-term rehabilitation setting for physical therapy conditioning and for stabilization of his diabetes and heart failure. He and his family are being educated about best practices to optimize conditioning and chronic disease management at home. This is his third admission in a year for acute decompensated heart failure attributed to ineffective self-management. In addition to Class C heart failure and hypertension, Mr. O's past medical history is significant for Type 2 diabetes, peripheral neuropathy, COPD, peripheral vascular disease, and chronic venous stasis. Mr. O had bilateral cataract removal 2 years ago. He has a 40 pack year history of smoking; he quit smoking 10 years ago. He has no history of alcohol or other substance abuse. Past family medical history is noncontributory. Mr. O resides with his wife, who at 70 years old is retired and in poor health. They both have demonstrated self-care neglect over the past several years. Mr. O has 2 older siblings who live in the same community. He has 2 daughters and 1 son; all live within a 2-hour drive. Mr. O is a retired bus driver with a high school education. He and his wife have lived in their second floor urban walk-up apartment for 30 years. He is sedentary and drives locally to do errands, keep medical appointments, and make occasional family visits. The couple attends the local senior center for lunch twice weekly. Mr. O receives social security, a pension, Medicare A and B, and has supplemental insurance.

Case Studies in Gerontological Nursing for the Advanced Practice Nurse, First Edition.
Edited by Meredith Wallace Kazer, Leslie Neal-Boylan.
© 2012 John Wiley & Sons, Inc. Published 2012 by John Wiley & Sons, Inc.

Over the last year, the children have encouraged their parents to move to a local senior congregate housing development. Both Mr. and Mrs. O are resistant to the idea of moving after his short-term rehabilitation stay, but eventually they acquiesce. The children are already working on the plan to transition their parents from their current apartment. Mr. O states that he "cannot wait to get home." Mrs. Ortiz states that her husband is "quite a handful". At the time of his hospital admission, Mr. O was taking glargine insulin, 20 units every night before bed, if blood glucose by finger stick is greater than 120; losartan, 150 mg daily; metoprolol succinate extended release, 200 mg daily; isosorbide dinitrate, 40 mg 4 times daily; spironolactone, 25 mg daily; tiotropium capsule, 2 inhalations daily; omeprazole, 10 mg daily. Mr. O will continue on these medications with the following additions: rapid-acting insulin, 5 units 15 minutes before each meal, and to a sliding scale 2 hours postprandial; furosemide, 20 mg daily. He is allergic to angiotensin-converting enzyme (ACE) inhibitors (cough).

OBJECTIVE

Mr. O's height is 5 ft 5 inches; weight: 175 lb; blood pressure: 154/92; heart rate: 74; respiratory rate: 24; oxygen saturation on room air: 98%; temperature: 98.6. Mr. O is awake, alert, and oriented to time, place, and person. He is in no apparent distress, pleasant, and interactive. Eyes: PERRLA; EOM intact. Oropharynx: Mucosa pink and moist; dentures intact and appear well fitting. Neck: No jugular vein distention apparent, no bruits, supple, no adenopathy. Lungs: Regular breathing pattern (RR = 24), no tripod position, good exchange, and clear to auscultation throughout all lung fields. Cardiac: Normal sinus rhythm, no murmurs, no rubs, no digital clubbing, pedal pulses present +2. GI: Bowel sounds of normal pitch in all quadrants, soft, nontender, no masses. Musculoskeletal: Equal grip, ambulates well with walker, one-assist to raise from chair, trace (nonpitting) edema in bilateral lower extremities.

ASSESSMENT

Chronic health issues: Mr. O is managing a number of chronic health issues including poorly controlled Type 2 DM; currently stable heart failure; well-controlled chronic venous stasis; stable COPD; impaired GFR; potential translocation stress; likely caregiver burden; and moderate physical deconditioning.

Self-care deficit: Due to numerous chronic health issues, living independently may no longer be possible. The patient and family need support for transitional care.

DIAGNOSTICS

Mr. O's fasting blood glucose by finger stick on the morning of hospital discharge was 158. Labs: HgAIc is 8%; CBC, BMP, and TSH are within the normal ranges. BUN and CR are also within normal ranges; GFR is 50.

CRITICAL THINKING

Using the elements of the Transitional Care Model, how can the advance practice clinician best support Mr. O's self-care deficit?

How does traditional discharge planning differ from the Transitional Care Model?

During the patient and family meeting, congregate housing is discussed. When Mr. O returns to his room, he asks the clinician what congregate housing is. What information does the clinician need to share with Mr. O?

Describe 5 specifically tailored interventions based on the transitional care model that the interdisciplinary team (coordinated by the agency discharge planner) might plan and/or facilitate as Mr. O and his wife transition to congregate housing.

How might Mr. O's ethnic, educational, or social history impact his adjustment to relocation in congregate housing?

What are some behaviors that may indicate that Mr. O is not making a good adjustment to congregate housing?

On what evidence would a discharge plan modeled on transitional care address the management of heart failure?

Are there any national guidelines that address relocation in cognitively intact elders?

What are the policy implications if the Transitional Care Model becomes more widely adopted as insurance coverage reimbursement becomes available in more states.

Explain how the middle range theory of transitions developed by Meleis et al. (2000) provides a framework or perspective for effective discharge planning. Identify the transitions the clinician believes Mr. O was experiencing.

RESOLUTION

Using the elements of the Transitional Care Model, how can the advance practice clinician best support Mr. O's self-care deficit?
The transitional care model is an evidence-based model that includes coordination and continuity of care; complication avoidance; timely treatment and management of acute and chronic illness; active involvement of patients, family, and informal caregivers; and sharing of information among health care providers (Naylor & Keating, 2008). For a more general overview of transitional care and practical application, see Burke (2009). Using the elements of the model, the clinician plans a meeting with the patient and family to determine options for improved self-care. The clinician can then work with other health care providers to coordinate a plan of care that includes supportive housing to facilitate continuity of care.

How does traditional discharge planning differ from the Transitional Care Model?
In traditional discharge planning, the nurse serves as a facilitator of home care needs post discharge, but does not physically follow the patient from hospital to home. Nor does the clinician continue to facilitate patient needs between home (with or without home care) and other providers. Within the Transitional Care Model, the clinician continues to follow the patient through all environments of care ensuring continuity of care. In the case of Mr. O, continuity of care could significantly impact further hospitalizations for preventable health problems.

During the patient and family meeting, congregate housing is discussed. When Mr. O returns to his room, he asks the clinician what congregate housing is. What information does the clinician need to share with Mr. O?
Congregate housing is a secure and semi-independent living arrangement in a community setting. Residents usually live in a private apartment and pay rent. It is not designed for individuals who need 24-hour supervision and assistance. Generally, one meal is provided in a communal setting along with housekeeping services. Some have service coordinators to help residents access community based services. Additional meals, transportation and recreational activities may be provided, but they may require additional fees. Congregate communities do not provide nursing or rehabilitative services, nor

monitor medication administration. There are differences in congregate housing resources between states (Housing Options, 2008).

Mr. O makes good progress in short term rehabilitation and is scheduled for discharge the following week. While no formal transitional care model is in place in this agency, many of the basic principles can be incorporated.

Describe 5 specifically tailored interventions based on the transitional care model that the interdisciplinary team (coordinated by the agency discharge planner) might plan and/or facilitate as Mr. O and his wife transition to congregate housing.

1. Reframe the move to congregate housing by focusing on the positive aspects of this transition or relocation. Discuss perceived losses and gains with Mr. and Mrs. O and their family. This will serve to lessen relocation stress.
2. Gather baseline data on activities of daily living (ADL) and instrumental activities of daily living (IADL) needs, medications, treatments, current sources of assistance and contact information for social supports at time of discharge.
3. Develop a seamless plan of care designed with the patient, family and providers, taking into account the information above.
4. Develop a clear emergency plan for early identification and intervention to prevent readmissions. Mr. or Mrs. O will know whom to call first.
5. Order a home care visit within 2 days of discharge to provide ongoing nurse evaluation of self-care management skills
6. Implement other community referrals as needed, including physical therapy and transportation.,
7. Communicate with the manager of congregate housing. Plan a family visit prior to moving in. Involve distant children in the plan of care.
8. Evaluate informal caregiving adequacy (Hertz, Rossetti, Koren, & Robertson, 2005; Naylor et al., 2004; Riegel et al., 2009).

How might Mr. O's ethnic, educational, or social history impact his adjustment to relocation to congregate housing?
Mr. O (and his wife) may have no experience with the concept of congregate housing. He is likely not to be an internet user and, therefore, not have easy access to information about congregate housing. Mr. O has been independent and has been the primary provider for himself and his family during his entire adult life. Congregate housing may threaten his perceptions of being independent, of being a good family provider, and of being healthy enough to live without assistance. He may have heard negative stories about congregate housing from his current neighbors.

What are some behaviors that may indicate that Mr. O is not making a good adjustment to congregate housing?

Mr. O (and his wife) will need several weeks to fully adjust to their new environment. This adjustment period may last longer if they have sacrificed long-held family belongings, furniture, and so on. Following a reasonable time for adjustment, behaviors that may indicate Mr. O has not made a successful transition to congregate housing include insomnia, lack of appetite, seclusion from family or the congregate housing community, anxiety, behavioral disturbances, incontinence, and unexplained aggression to staff. There also may be evidence of physiologic changes related to his multiple comorbidities, suggesting ineffective self-management.

On what evidence would a discharge plan modeled on transitional care address the management of heart failure?

The American Heart Association and the American College of Cardiology Foundation jointly sponsored the *2009 Focused Update: ACCF/AHA Guidelines for the Diagnosis and Management of Heart Failure in Adults* (Jessup et al., 2009). A link to these guidelines and other numerous easily accessible heart failure references in PDF format are available. (Heart failure, 2010).

Are there any national guidelines that address relocation in cognitively intact elders?

The Management of Relocation in Cognitively Intact Older Adults Guidelines (2005) is available at the National Clearing House Web site. This guideline is based on work from the University of Iowa Gerontological Nursing Interventions Research Center (Hertz et al., 2005).

What are the policy implications if the Transitional Care Model becomes more widely adopted as insurance coverage/reimbursement becomes available in more states?

The Transitional Care Model (TCM) is formally in use in only some states at this time (e.g., CA and PA), but it has potential for more widespread use as insurance coverage/reimbursement becomes more available for this. The federal government also has recently offered funding for Nurse Managed Health Centers, which offer a ready model for implementing the TCM. For elders with chronic health problems and multiple comorbidities, the TCM has shown to reduce hospital readmissions, enhance satisfaction of consumers, and reduce health care costs. To extend the question, students may be asked to compare the TCM to the Medical Home Concept (Transitional Care Model: Quality, Cost, and Value, 2008–2009).

Explain how the middle range theory of transitions developed by Meleis et al. (2000) provides a framework or perspective for effective discharge planning. Identify the transitions the clinician believes Mr. O was experiencing.

Meleis describes the process and outcomes of transitions, and types of transitions (developmental, situational, health/illness, or organizational). She also describes patterns and characteristics of transitions. Transitions present both a threat to personal identity as it relates to health and vulnerabilities in beliefs regarding health practices for patients and families. Much depends on personal meanings, cultural beliefs, socioeconomic status, knowledge, and the support of family, community, and society. Positive outcomes include mastery of the transition by the individual and family, as revealed by feeling connected and confident in their coping skills. Knowledge of this theory helps the clinician to better understand the experience of Mr. O's transitions and better plan interventions to assure better outcomes (Meleis et al., 2000).

Mr. O is experiencing a health-illness transition. He is coping with multiple comorbidities and a worsening of his heart failure. He has also experienced a situational transition with his discharge from acute care to short-term rehabilitation and his move to congregate housing.

REFERENCES

American Heart Association. (2010). Heart failure. Retrieved from http://www.americanheart.org/presenter.jhtml?identifier=3004550

Burke, M. (2009). Transitional care: What does it mean for nurses? *Journal of Gerontological Nursing, 35*, 3–4.

Hertz, J. E., Rossetti, J., Koren, M. E., & Robertson, J. F. (2005). *Management of relocation in cognitively intact older adults.* Retrieved from http://www.guideline.gov/summary/summary.aspx?doc_id=8110&nbr=004517&string=relocation

Jessup, M., Abraham, W. T., Casey, D. E., Feldman, A. M., Francis, G. S., Ganiats, T. G., . . . Yancy, C. W. (2009). 2009 focused update: ACCCF/AHA guidelines for the diagnosis and management of heart failure in adults: A report of the American College of Cardiology Foundation/American Heart Association Task Force on Practice Guidelines. *Circulation, 119*, 1977–2016. doi: 10.1161/CIRCULATIONAHA.109.192064.

Meleis, A. I., Sawyer, L. M., Im, E., Messias, D. K., & Schumacher, K. (2000). Experiencing transitions: An emerging middle range theory. *Advances in Nursing Science, 23*, 12–28.

Naylor, M., Brooten, D., Campbell, R., Maislin, G., McCauley, K., & Schwartz, J. (2004). Transitional care of older adults hospitalized with heart failure: A randomized controlled trial. *Journal of the American Geriatrics Society, 52*, 675–684.

Naylor, M., & Keating, S. (2008). Transitional care. *Journal of Social Work Education, 44*, 65–73.

Naylor, M. D. (2008–2009). Transitional care model: Quality, cost, and value. Retrieved from http://www.transitionalcare.info/ToolQual-1801.html

Riegel, B., Moser, D. K., Anker, S. D., Appel, L. J., Dunbar, S. B., Grady, K. L., & Whellan, D. J. (2009). State of the science: Promoting self-care in persons with heart failure: A scientific statement from the American Heart Association. *Circulation, 120,* 1141–1163. doi: 10.1161/CIRCULATIONAHA. 109.192628.

State of Connecticut Department of Social Services, Aging Service Divisions State Unit on Aging. (2008). Housing options. Retrieved from http://www.ct.gov/agingservices/cwp/view.asp?a=2513&q=313066

Case 4.6 Shifting the Focus of Care

By Alison Kris, PhD, RN

Mrs. B is a 65-year-old woman diagnosed with stage IV ovarian cancer, who has been admitted to a nursing home. For the past 5 years, she has undergone aggressive treatment for her cancer at a local academic medical center. She failed 6 cycles of carboplatin and paclitaxel (Taxol) and 1 round of high-dose chemotherapy accompanied with autologous bone marrow transplantation (ABMT). Prior to admission, she had debulking surgery to help ease pain and to alleviate gastrointestinal distress. Before her diagnosis with ovarian cancer, her health was excellent; and she regularly participated in triathlons. She is divorced and has no contact with her former spouse. She has 2 young sons aged 24 and 28, who visit her regularly in the nursing home. Her parents are deceased. Despite the fact that she has sold her home in order to pay for her nursing home stay, she worries that an extended stay in the nursing home will quickly exhaust her resources. Her children are not in a position to help pay for her nursing home care. Her ovarian tumor has rapidly regrown following her debulking surgery and is now completely occluding her intestine. She has a nasogastric (NG) tube to suction for decompression and is NPO (nothing by mouth) receiving TPN (total parenteral nutrition) through a central line for nutrition. Her orders include morphine sulfate, 2 mg every hour as needed for pain; TPN, 6 mL/h, 1 bag every 24 hours; daily weights; I/O (intake and output); finger sticks every 6 hours; weekly labs; central line dressing changes per protocol; oxygen 2 L, NC (nasal cannula), as needed; NG tube to suction; and V/S (vital signs) every shift. She has no known allergies.

Case Studies in Gerontological Nursing for the Advanced Practice Nurse, First Edition.
Edited by Meredith Wallace Kazer, Leslie Neal-Boylan.
© 2012 John Wiley & Sons, Inc. Published 2012 by John Wiley & Sons, Inc.

OBJECTIVE

Mrs. B is sitting in her nursing home bed. She has short gray hair and looks significantly younger than her stated age. On her wall are drawings and other artwork by her nieces and nephews. Her physical exam reveals increasing generalized edema (anasarca). Over the past week, her weight has increased from 127 to 145 pounds. She is slightly tachypneic (respiratory rate = 25) and tachycardic (pulse = 100); she is afebrile. Her oxygen saturation is 98% on room air. Her mouth is dry; and she is NPO, although she tells the clinician that she is often not compliant with the NPO orders because she still experiences hunger and derives pleasure from eating. She has an NG tube to suction for decompression, and she says that it had previously been helpful with her feelings of nausea, although more recently she is feeling nauseous despite the NG tube. She is dizzy when she stands, and she complains that her legs have gotten so heavy that it is difficult to walk. She wanted to take a shower earlier in the day, but she was not able to make it down the hall to the shower without stopping. She ultimately became so dizzy and fatigued that she decided to return to her room to lie down. Her skin is taut from the severe edema, although it is grossly intact. She complains of worsening pain in her back. The I/O log is incomplete, so it is unclear if her urinary output is decreasing. The clinician notes that she has received her as-needed MS 8 times in the past 3 days.

ASSESSMENT

Tachypnea: Mrs. B is experiencing SOB (shortness of breath) on exertion and is slightly tachypneic at rest. She has an order for as-needed oxygen; however, she does not like to wear her oxygen. The clinician understands that her shortness of breath may increase as she moves toward the end of life.

Oral health care: Because Mrs. B is NPO, excellent oral health care is extremely important. Additional education with the nursing home staff may be necessary to address this issue. Oral swabs every 2 hours should be ordered once Mrs. B is no longer able to be independent with oral health care. Clinicians should ensure access to mouthwash and dental supplies as needed.

Pressure ulcer prevention: Due to the extreme generalized edema, Mrs. B is at high risk of developing pressure ulcers. As her illness progresses, she will become gradually less mobile and will become increasingly dependent on the nursing staff for repositioning.

Fall prevention: Mrs. B is at high risk of falling due to her recent increases in edema and dizziness. While it is important that the nursing staff help Mrs. B maintain as much independence as possible, a clinician may need to frequently reevaluate her ability to move independently and consider what level of assistance is appropriate to prevent a fall.

Pain management: Due to the progressive nature of the disease, it is likely that pain levels will increase over time.

Nausea: Mrs. B is experiencing nausea due to the pooling of gastric secretions. She may also be experiencing fluctuating levels of opioid narcotic, which can contribute to her nausea due to the dependence on as-needed medications to manage pain levels.

DIAGNOSTICS

It is important to evaluate the benefit of additional intervention and to consider which treatments should be continued and which might be eliminated. Because Mrs. B is receiving TPN, she is not eligible for hospice care services. As is typical of hospice care companies, none in her community will accept a patient who wants to continue TPN. Mrs. B, however, feels that discontinuing TPN would have been an act of suicide since she was unable to take any food or fluid by mouth. Therefore, in this case formal hospice care from a hospice care company is not possible; instead, essential components of hospice care (symptom management, psychological and spiritual support, and bereavement services for the family) must be provided by the nursing home staff.

CRITICAL THINKING

Upon reviewing Mrs. B's orders, which might the clinician change and why?

How might the clinician be able to help Mrs. B's young sons?

What specific instructions might the clinician give to the nursing assistants who are caring for Mrs. B?

What conversations might the clinician initiate with Mrs. B?

RESOLUTION

Upon reviewing Mrs. B's orders, which might the clinician change and why?

When Mrs. B and her family decide to move towards hospice care, the goals of care should shift to palliation of distressing symptoms. This may include the following:

1. **Orders to discontinue:** All painful and unnecessary treatments should be discontinued. Finger sticks can be discontinued at this point, as can daily weights and vital signs. Since Mrs. B has an NG tube to intermittent suction, strict adherence to NPO is not necessary; and she should be able to consume foods as tolerated to enhance her quality of life. Diet can be advanced as tolerated to the extent that it does not create any additional nausea. Any food ingested will be removed by gastric suction, and this will allow the patient to experience the pleasure of eating.

2. **New orders to consider:** The fact that she has asked for her as-needed MS 8 times over the past 3 days implies that her pain management is subadequate. In reviewing WHO guidelines for pain management, it is clear that a basal dose of pain medication is needed with a prescription for additional bolus doses as needed for pain control. Mrs. B should have a basal dose of an as-needed opioid to help control her pain. Since Mrs. B already has central venous access, a PCA pump may be a reasonable solution. Alternatively, the use of fentanyl patches would provide stable pain relief over several days and would allow the IV to be discontinued in the last days of life. In addition, medications should be ordered to help control sensations of nausea. Nursing orders should include a mandate to provide assistance with oral health care as needed on each shift and a reminder to help the patient reposition frequently.

How might the clinician be able to help Mrs. B's young sons?

When her sons come into the facility, it will be important for the clinician to communicate with them frequently about their mother's care. In addition, there is an opportunity to serve as a resource for information and support for the staff nurses and nursing assistants working on Mrs. B's unit.

Often nurses working in long-term care have had limited hospice and palliative care experience; therefore, the clinician has an important role in staff education and supervision. The nurses on the unit should be encouraged to express concern for the well-being of Mrs. B's family. Teaching the staff can include the following points:

- Ensure that there are enough chairs in Mrs. B's room so that there is enough room sit comfortably.
- Offer the family something to eat or drink if at all possible. Encourage the sons to sit physically close to their mother.
- If possible, provide for a private room for Mrs. B. The nurses may be able to provide some additional resources (see resources) to help with the grief and bereavement process.
- In daily conversations with Mrs. B, talk to her to find out if there are any small items that might make her stay more comfortable. Special food items, nicely scented lotions, and lip balm are often appreciated by terminally ill patients in long-term care institutions. Encouraging the sons to bring those items in for their mother will help them to feel that they are helping to provide care for her.
- Explain to the family that visiting hours do not apply to family members of patients who are seriously ill and that they should feel free to call or to come into the facility at any time of the day or night.

What specific instructions might the clinician give to the nursing assistants who are caring for Mrs. B?

As a clinician, education of the nursing home staff should extend to the level of the nursing assistants. The importance of maintaining a pleasant environment of care should be emphasized. Encourage the nursing assistants to brighten up the room and to keep it clean. Because Mrs. B is experiencing nausea, it is important that items with strong odors be removed from her room quickly. Staff development and education can provide demonstrations about the provision of oral health care. Teach the nursing assistants to engage in conversations with Mrs. B about what type of swabs and mouthwashes she prefers. This will be important information at the point when she is no longer able to communicate her preferences. In addition, clinicians with experience in end-of-life care should role model and simulate conversations that might occur with patients at the end of life.

What conversations might the clinician initiate with Mrs. B?

The clinician may be able to ask Mrs. B if she has thought about the end of life. The clinician might ask her what she imagines it to be and discuss with her how any distressing symptoms might be managed, who should be called, and whether she would like her sons to be present. The clinician may ask if there is anything that could be done to make the environment more comfortable (music, photos from home, etc.). If Mrs. B does not currently have DNR orders in place (there is no indication of this) these orders should be discussed and initiated. Also, if there is a living will or DPA, these documents should be placed in her chart.

ADDITIONAL RESOURCES

Hartford Institute for Geriatric Nursing: ConsultGeriRN. http://consultgerirn. org Hospice and Palliative Care Nurses Association. http://www.hpna. org/

Resources for families: Information about nearing the end of life from the American Cancer Society. http://www.cancer.org/Treatment/ NearingtheEndofLife/NearingtheEndofLife/index.

Case 4.7 Without a Home

By Mary Shelkey, PhD, ARNP

Mr. A is a 58-year-old male who presents during the clinic's evening walk-in hours. The receptionist pages the clinician for clearance to register him because of his poor personal hygiene and his lack of a permanent address. He states that he is homeless but that he has a state voucher for medical care. He is complaining of the right lower leg pain. He has never been seen in the clinic and states that has no primary care physician but usually visits walk-in clinics or the emergency room (ER) when his legs "get bad". He has a rumpled discharge note from his last ER visit which lists his discharge diagnoses as chronic obstructive pulmonary disease, chronic alcohol abuse, and peripheral vascular disease with venous stasis ulcers. Discharge instructions included a referral to a day alcohol treatment program, a referral to a wound center for treatment of his venous stasis ulcers, smoking cessation instructions, and a prescription for an albuterol inhaler, 2–4 puffs (36–72 mcg) every 6 hours, and dicloxacillan, 250 mg every 6 hours for 7 days. He states that he received the medications at the hospital pharmacy, took them for a few days, but then lost them. He does not take any over-the-counter medications and states, "I can't afford any medications." Ten years ago, Mr. A moved to this city from the Midwest hoping to find permanent work. He claims he has been homeless for 2 years since he lost his job working odd jobs at construction sites. Prior to that, he drove taxis and served 2 years in the military as a young adult. He admits to over 40 years of drinking and smoking. He denies

Case Studies in Gerontological Nursing for the Advanced Practice Nurse, First Edition.
Edited by Meredith Wallace Kazer, Leslie Neal-Boylan.
© 2012 John Wiley & Sons, Inc. Published 2012 by John Wiley & Sons, Inc.

any other recreational/illicit drug use. He states he has lost a great amount of weight over the last year; he does not know how much but states that he used to weigh 145 lb.

He is estranged from his family, uncertain about family medical history, and has only a few friends whom he refers to as "my buddies on the street". He denies any prior psychiatric treatment/hospitalizations or any sad or anxious mood symptoms. He denies any drug or food allergies.

OBJECTIVE

Mr. A's general appearance is disheveled, with dirty clothing that is very malodorous. He presents as cognitively intact; alert; and oriented to person, place, and date. His mood is pleasant, without sad or anxious symptoms. His vital signs are oral temperature: 98.4 degrees Fahrenheit; blood pressure: 146/88; pulse: 88; respirations: 16 and unlabored; and SaO_2: 96%. His height is 5 ft 10 inches, and his weight is 120 lb, with a body mass index of 17.2 (underweight). Examination of his mouth reveals poor hygiene with obvious caries and broken teeth. His heart sounds are normal. His chest configuration is mild barrel chest, and his lungs sounds are generally clear with some scattered expiratory wheezing. His abdominal exam is normal with no organ enlargement. Gross neurologic function, including cranial nerves and deep tendon reflexes, is intact. His musculoskeletal exam is normal with full active range of motion of all joints. Upper (bilateral brachial, radial) and lower extremity pulses (bilateral posterior tibial, dorsalis pedis) are all 2+ (normal). His skin exam is normal except for bilateral 2+ lower extremity edema with an anterior right lower extremity, oval 4 cm × 5 cm × 1 cm ulcer, with serosanguinous drainage and mild erythema of surrounding skin (Fig. 4.7.1).

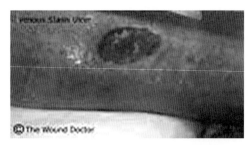

Figure 4.7.1. Venous stasis ulcer showing good granulation (The Wound Doctor, 2011).

ASSESSMENT

Right lower extremity venous stasis ulcer: This patient has a history of peripheral vascular disease and chronic venous stasis ulcers. Homelessness typically exacerbates medical conditions and causes homeless older adults to experience higher rates of morbidity and mortality compared to older adults with adequate housing. Premature death most often results from acute and chronic medical conditions aggravated by homelessness, rather than either mental illness or substance abuse (National Coalition for the Homeless, 2009).

Peripheral vascular disease—venous: Surgical treatment is not typically indicated for this disorder. Elevating the legs and applying compression hose are the most appropriate methods for reducing this edema. Homeless elders do not typically have the resources to buy or maintain compression hose. As well, malnutrition and low albumin levels often worsen the edema as fluid escapes from the intravascular space into the interstitial space and causes edema.

Chronic Obstructive Pulmonary Disease (COPD): The primary approach to arrest this disease is smoking cessation. Medication therapy includes inhalers or nebulizers to maximize keeping the small airways patent. Health promotion measures, such as influenza and pneumococcal immunizations, are critical in preventing complications of this disease. With the decreased monies to public health over the last decade, fewer health maintenance resources are available to all poor individuals, including the homeless.

Chronic alcohol use: Alcoholism is a growing and often undetected problem among older adults. Treatment approaches are generally the same across the life span, including alcohol treatment programs, counseling, and individual and family therapies. Treatment of the disorder will be complicated and likely unsuccessful if an underlying cause is not addressed (e.g., depression).

Tobacco use: Cigarette smoking is the most common cause of COPD in America and Western Europe (McPhee & Papadakis, 2010). Additionally, smoking increases the risk of fatal heart disease, lung cancer, and other cancers such as cancer of the mouth, throat, pancreas, esophagus, kidney, bladder, and cervix. Therapeutic approaches to smoking cessation include strong, clear encouragement by a clinician to stop smoking at each health encounter. Planning behavioral strategies, such as eliciting the support of family and friends and removing cigarettes from the environment, can be very helpful. Nicotine gum and patches may also be used but can be expensive.

Homelessness: In the United States, homelessness in older adults is reported to be increasing at an alarming rate due to the national economic downturn as well as other challenges, such as medical problems and mental illness. Although older adults are reported to have the lowest rate of homelessness, they suffer disproportional rates of chronic illness and premature death. Although there is no consensus regarding the age that defines a homeless older adult, there is a growing agreement that people aged 50 and over should be included in this category (National Coalition for the Homeless, 2009). Homeless people rarely live beyond 65 years of age. The average age of death among homeless men has been reported to be between 51 and 53 years old (Wright, 1989). The Hearth Foundation, a Boston, Massachusetts–based advocacy group serving homeless older adults, conducted a survey of homeless older adults (Hearth Foundation, 2009). These homeless older adults reported multiple challenges. Many of them, most in their fifties, had chronic health problems associated with old age, making it unlikely to obtain employment. They reported the following multiple causes for their homelessness: mental health problem (36%), physical health problem (30%), family and friends ask them to leave (28%), addictions (19%), eviction (14%), loss of family member providing home or care, (9%); loss of housing unit (6%), domestic violence or elder abuse (4%), and self-neglect (4%). The most common physical problems reported were circulation/heart (69%), hypertension (61%), diabetes (52%), arthritis (52%), vision problems (32%), lung problems (28%), dental problems (21%), hearing problems (20%), and skin problems (20%). The most commonly reported psychiatric problems were a past history of alcohol use (25%), schizophrenia (22%), depression (20%), AD and dementia (13%); paranoia (8%), and bipolar disorder (5%). Developmental disabilities (10%) were also reported, but current substance use was not reported. Many of these older adults required assistance with instrumental activities of daily living (e.g., medication administration) and activities of daily living (e.g., cooking, hygiene).

Elderly homeless persons are more prone to victimization and more likely to be ignored by law enforcement. In 2006, 27% of the homeless victims of violent crimes were between 50 and 59 years of age (National Coalition for the Homeless, 2009). Despite their multiple health needs, homeless older adults face numerous barriers in accessing adequate medical care.

DIAGNOSTICS

Diagnostic testing for Mr. A's lower extremity venous stasis ulcer will include a complete blood count to gauge the severity of the infection.

If the ulcer has a very toxic appearance, laboratory testing for an elevated creatinine kinase level should be added to rule out rhambdomyolysis. If the venous stasis ulcer has drainage, a culture and sensitivity might be considered. If suspected, a culture specifically testing for methicillin-resistant *Staphylococcus aureus* should be done.

Given Mr. A's homelessness, chronic alcohol abuse, and low body mass index, malnutrition needs to evaluated. Protein-energy malnutrition is typically divided into the following 2 distinct syndromes; **Kwashiokor**, which is caused by a deficiency of protein in the presence of adequate energy, and **Marasmus**, which is caused by combined protein and energy deficiency. Serum albumin levels will be needed to determine Mr. A's protein stores. Additionally his chronic alcoholism may have caused hepatic dysfunction; therefore, a complete metabolic panel is indicated.

The CBC was normal. The culture and sensitivity test was done and is pending, although it is uncertain that Mr. A will return to the clinic or be able to call for follow-up results. The complete metabolic panel was essentially normal except for the serum albumin, which was 2.8 g/dL, which signifies protein calorie malnutrition.

CRITICAL THINKING

What is the most likely diagnosis and why?

What is the plan of treatment for Mr. A?

What is the plan for follow-up treatment?

Does the patient's psychological history impact the way the clinician treats this patient?

What should be done if the clinician is concerned about tuberculosis?

What are the best treatment options for Mr. A considering the differentials listed?

Are there any standardized guidelines that the clinician should use to assess or treat this case?

RESOLUTION

What is the most likely diagnosis and why?

Cellulitis: Two life-threatening entities that present in similar ways to cellulitis include necrotizing fasciitis and deep venous thrombosis

(DVT). The diagnosis of necrotizing fasciitis should be considered in a very toxic appearing patient. It should also be considered in a patient with bullae, crepitus, or anesthesia of the involved skin; overlying skin necrosis; and elevated CK. These findings may also be present in severe cellulitis and bacteremia, but it is essential to rule out necrotizing fasciitis, as immediate surgical debridement would be necessary (Berger, 2010).

Deep vein thrombosis should be suspected for patients with a history of cancer, recent limb immobilization, or recent confinement to bed. Color duplex ultrasonography may be performed on patients with no obvious cause of lower extremity swelling, since DVT is difficult to exclude on clinical grounds (Gonzales & Nadler, 2010).

Weight loss: The history is very important in establishing the causes of unintentional weight loss. It is important to consider decreased intake, impairment in absorption, and excess demand. Excessive alcohol use can contribute to malabsorption, as well as other conditions such as hepatitis, poor dentition, renal or liver disease, and mood disorders (Goroll & Mulley, 2009). A difficult diagnostic issue in the evaluation of weight loss is the possibility of an occult malignancy. However, by the time weight loss has occurred, most malignancies are advanced with a median survival about 2 months; few live longer than a year. A simple panel of blood tests complete blood count, erythrocyte sedimentation rate, aspirate amino transferase, alanine amino transferase, gamma-gutamyl transpeptidase, alkaline phosphatase, and serum albumin have been found to have a high sensitivity (95%) but low specificity (35%) for diagnosis of cancer in older adults with unexplained weight loss.

What is the plan of treatment for Mr. A?

The most difficult problem in dealing with Mr. A's treatment plan is his current homelessness, chronic alcoholism, and malnutrition. Treatment of his venous stasis wound is more straightforward as his previous prescription of dicloxacillan, 250 mg every 6 hours for 7 days, had slightly improved the condition of his wounds. However, he had not finished the course of medication treatment and was unable to get regular wound dressing changes. The clinician prescribes the antibiotic again and educates Mr. A regarding the importance of completing the course of the antibiotics. His wounds will need daily dressing changes and evaluation.

Additionally, his low serum albumin is likely worsening his lower extremity edema, as his intravascular fluid is leaking into the interstitial spaces of his lower extremities. The clinician is reluctant at this point to do an aggressive workup for an occult malignancy because of the poor prognosis if positive and the likelihood that his poor nutritional intake may be the primary cause of his weight loss.

What is the plan for follow-up treatment?

The clinician consults with the clinic social worker, and he is able to locate a church near the soup kitchen where Mr. A typically eats. There is a parish nurse who is willing to change the lower extremity dressing every day. She also agrees to speak to the workers in the soup kitchen and request that they encourage Mr. A to increase his protein intake.

The social worker develops a treatment plan for Mr. A to return to the clinic every 3 days for evaluation of his wound and medication adherence. The social worker is able to arrange for a meal voucher and a free shower in the emergency room, and Mr. A is extremely pleased with this arrangement and agrees to return to the clinic. The social worker schedules a weekly follow-up visit with Mr. A with the goal of alcohol-abuse and job counseling. Mr. A and the social worker will work together to explore community availability of permanent housing. A nearby hospital has an alcohol support group that has many veterans and occasionally some homeless men, and the social worker has encouraged Mr. A to attend.

Does the patient's psychological history impact the way the clinician treats this patient?

The physical, psychological, and social problems associated with this case make it a complex treatment plan. The patient has no previous history of psychiatric illness but has been chronically abusing alcohol. As some older adults self-medicate their depression with alcohol, this is an important area of inquiry with this patient. As medication costs and compliance are important barriers to antidepressant treatment, counseling and support groups would be important treatment options to explore with this patient. Again, the clinic social worker is a valuable resource in providing or accessing these services.

What should be done if the clinician is concerned about tuberculosis?

If the patient complains of night sweats and cough, in addition to unintentional weight loss, tuberculosis (TB) would need to be considered. The tuberculin skin test is the most sensitive test for the diagnosis of infection with *Mycobacterium tuberculosis*, far more sensitive than a chest x-ray.

Approximately 20% of newly recognized cases of TB are extrapulmonary and are largely among HIV-positive patients. It might be necessary in patients with HIV exposure to test for this infection as well (Davis, 2009).

What are the best treatment options for Mr. A considering the differentials listed?

The most important treatment option for Mr. A is to establish a treatment plan that can assist in dealing with his overwhelmingly adverse social situation. Immediate treatment of his cellulitis can only be successful with collaboration of the social worker who will assist in negotiating a feasible plan for follow-up including accessing community resources to increase Mr. A's access to appropriate medical and nursing care.

Oral antibiotics for his lower extremity are the first-line treatment; they are the least invasive, and most cost effective. If the outpatient plan does not work, an inpatient stay for intravenous antibiotics may need to be considered. Dressing changes, as well as evaluation if the healing process, need to be done on a regular basis in order to prevent further contamination of the wound.

Involving the social worker, who can then access community resources, is the best option for addressing the patient's weight loss. Alcohol consumption reduction or cessation, with improved nutritional intake, should increase the patient's weight, albumin status, and vitamin and mineral intake unless another underlying occult process is responsible. An increase in serum albumin should decrease the loss of intravascular fluid into the interstitial spaces, thereby decreasing the lower extremity edema. Long-term goals for this patient will be to assist him in alcohol and smoking cessation and assist him in obtaining employment and permanent housing.

Are there any standardized guidelines that the clinician should use to assess or treat this case?
The National Clearing House has a clinical guideline for the diagnosis and management of skin and soft tissue infections at http://www.guideline.gov/content.aspx?id=8206.

The National Clearing House also has a guideline for unintended weight loss in older adults at http://www.guideline.gov/content.aspx?id=15436.

REFERENCES

Berger, T. G. (2010). Dermatologic disorders. In S. J. McPhee, M. A. Papadakis (Eds.), *2010 current medical diagnosis and treatment* (pp. 94–150). New York: McGraw Hill Medical.

Davis, B. T. (2009). Management of tuberculosis. In A. H. Goroll, A. G. Mulley (Eds.), *Primary care medicine: Office evaluation and management of the adult patient* (6th ed., pp. 403–408). Philadelphia: Wolters Kluwer: Lippincott Williams & Wilkins.

Gonzales, R., & Nadler, P. (2010). Common symptoms. In S. J. McPhee, M. A. Papadakis (Eds.), *2010 current medical diagnosis and treatment* (pp. 22–48). New York: McGraw Hill Medical.

Goroll, A. H., & Mulley, A. G. (2009). *Primary care medicine: Office evaluation and management of the adult patient* (6th ed.). Philadelphia: Wolters Kluwer: Lippincott Williams & Wilkins.

Hearth Foundation (2009). *Ending elder homelessness*. Retrieved from http://hearth-home.org/.

McPhee, S. J., & Papadakis, M. A. (2010). *2010 current medical diagnosis and treatment*. New York: McGraw Hill Medical.

National Coalition for the Homeless (2009). *Homelessness among elderly persons*. Retrieved from http://www.nationalhomeless.org/factsheets/Elderly.pdf.

The Wound Doctor.*Venous stasis ulcer showing good granulation*. Retreived June 10, 2011, from http://www.thewounddoctor.com/venousulcer.htm

Wright, J. D. (1989). *The homeless in America: Social institutions and social change*. New York: Aldine de Gruter.

ADDITIONAL REFERENCES

U.S. Census Bureau (2007). Income, poverty, and health insurance coverage in the United States: 2007. Current Population Reports, p. 60–235. U.S. Government Printing Office. Washington, DC.

U.S. Department of Housing and Urban Development (2010). The 2009 annual homeless assessment report. Retrieved from http://www.huduser.org/portal/Publications/pdf/5thHomelessAssessmentReport.pdf

U.S. Interagency Council on Homelessness (2010). Opening doors: Federal plan to prevent and end homelessness. Retrieved from http://www.ich.gov/

U.S. Social Security Administration (2009). Supplemental Security Record. Washington, DC.

Case 4.8 A Place Called Home

By Kelly Smith Papa, MSN, RN, and
Eileen O'Connor Smith, BSN, RN-C

It has been 3 months since Mrs. R moved into the Meadow Ridge Health Care Center. Over the past month, she has usually been found sitting alone in her reclining chair, facing the window in her dark semi-private bedroom. Her space is sparsely decorated with one framed painting, a couple of greeting cards, a stuffed teddy bear, and a shared television that is rarely turned off. Her bed is covered with a blush-pink quilt. The bedroom privacy curtain is partially drawn in the center of the shared space, and the room lights are usually off.

Mrs. R has Alzheimer disease. Her short-term memory loss is evident when speaking with her, and at times she needs assistance with personal care. When asked about the experience of living at Meadow Ridge, Mrs. R shares, "I'll have to be here for the rest of my time; I'm 91. In November, I will be 92; so I just can't 'go' anymore. I am never going home; I have to get use to it." She describes how it was getting harder for her to care for herself, especially to make her own meals while living in her own apartment and that she did not want anyone to come and live with her. Mrs. R cared for her husband when he was suffering from Alzheimer disease in their home. She states, "I did for him. I always promised I would not put him into a nursing home; now I am here." It has been 2 years since her husband's death. She has 3 daughters and states that she wishes she could live closer to them and to her church.

Mrs. R has had a hard time adjusting to having a roommate, who she feels dislikes her. She states that she made the decision to "overlook" her roommate's unfriendly behaviors. "I just ignore her. If she

Case Studies in Gerontological Nursing for the Advanced Practice Nurse, First Edition.
Edited by Meredith Wallace Kazer, Leslie Neal-Boylan.
© 2012 John Wiley & Sons, Inc. Published 2012 by John Wiley & Sons, Inc.

wants to speak, I'll talk to her; but I don't hold it against her. I don't think she remembers."

Care partners on the Meadow Ridge care team are concerned with the changes they have seen in Mrs. R's personality over the past 2 months. When she first arrived, she smiled and greeted others, asked them about their lives, and enjoyed spending time with other residents. Over the past 2 months, she has appeared to those around her to be increasingly sad, anxious, easily annoyed; has lost interest in things she once enjoyed; and has required more assistance with dressing and bathing. One morning last week, she became very angry and yelled at a care partner who offered to help Mrs. R get out of bed and get ready for the day. Mrs. R currently eats about half of each of her meals and has lost 6 lb in the past month. Her care partners report that she does not like to leave her bedroom and is quick to leave the dining room after a meal.

Recently one of Mrs. R's daughters called the charge nurse and shared that her mother had told her not to come and visit anymore. This change in behavior was very concerning to her daughter because she felt that her mom was always very social and enjoyed being with her family. Mrs. R's family described her as a kind and gentle person who always liked to make new friends, eat good food, laugh, and have a good time. Her family wonders if the changes in personality are part of the progression of her Alzheimer disease or results of something else?

Mrs. R's medications include Aricept, 10 mg by mouth daily; Namenda, 10 mg by mouth twice daily; Diovan with HCTZ, 80/12.5 mg by mouth daily; Lipitor, 10 mg by mouth daily; ASA, 81 mg by mouth daily; health shake nutritional supplement drink, 240 cc/8 oz 3 times daily; Tylenol, 650 mg by mouth every 4 hours as needed for pain; and an as-needed bowel regime including Milk of Magnesia, Dulcolax Suppository, and Fleet enema. She has no known allergies (NKA).

OBJECTIVE

Mrs. R presents as alert, forgetful, and oriented to place. Her vital signs are BP: 110/80; pulse: 70; respirations: 12; O_2 sat on room air: 99%; afebrile. She is 5 ft 6 inches tall and weighs 122 lb. Her pupils are equal, round, and react to light and accommodation (PERRLA). Mrs. R wears glasses and has mild wax buildup in her bilateral ears. Her oral mucosa is pink and moist. Her lung sounds are clear. Her abdomen is soft, nontender, with positive bowel sounds in all 4 quadrants. Mrs. R's skin is pink and intact, with dry skin on her legs and arms. She has no edema. Range of motion (ROM) is within normal limits. Test of muscle strength indicates slight weakness upon resistance.

ASSESSMENT

Cognitive cause for behavior change: Depression is very common among people with dementia, yet frequently unrecognized and untreated. Memory loss, forgetfulness, withdrawal, anger, changes in personality, and impaired ability to communicate can result in unrecognized and undertreated depression.

Physical causes for behavior change: Individuals with dementia are at a high risk for unidentified, undertreated, or untreated pain (Miller, Nelson, & Mezey, 2000). The clinician should assess for infections (urinary tract infections), gastrointestinal causes, and side effects of medications. It is also important to assess the amount and quality of uninterrupted sleep, as well as her fluid and nutritional intake.

Caregiver approach and/or environmental causes for behavior change: Due to cognitive, visual, and auditory deficits, the person with dementia may misinterpret the approach of the caregivers or the chaos in their environment. The person with dementia may be overwhelmed by the speed of the caregivers' approach, by not being able to see or hear their caregiver, or by the feeling of loss of physical and/or emotional control. The noise level or stimulation of the environment (including intercoms, other residents, televisions, inappropriate music, rushing staff, clutter, lack of light or personal connection) can also cause the person with dementia to have increased confusion.

Needs for purposefulness, relationships, and meaningful activities: Beyond our basic needs of food, clothing and shelter are the needs for connections to others and purposefulness in our lives. It is possible to feel loneliness even in the presence of others and boredom while being entertained.

DIAGNOSTICS

The following assessments were completed and results are as follows: pain assessment for advanced dementia (PainAD) score of 2. Cornell Scale for Depression in Dementia (CSDD) score is 14. The CSDD is used rather than the Global Depression (GD) scale because it has been found to be more reliable for people with Alzheimer disease. A score of 12 or higher indicates severe depression. The GD can be used for people with mild cognitive impairment with effect; but for people with , the CSDD is more reliable (Debruyne et al., 2009). Mini-mental State Examination (MMSE) score is 19. Functional Assessment Staging Tool (FAST) score is 6b.

A nursing assessment should track the hours and quality of sleep and wake patterns over a week. What is keeping her from getting restful uninterrupted sleep? What time is she waking up? Is she waking numerous times during the night? In fact, Mrs. R was waking up 3–4 times a night and sleeping for about 2–3 hours at a time. Her bedtime and the time she woke up in the morning have been different from her sleep wake cycle prior to living at Meadow Ridge. The following laboratory tests were ordered: urinalysis (UA) with microscopy; complete blood count (CBC); comprehensive metabolic panel (CMP); thyroid stimulation hormone (TSH); folic acid level; cholesterol; lipid panel; and 25-hydroxyvitamin D. The test results showed that the UA was negative for infection. CBC, CMP, TSH and folic acid levels were all within normal limits. Cholesterol levels were high. Mrs. R's vitamin D level was found to be insufficient at 27 ng/mL. Normal range is 20–80 ng/mL, <20 ng/mL is considered deficient, 20–30 ng/mL is insufficient, and >32 ng/mL is optimal.

CRITICAL THINKING

What is the most likely cause of Mrs. R's changes in personality?

What is the plan of treatment?

In a person-centered skilled nursing facility, how does a person's life story impact their plan of care?

What is the role of the advanced clinician in a person-centered skilled nursing facility? What impact can the clinician have on creating person-centered care environments?

What steps can be taken to help Mrs. R build relationships with others and feel more comfortable in her new home?

How should the care environment be modified to meet the needs of people with dementia who live there?

RESOLUTION

What is the most likely cause of Mrs. R's changes in personality?
- It is important to consider the multiple causes of Mrs. R's personality changes. Her CSDD score of 14 indicates that depression needs to be assessed and treated. Changes in personality are symptoms of Alzheimer disease.

- Moving away from her home decreases the compensatory strategies that a home environment creates to keep the person with Alzheimer's successful and independent. Mrs. R could be noticing changes in her memory as she is adjusting to her new room, bathroom, and dining room. It is no wonder that an awareness of this memory loss is frightening.
- The third area to consider as a cause of her personality change is to look at how she is coping with the transition from home into a skilled nursing environment. A transition into a nursing home is a major life event, one filled with many emotions including grief. The clinician should consider how she is coping with being away from home, suffering from short-term memory loss, meeting new people each day, and other life changes she is experiencing.

What is the plan of treatment?
- To treat Mrs. R's depression, she would need to have a comprehensive psychiatric evaluation and follow-up care with orders that could include placing her on an antidepressant. The psychiatric team might consider Remeron because it is an antidepressant and it stimulates appetite.
- She has had significant weight loss. Care partners reported that she is quick to leave the dining room. Further assessment needs to look at the reasons why she is not completing her meal and is rushing to leave. Is it the environment? Is it too noisy or chaotic? Does she know the people she is dining with? Is the food appetizing? Her orders include drinks 3 times a day to supplement her dietary intake. Are they filling her up and, therefore, she is not eating? What foods does she enjoy? How the dining experience be made to be more meaningful to her?
- The clinician should consider the physical environment that she is living in—her bedroom and the community of which she is a part. What does it look like? Does it look like her home, a hotel, or a hospital? Her bedroom space should be made like her home—not home-like—but her home. By decorating it with her personal touches, the bedroom space becomes the patient's home. Arrange to bring in her furniture, precious personal mementos, and framed family photographs. If possible, ask her to select the paint color and a bedspread. These personal touches to her room help her care partners learn more about her and the stories of her life.
- To help treat Mrs. R and the other residents that live in her community who are most likely experiencing the same emotions, the clinician may assist with offering many ways for care partners to learn about person centered care approaches and practices. Care partners include all team members and the leaders who create the culture of the home.

In a person-centered skilled nursing facility, how does a person's life story impact their plan of care?
The clinician should get to know the person's life story. The more the clinician knows about the person, the easier it is to transcend from caring **for** a person to caring **about** a person. This shift impacts how people prefer to live, knowing that they are a person first and not solely a task to be completed. There are many ways to learn about a person. The clinician could begin by asking open-ended questions that encourage reflection of life experiences. From the moment the person walks in the door of the home, opportunities to learn and share the stories with all care partners exist. Begin with and build the care plans around these life stories. This will help to build a relationship between residents and consistent care partners. As the person progresses in their disease, it is reassuring to them to hear a story from their past.

Avoid asking questions that have one correct answer or test memory. People with Alzheimer disease have so much to share, and facilitating this sharing helps build the relationship as collaborative, not one sided. Clinicians may help to build meaningful reciprocal relationships by asking about personal beliefs and values or by asking for advice. Instead of saying, "How many kids do you have?" which would test memory, the person may be asked, "My daughter is turning 2, and we are potty training her. What parenting advice do you have?" Conversations that offer personal thoughts and reflection are filled with the wisdom of their lives, personal philosophies, and a tie to the moment they are living.

What is the role of the advanced clinician in a person-centered skilled nursing facility? What impact can the clinician have on creating person-centered care environments?
As a clinician in a person-centered skilled nursing facility, the role goes beyond physical assessments and ordering lab work or medications. The clinician is a leader and a teacher who values the work of each team member necessary for the people who live in a person-centered care home. The role includes creating environments that people are proud to live and work in. The clinician helps the care team to always place the person before the task by role modeling this approach. The clinician asks the right questions, ones that help team members reflect with empathy on their actions and their hopes for the people who live there. The clinician should find ways to hire the right team members, hire for compassion and empathy, help to train, and evaluate their skills. They should utilize auditing tools to evaluate that person-centered approaches are not just talked about, but that they are being lived out each day during ADL, meals, activities, and with families.

What steps can be taken to help Mrs. R build relationships with others and feel more comfortable in her new home?
The antidote to loneliness and boredom is found in relationships. Mrs. R comes into contact with many people each day; but a relationship is

a friendship, a partnership between two people who know each other. A relationship is developed when people share life stories, have similar interests, live in the moment, share thoughts, and find ways to enjoy the other's company. It is important to seek ways in which to connect residents with like interests and in guiding the care team as they find methods to learn more about life stories and how to incorporate them into the day's events. The clinician should assist in developing examples of open-ended questions to spark the creative process of relationship building. For example, a discussion to reminisce on summertime memories may begin with "What were things you enjoyed doing in the summer before you went to bed?" Ask the family members to share their memories of things they did as a family in the summer (Spence, 1997).

It is important to introduce the patient to the people with whom she is dining or with whom she is engaging in social events? Her short-term memory loss may cause her to think that the people she sees each day are strangers? Dining is social; the more a person is engaged socially at a meal, the better they may eat. Many times we fail in our attempts to connect with others because we take too little time to sense and understand their needs. We assume too much, or we place our needs before theirs. We want them to get up, use the toilet, get dressed, take their medications, or eat. We must first seek to understand their feelings and needs by listening to their body language, words, and tone.

How should the care environment be modified to meet the needs of people with dementia who live there?

As the clinician reflects on the physical environment and what it looks like, they should think about the words used to describe the people who live in the home. Are they words of empathy or words that describe a task or a disability rather than a person? The language and words we use are powerful. How would Mrs. R feel if she heard people refer to her by using phrases such as "she refused," "she is resistive," "she's a walky-talky," "(Room number) 214 is easily agitated" or "she's a total," "she's a wanderer"? What image or symbol comes to mind when these words are used? As a nursing leader, the clinician can help to create a dignified home for the people who live there by considering language (Smith, Smith, & Papa, 2010).

Meadow Ridge and other skilled nursing facilities around this country are home to millions of people; however, in many cases a skilled nursing facility symbolizes something not friendly or home-like in our culture, but more of a mini-hospital. It is the role of all leaders in person-centered skilled nursing facilities to seek ways to lead a culture change and to improve the lives of the people who live and work in the home. This can be done on many levels; the first step is asking yourself, "Would I be proud to live here? Would I call this place home?"

REFERENCES

Debruyne, H., Van Buggenhout, M., Le Bastard, N., Aries, M., Audenaert, K., De Deyn, P., & Engelborghs, S. (2009). Is the geriatric depression scale a reliable screening tool for depressive symptoms in elderly patients with cognitive impairment? *International Journal of Geriatric Psychiatry, 24,* 556–562.

Miller, L., Nelson, L., & Mezey, M. (2000). Comfort and pain relief in dementia. *Journal of Gerontological Nursing, 26*(9), 32–40.

Smith, M., Smith, E., & Papa, K. (2010). Emotional memory. *Advance for Long-term Care Management, 13*(5), 51–52 & 69.

Spence, L. (1997). *Legacy.* Athens, Ohio: Swallow Press/Ohio University Press.

Case 4.9 Aging in Place

By Karen Dick, PhD, GNP-BC, FAANP

Mr. J is an 87-year-old retired engineer who has been a resident of The Pine Grove continuing care retirement community (CCRC) for the past 3 years. He has been followed by his long-term care clinician for the last 15 years; but since he is no longer driving into the city where his clinician is located, he has made the decision to join the primary care practice at the CCRC. He has a long and complex list of medical problems which include degenerative joint disease (DJD) of the lumbar and cervical spines with significant stenosis at L4-5 (last epidural steroid injection 2 years before), bilateral knee DJD, status post bilateral total knee replacement (TKR). He also has a history of inflammatory/rheumatoid arthritis, asthma, dysfunctional voiding syndrome, anxiety/depression, gout, hypertension, gastroesophageal reflux disease (GERD), venous insufficiency, peripheral neuropathy, restless leg syndrome, chronic constipation, and chronic insomnia. He reports that he had a fall last night while in the kitchen making cocoa. He landed on his buttocks and denies hitting his head or losing consciousness. Upon close questioning by the clinician, Mr. J and his companion admit that he has had 6 falls in the last 6 months, all occurring in the middle of the night. The patient volunteers that he has avoided additional falls by reaching out to hold onto something to break those falls. None of the falls were associated with precipitating events or syncope. Further questioning revealed that Mr. J was taking his companion's tramadol for back pain (which did help), that the Ambien was no longer helping him sleep, and that he has had an increase in urinary urges throughout the night without being able to void.

Mr. J is divorced and has 3 grown children. He decided to move into the CCRC as his companion of many years had moved in the year

Case Studies in Gerontological Nursing for the Advanced Practice Nurse, First Edition.
Edited by Meredith Wallace Kazer, Leslie Neal-Boylan.
© 2012 John Wiley & Sons, Inc. Published 2012 by John Wiley & Sons, Inc.

before. Mr. J does not smoke and reports drinking 1 glass of wine daily. He has recently stopped driving long distances but still has a car on the premises and admits to short trips to the grocery and for other errands. On the review of systems, he admits to decreased hearing despite wearing bilateral hearing aides. He reports that he is still dealing with depression and that "nothing has ever really helped". He describes an ongoing problem with insomnia and a dependence upon Ambien. He is up frequently during the night to urinate, which also impacts his ability to get adequate sleep. He has ongoing pain in his back and knees bilaterally that has affected his ability to walk. He has had an increase in the frequency of falling in the past 6 months and has been using his cane more consistently. He denies dyspnea on exertion (DOE), shortness of breath (SOB), and chest pain (CP); and he has no edema. He also reports being constipated over the last 3 days and admits to using his companion's Miralax this morning without any movement of his bowels. This, too, has been a long-term problem. His medications include lisinopril, 40 mg by mouth daily; ASA, 81 mg by mouth daily; allopurinol, 300 mg by mouth daily; omeprazole, 20 mg by mouth daily; finasteride, 5 mg by mouth daily; Flomax, 4 mg by mouth daily; Ambien CR, 12.5 mg by mouth hs as needed; melatonin, 3 mg by mouth at bedtime as needed; Os Cal with vitamin D, twice daily; Amitiza, 24 mcg by mouth daily; Sanctura, 20 mg by mouth daily; albuterol inhaler, as needed; and Tylenol, as needed. He is allergic to codeine, which causes him a headache.

OBJECTIVE

Mr. J is alert and oriented and in no acute distress. His vital signs are as follows: BP: 118/62; HR: 74; O_2 sat: 92%. He weighs 185 lb and is 5 ft 8 inches tall. His HEENT assessment reveals no thyromegaly and no lymphadenopathy. His heart rate is regular S1, S2, with no murmurs, rubs, or gallops. His lungs are clear to auscultation. Mr. J's abdomen is soft and nontender. There is no distension and no hepatosplenomegaly. His extremities reveal no edema. His skin assessment reveals several actinic keratoses of the hands and forearms. His gait is antalgic with short steps. The neurological exam is within normal limits. Past laboratory results are reviewed in his records.

ASSESSMENT

Potential fracture: Since Mr. J fell and landed on his buttocks, it is possible that he sustained a fracture. Continued reports of pain further support this as a possible differential diagnosis.

High risk for falls: Mr. J has had a number of falls over the past several months. The greatest risk factor for falls is a history of a prior fall. It is essential that the clinician consider referring him to the onsite fitness director for an exercise prescription to aide in strengthening and stability and obtain records from his neurologist in regard to his back pain. Records from his urologist were also requested.

Aging in place: Given Mr. J's long list of medical problems and current safety concerns, his future residential requirements must be considered. Aging in place is a concept that describes older adults' wishes to stay in familiar locations/environments as they age. Continuing care retirement communities (CCRCs) such as the one in which Mr. J currently resides provide older adults with the ability to maintain autonomy and to increase social engagement as they age (Heisler, Evans, Moen, 2004) The CCRC is a hybrid institution that provides housing, health care, and other social services for older adults along a continuum that begins with independent living and typically extends through assisted living and skilled nursing care. CCRCs often have a primary care practice. Residents of the CCRC are able to access (and pay privately for) independent providers who rent space at the CCRC and provide services such as massage, Reiki, and acupuncture services.

DIAGNOSTICS

Although Mr. J has some lab work from his previous provider in his chart, updated laboratory results should be ordered including a complete blood count (CBC) and metabolic profile. Since this latest fall has left Mr. J in acute pain, likely imaging and other diagnostics based on the history and physical exam would be ordered. An x-ray of the pelvis and spine should be ordered to determine the possibility of fractures from his recent falls. Further fall assessment, such as the get-up-and-go test, and examination of gait and neuropathy should also be conducted. The laboratory findings are all within normal limits. However, the x-ray shows an acute T12 compression fracture and a nondisplaced coccyx fracture.

CRITICAL THINKING

What factors are contributing to his risk of falls?

How can Mr. J's pain be best managed without increasing his risk for falls?

What would the next steps in a workup be?

What if Mr. J's health status and living situation continue to decline?

What guidelines are available to help with assessing an individual's need for assisted living?

RESOLUTION

What factors are contributing to his risk of falls?
This patient's impaired sleep and use of a hypnotic, along with an inadequate pain regime that has led to indiscriminate use of his companion's pain medication with subsequent side effects and coupled with urinary frequency at night, have all likely contributed. A detailed history and physical exam is needed to help identify what other factors (cardiovascular, neurological, musculoskeletal, infectious) could be contributing, so as to not draw a premature conclusion about the cause of these falls. Falls generally have multifactorial etiologies, and each potentially contributing etiology must be explored.

How can Mr. J's pain be best managed without increasing his risk for falls?
Given his strong pain complaints, Mr. J is initially prescribed a pain regime that includes oxycodone, 5 mg 3 times daily, with supplemental extra strength (ES) Tylenol. He is seen by neurosurgery, which recommends bracing and physical therapy. After a month, the patient is able to be weaned off the oxycodone; and his pain managed by tramadol and applications of ice alternating with heat. His bowel regime is changed to include a stool softener and daily Miralax. Ambien is discontinued, and he is started on trazodone, 50 mg by mouth at bedtime, with initial positive effects. He completes a trial of home physical therapy and is able to ambulate with a rolling walker. Of note, the physical therapist tells the clinician during the weekly team meeting that Mr. J's companion admitted to her that they shared medications and that this had been their practice for many years. Each "borrowed" each other's pain and sleeping medications.

What would the next steps in a workup be?
Mr. J needs an updated assessment of his mood. In this instance, the Geriatric Depression Scale (GDS; Yesavage et al., 1983) is used, as the practice does annual screening with patients to establish a baseline. His score is 7/15, which then leads to a referral to both the MSW to explore conflicts with his companion that Mr. J discussed and to the psychiatrist for further evaluation and treatment of his depressed mood. Since Mr. J's physical and emotional problems are contributing to his declining health status, the medical, rehab services, social work,

and psychiatry staff need to meet to establish an interdisciplinary plan of care with goals of improving pain relief, mood, and function.

What if Mr. J's health status and living situation continue to decline?
Four months later, Mr. J's companion calls for emergency help as she has found Mr. J on the floor next to his bed at 3 a.m. He is awake and talking but is found to be delirious, asking about "his meeting later in the day with the general." His companion reports that she has been giving him meclizine (an old prescription she had in the medicine cabinet) for recurrent dizziness without effect. Also, Mr. J had been seeing a neurologist outside the practice and had been started on Neurontin, 200 mg at hs, for leg pain, which he had been taking without letting the practice know. He is sent to the ER at the local community hospital. A workup is negative for any acute process, and the Neurontin is discontinued (likely causing dizziness). However, the delirium continues, and he is sent to the skilled nursing facility within the CCRC until the delirium resolves and he is safely able to return to independent living. Physical therapy works with him and finds his gait remains unsteady despite the use of a rolling walker. After several weeks in the SNF, he is discharged back to independent living. A private home health aide is hired to assist Mr. J in the morning with his shower, dressing, and meal preparation. He continues to spend time with his companion, going between the two apartments when able.

Over the next year, Mr. J is seen in clinic frequently with continued complaints of leg pain, fatigue, depression, and insomnia. The clinician is working with colleagues to consistently assess his medication use, alcohol intake, mood, and function. Various medications are trialed for these problems, and the patient is followed intermittently on site by both psychiatry and social work. His mood is better with the addition of Celexa. He is sleeping better with the use of trazadone; but the home health nurses report that his medication box is often filled incorrectly or not at all by his companion, leading to missed doses. He has also found some pain relief with massage and acupuncture, but his function deteriorates to the point where he needs more assistance with his ADL. He also neglects to use his walker, relying on a cane, which has led to some noninjurious falls. His companion has had her own health issues over this last year and is no longer able to provide consistent assistance. There have been reports by home care staff of Mr. J and his companion yelling and shoving in the hallways of the building. Meetings are held with the CCRC administration, and family members of both Mr. J and his companion to sort out the living situation and plan the next steps.

Eventually the CCRC team, in conjunction with Mr. J and his family, meet to consider a move to the assisted living (AL) unit, where he can receive additional personal care assistance and some distance from his companion. Mr. J is also in need of a consistent medication management system. The relationship between an impaired ability to safely self-administer medications and the need for assisted living has been described by some authors (Lieto & Schmidt, 2005). The assisted living unit can provide the supervision and care that he needs while he still has some capacity for self-care. It maximizes independence by filling a niche between independent living and the high degree of care required by those on skilled nursing units.

Mr. J agrees to move to the AL, admitting that he knew he needed more help and supervision. His children assist with the move, and he settles in without incident. The staff reports that he seems calm and upbeat, more content, enjoying the daily bridge/chess games with other residents. He no longer drinks alcohol. He uses his walker more consistently, and he does occasionally visits his companion in her independent living apartment. The staff contracts with him regarding his need to report any verbal or physical mistreatment by his companion that occurs during those visits. He has had no falls since being on the unit. He celebrated his 89th birthday surrounded by staff and other residents recently.

What guidelines are available to help with assessing an individual's need for assisted living?

At this time, there are no established guidelines for determining placement decisions in CCRCs in the transition from independent living to assisted living. One example of an assessment tool that has been described by Anderson and Tom (2005) that may be useful in measuring a resident's need for a higher level of care in the CCRC is the Geriatric Functional Rating Scale (GFRS). Some CCRCs may use formalized assessments of mood, function, cognitive status, and medication management that are done by the medical staff at regular intervals (annually, semiannually, and with any change in status) that can help establish a change from baseline over time. Ongoing interdisciplinary assessment and collaboration are keys to monitoring residents over time.

REFERENCES

Anderson, B., & Tom, L. (2005). Transition through the continuum of care in a continuing care retirement community: Can a functional rating scale be a decision making tool? *Journal of the American Medical Directors Association*, 6(3), 205–208.

Heisler, E., Evans, W., & Moen, P. (2004). Health and social outcomes of moving to a continuing care retirement community. *Journal of Housing for the Elderly*, 18, 5–24.

Lieto, J., & Schmidt, K. (2005). Reduced ability to self administer medication is associated with assisted living placement in a continuing care retirement community. *Journal of the American Medical Directors Association*, 6, 246–249.

Yesavage, J., Brink, T., Rose, T., Lum, O., Huang, V., Adey, M., . . . Leirer, V. O. (1983). Development and validation of a geriatric depression screening scale: A preliminary report. *Journal of Psychiatric Research*, *17*, 37–49.

ADDITIONAL RESOURCES

American Assisted Living Nurses Association. http://www.alnursing.org
Assisted Living Federation of America. http://www.alfa.org/alfa/default.asp
Center for Excellence in Assisted Living. http://www.theceal.org/
National Center for Assisted Living. http://www.ahcancal.org/ncal/Pages/ default.aspx

Section 5

Cognitive and Psychological Issues in Aging

Case 5.1 The Diabolical Ds

By Kathleen Lovanio, MSN, APRN, F/ANP-BC,
Patricia C. Gantert, MSN, RN-BC,
and Susan A. Goncalves, DNP(c), MS, RN-BC

Mrs. S, an 86-year-old woman, arrived by ambulance in the emergency department (ED) after an unwitnessed incident at home. She could only remember that she was rushing to go to the bathroom and the next thing she remembered was hearing her daughter calling out, "Mom, Mom, are you okay? What happened?" Her daughter stated that she found her mother lying on the floor in a puddle of urine near the bathroom and called 911.

Mrs. S is 86 years old and lives alone in a retirement community for the past 5 years since the death of her husband. She is independent in all activities of daily living (ADL). When her husband was alive, he managed all the finances; and since his death, Mrs. S refuses to take on this responsibility and relies on her daughter to manage her finances. However, she still drives, does the grocery shopping, and cooks her own meals. Her daughter lives nearby and either visits or calls her mother daily. Up until about 2 months ago, Mrs. S participated in many community activities (attending church daily, playing bingo weekly, and taking exercise classes at the local senior center); however, she has slowed down considerably. Her daughter attributes the slowdown to her mother's "aging". Her daughter notes that Mrs. S has been repeating herself more often and has needed reminders for upcoming events. Mrs. S has noticed some memory issues, but appears happy, content, and not worried. "What do you expect at my age?"

In spite of these concerns, Mrs. S has been in relatively good health, although she has both vision and hearing impairments for which she wears bifocals and hearing aids. Her medical history includes

Case Studies in Gerontological Nursing for the Advanced Practice Nurse, First Edition.
Edited by Meredith Wallace Kazer, Leslie Neal-Boylan.
© 2012 John Wiley & Sons, Inc. Published 2012 by John Wiley & Sons, Inc.

hypertension (HTN), osteoarthritis, hypercholesterolemia, and atrial fibrillation (A-fib). Her medications include metoprolol XL, 50 mg daily; hydrochlorothiazide, 50 mg daily; Lipitor, 40 mg daily; Coumadin, 2.5 mg on Monday, Wednesday, and Friday; Coumadin, 5 mg on Sunday, Tuesday, Thursday, and Saturday; and Extra Strength Tylenol as needed. She is allergic to sulfa drugs.

On Friday evening while in the ED, Mrs. S was alert, oriented, and anxious to leave the hospital to go home. However, the results of her telemetry tracings noted atrial fibrillation with heart rate in the 110s, so it was decided to admit Mrs. S to the telemetry unit for further workup and possible medication adjustment. All diagnostic and laboratory results while in the ED were unremarkable with the exception of the UA which came back positive for a UTI, and amoxicillin-clavulanate was ordered. Mrs. S spent the night in the ED waiting for a bed on the telemetry unit. She complained of moderate pain in her right knee (5/10); and Demerol, 100 mg every 3–4 hours as needed, was prescribed by the new resident on call. The nurse administered Demerol, 100 mg, at 2400 and again at 0300 with good effect. In addition, the resident wrote an order for complete bed rest for Mrs. S. On Saturday afternoon, 16 hours after Mrs. S arrived at the ED, she was transported to a bed in the telemetry unit. Her daughter came to visit and stayed only a short time, noting that her mother appeared extremely tired and thought it was best for her to catch up on her sleep. The daughter called the nursing station that evening and was told that her mother was stable, resting comfortably, and continuing to take Demerol for pain relief.

When Mrs. S's daughter arrived the next day, she found her mother lying in bed, lethargic, and confused. She had difficulty focusing her attention and answering her daughter's questions. Her speech was slow, and conversations were disorganized and unclear. She noticed that her mother was wearing an adult disposable brief and asked the nurse why. The nurse stated that she arrived on the unit wearing a brief; and since her mother never asked to be assisted to the bathroom, they assumed that Mrs. S was incontinent. Her mother had not been out of bed since her arrival to the ED Friday evening. Her hearing aid and glasses were nowhere to be found. At this point, the daughter became angry and shouted at the nurse, "What are you doing to my mother?"

OBJECTIVE

Mrs. S is lying in bed lethargic, confused, unable to follow commands, and dependent in all activities of daily living (ADL). Her vital signs are as follows: temperature: 99.8 oral; BP: 100/60; P: 108 irregular; RR:

18 shallow. Tenting skin turgor on the forehead and absence of axillary moisture are noted. Her oral cavity reveals dry mucous membranes and longitudinal furrows on tongue; lips are dry and cracked. Her lungs are clear to auscultation (CTA). There are no adventitious breath sounds. Her appetite is poor. There is no nausea or vomiting. The abdomen is distended and slightly tender; bowel sounds are positive. Mrs. S is incontinent of urine, and no bowel movement (BM) has been noted during the hospital course. There is marked upper body muscle weakness bilaterally. Her lower extremities show no obvious deformities. There is a bruise on her left knee and lateral thigh. Mrs. S is guarded when palpating the bruised area. There is no swelling. Her skin is dry and intact.

ASSESSMENT

Dehydration: Dehydration can be defined as a clinically significant decrease of an individual's optimal total body water (TBW) and may occur with or without the loss of electrolytes. It is a common occurrence in the older adult population and extremely prevalent in hospitalized older adults. Lipschitz (2006) reports that dehydration is the single most common cause of acute confusional state and is primarily associated with the age-related decline in the thirst mechanism. Moreover, older individuals have a decreased ability to respond to fluid deprivation in a state of illness, such as a respiratory or urinary tract infections. The mortality of patients with dehydration is high if not treated appropriately. Confusion, constipation, and falls are often atypical presentations of dehydration in the older adult population.

Delirium: The American Psychiatric Association (2000) defines delirium as a disturbance of consciousness with reduced ability to focus, sustain, or shift attention; a change in cognition or the development of a perceptual disturbance that occurs over a short period of time and tends to fluctuate over the course of the day. Psychotic symptoms, such as hallucinations and paranoia, and behavioral problems are frequently exhibited. An altered sleep cycle is common in delirium, and symptoms are worse at night. The incidence of delirium increases with age, cognitive impairment, frailty, illness severity, and comorbidities. In addition, delirium can occur with a trauma (i.e., a fall) or merely sudden environmental changes such as hospitalization. Inouye (2006) noted emergency departments and hospitals as having the highest rates of delirium with new cases arising during hospitalization as much as 6%–56%. Sensory impairments such as vision and hearing loss can also contribute to delirium. Common symptoms of a urinary tract infection (UTI)—frequency, urgency, and incontinence—may be absent in the older adult. Changes in the person's orientation, acute confusion, and cognitive disturbances, often leading to falls, can be the first signs of infection. If untreated, a UTI can cause a delirium.

Dementia: The national prevalence of dementia in individuals 71 years and older is estimated to be about 13.9% and accounted for 3.4 million individuals in the U.S. in 2002 (Plassman et al., (2007). This study demonstrated that the dementia prevalence increased with age, from 5% of those aged 71–79 years to 37.2% of those aged 90 and older. The American Psychiatric Association (2000) established standard criteria for the diagnosis of dementia. This standard describes dementia as multiple cognitive deficits that include memory impairment and at least one of the following cognitive disturbances: agnosia, aphasia, apraxia, or a disturbance in executive functioning. The deficits must be sufficient to cause functional impairment in home or work life.

DIAGNOSTICS

There is no "gold standard" to assess the fluid status of an older adult. Faes, Spigt, and Olde Rikkert (2007) emphasize that the diversity in dehydration episodes and the heterogeneity of the older adult population rule out a "one size fits all "approach to diagnosing dehydration. As a rule, serum creatinine, blood urea nitrogen (BUN), and the BUN-to-creatinine ratio are advocated as laboratory measurements for detection of dehydration, with creatinine being the most sensitive measure (Faes et al., 2007). The loss of fluids also causes an increase in the concentration of solutes in the blood that leads to increased serum osmolality (Mentes, 2006). It is important to assess Mrs. S's kidney function, since kidney function is adversely affected by dehydration. The 24-hour creatinine clearance (CrCl) test is used to determine glomerular filtration rate (GFR); but in this case it is not a feasible option. The National Kidney Foundation (NKF) recommends estimating GFR from serum creatinine. Two commonly used equations are the MDRD study equation and the Cockcroft and Gault equation. Both equations use serum creatinine in combination with age, sex, weight, or race to estimate GFR. Persistent reduction in GFR to below $60\,mL/min/1.73\,m^2$ for ≥3 months is defined as chronic kidney disease.

The Confusion Assessment Method (CAM) is an instrument and diagnostic algorithm for the identification of delirium. The CAM assesses the presence, severity, and fluctuation of 9 delirium features: acute onset, inattention, disorganized thinking, altered level of consciousness, disorientation, memory impairment, perceptual disturbances, psychomotor agitation or retardation, and altered sleep-wake cycle. The CAM is based on the following 4 cardinal features of delirium: 1) acute onset and fluctuating course, 2) inattention, 3) disorganized thinking, and 4) altered level of consciousness. A diagnosis of delirium according to the CAM requires the presence of features 1 and 2; and either 3, or 4. Patients with delirium can exhibit a wide range of abnormal behaviors. At least 3 clinical subtypes of delirium have been identified: hyperactive-hyperalert (agitated), hypoactive-hypoalert (somnolent), and mixed. One study concluded that patients with hypoactive delirium were sicker on admission, had the longest hospital stay, and were most likely to develop pressure sores; in contrast, patients with hyperactive delirium were most likely to fall in the hospital (O'Keeffe & Lavan, 1999).

Early recognition of cognitive impairment and identification of potentially reversible causes contributing to cognitive impairment are paramount in the assessment. Many tools are available to conduct a mental status evaluation. The Mini-Mental State Examination (MMSE) has been validated and is nationally recognized as the standard of care. Concerns have been expressed due to the length of time to administer the MMSE, high false positive rates for those with little education, and the lack of sensitivity in detecting early or mild dementia (Zwicker & Fulmer, 2008). The Mini-Cog exam is another useful clinical tool to assess an individual's registration, recall, and executive function and can be administered in various settings, including acute care. The Mini-Cog is composed of 3-item recall and the Clock Drawing Test (CDT). In comparison to the MMSE, the Mini-Cog is quick to administer, has less language and educational bias, and is more sensitive in identifying milder stages of cognitive impairment (Capezuti et al., 2008). CBC, TSH, B12, and electrolytes are recommended laboratory tests for the evaluation of cognitive impairments (Reuben et al., 2009). Depression can present as cognitive impairment in this population and often accompanies dementia in the beginning stages, so the Geriatric Depression scale should be administered. Due to the abrupt onset, the rapid decline of cognitive impairment, and the recent fall, neuroimaging studies will be repeated.

With the exception of the following, results all other diagnostics, including neuroimaging were within normal limits (Table 5.1.1).

Due to Mrs. S's lethargic state, screenings for dementia (MMSE and/ or Mini-cog) and depression (GDS) were unable to be performed at this time. On the CAM, Mrs. S scored positive for acute onset and fluctuating course, inattention, disorganized thinking, and altered LOC.

CRITICAL THINKING

What is the most likely differential diagnosis?

What is the plan of care?

TABLE 5.1.1. Laboratory Test Findings.

Test	Normal	Result
BUN	60 plus; 8–23 mg/dL	48 mg/dL
Serum Cr	Adult women: 0.6–1.1 mg/dL	1.4 mg/dL
Estimated Cr/Cl ratio	10:1–20:1	34:1
Serum osmolality	280–295 mOsm/kg H20	321 mOsm/kg H2O
Estimated GFR	Average estimated GFR: 70 plus; 75	65
INR	2–3	5

Could the delirium have been prevented?

Are referrals needed?

What should the clinician consider before prescribing medications for older adults?

When prescribing an antibiotic to treat this patient's UTI, what is important to consider?

Are there any evidenced-based guidelines available?

RESOLUTION

What is the most likely differential diagnosis?
Based on Mrs. S's stated lab results and physical assessment (decreased BP, increased pulse, poor skin turgor on her forehead, dry skin on axillary, dry mucous membranes, furrows on tongue, and dry cracked lips), dehydration has been ruled in as one of her diagnoses. Her acute changes in baseline function and mental status and the screening results of the CAM establish delirium.

What is the plan of care?
Acute confusional states, as in delirium, always have a cause and should not be interpreted as a disease. Once a delirium diagnosis has been established, the goal of management is to determine the underlying pathology, manage symptoms, prevent complications, and promote a safe environment for the patient and staff. Interventions involve the use of interprofessional protocols directed toward improving cognitive impairment. Eliminate or minimize risk factors by treating infections, prevent and treat dehydration and electrolyte disturbances, provide adequate pain control, regulate bowel and bladder function, and provide adequate nutrition. Clinicians should encourage a therapeutic environment by utilizing calendars, clocks, and caregiver

identification; explaining all activities; and communicating clearly. Providing appropriate sensory stimulation such as a quiet room, adequate light, and noise reduction strategies, eyeglasses and other devices that assist sensory perception should be used whenever possible and should not be put away during a delirious episode. One of the most helpful interventions is having family members stay with the patient. Family members should also be encouraged to bring personal effects from home, because some patients with delirium are greatly comforted by the presence of familiar photographs or objects. Facilitate sleep by providing back massage, warm milk or herbal tea at bedtime, and relaxation music tapes and avoid waking patients for procedures during the night when possible. Maintain consistency of caregivers and minimize relocations. Maximize mobility, and ambulate at least 3 times daily. Mobility assists with orientation. All nonpharmacological interventions should be implemented before pharmacological interventions. Pain, sleep, and anxiety medications should be used judiciously because these medications can exacerbate delirium (Capezuti et al., 2008). Physical restraints, once a mainstay in the treatment of delirium, are now used only when all pharmacologic and nonpharmacological interventions have failed.

Could the delirium have been prevented?

Delirium is multifactorial with predisposing and precipitating factors contributing to its development. Predisposing factors include cognitive or functional impairments, deconditioning, severity of illness, advanced age, depression, and vision and/or hearing impairments. Mrs. S presented to the ED with advanced age and UTI and had both visual and hearing impairments; yet a delirium protocol was not put in place. Precipitating factors during hospitalization may include use of physical restraints, indwelling bladder catheter, metabolic disturbances such as azotemia, pH alterations, nutritional deficiencies, polypharmacy, pain, infection, dehydration, electrolyte imbalances, immobilization, environmental factors, anxiety, and lack of sleep (Sendelbach & Guthrie, 2009). The goal of nursing care is to eliminate or minimize the severity of all potential precipitating factors unique to each patient's condition and circumstance. Mrs. S was in the ED for 16 hours before being transferred to a hospital room. This is not a therapeutic environment. Her glasses and hearing aid were not in use, she became dehydrated, an inappropriate medication was ordered for pain, and a complete bed rest order was unnecessary. This is a good example of cascade iatrogenesis that leads to the development of adverse events in hospitalized older adults. Nursing staff is crucial in preventing delirium and detecting delirium during hospitalization. Close monitoring of the older adult patient and quick response to mental status changes are vital. Taking a proactive approach to ensure that the patient's needs are met is the cornerstone of high quality nursing care.

Are referrals needed?

Unfortunately, Mrs. S was unable to be discharged to her home due to deconditioning (functional decline) that resulted from her hospital course and was transferred to a short-term care rehabilitation facility. Deconditioning is a complex process of physiological change following a period of inactivity, bed rest, or sedentary lifestyle. It is frequently associated with hospitalization and may occur after as little as 2 days of bed rest (Hirsch, Sommers, Olsen, Mullen, & Winograd, 1990). In combination with the decrease in age-related muscle mass and strength, deconditioning can lead to dependency in ambulation and other activities of daily living. Prevention of deconditioning requires ongoing assessment of patients by clinicians and interventions to promote functional mobility in this population. Mrs. S will also be referred for a comprehensive geriatric assessment after discharge from the hospital for mood and memory assessments.

WHAT should the clinician consider before prescribing medication for older adults?

Older adults often have numerous comorbidities for which they are prescribed multiple medications, thereby increasing the risk for adverse drug reactions (ADR). The risk is heightened by age-related physiological changes that influence pharmacokinetics and pharmcodynamics. It is estimated that medication-related problems cause 106,000 deaths annually; and if medication-related problems were considered a disease, it would be the fifth leading cause of death in the United States (Lazarou, Pomeranz, & Corey, 1998; Perry, 1999). The Beers Criteria is a consensus-based guideline that looks specifically for potentially inappropriate medications in the older adult population and is widely used (Fick et al., 2003). The Screening Tool of Older Persons' potentially inappropriate prescriptions (STOPP) and Screening Tool to Alert doctors to the Right Treatment (START) are new screening tools designed to detect instances of potentially inappropriate medication use and underprescribing of clinically indicated medications in older patients (O'Mahony & Gallagher, 2008). Prescribers should be aware that these references exist and refer to them to prevent ADR in the older population. In this case, Mrs. S's first noxious insult began in the ED when the new resident prescribed an inappropriate medication, meperidine (Demerol). Beers criteria listed meperidine as a high risk medication that may cause confusion, not an effective oral analgesic.

When prescribing an antibiotic to treat this patient's UTI, what is important to consider?

Antibiotics as well as many other classes of drugs can dangerously interfere with an anticoagulant medication such as warfarin (Coumadin). An increased INR secondary to warfarin interactions with various antibacterial agents is a known phenomenon. An increased awareness of warfarin and amoxicillin/clavulanate (AM/CL) interaction and appropriate monitoring are essential to control the INR levels and prevent bleeding complications (Davydov, Yermolnik, & Cuni, 2003). An international normalized ratio (INR) measures the time it takes for the blood to clot and compares it to an average; it is used to monitor the impact of anticoagulant medicines, such as warfarin (Coumadin). Levels should be between 2.0 and 3.0 for patients with atrial fibrillation. An elevated INR such as INR = 5 indicates that there is a high chance of bleeding; whereas, if the INR = 0.5, then there is a high risk of developing a clot.

Are there any evidenced-based guidelines available?
Three evidence-based guidelines for delirium are available on the Agency for Healthcare Research and Quality (AHRQ) National Guideline Clearinghouse Web site at http://www.guideline.gov: *Evidence-based practice guideline: Acute confusion/delirium,* (2009), University of Iowa Gerontological Nursing Interventions Research Center (Sendelbach, Guthrie, and Schoenfelder (2009); *Delirium and acute problematic behavior in the long-term care setting,* (2008), American Medical Directors Association; and *Delirium, prevention, early recognition, and treatment in: Evidence-based geriatric nursing protocols for best practice* (2008), Hartford Institute for Geriatric Nursing.

REFERENCES

American Psychiatric Association (2000). *Desk reference to the diagnostic criteria from DSM- IV-TR.* Washington, DC: American Psychiatric Association.

Davydov, L., Yermolnik, M., & Cuni, L. J. (2003). Warfarin and amoxicillin-clavulante drug interaction. *The Annals of Pharmacotherapy, 37*(3), 367–370. Retrieved from http://www.theannals.com/cgi/content/abstract/37/3/367

Faes, M. C., Spigt, M. G., & Olde Rikkert, M. G. (2007). Dehydration in geriatrics. *Geriatrics and Aging, 10*(9), 590–596.

Fick, D. M., Cooper, J. W., Wade, W. E., Walter, J. L., Maclean, J. R., & Beers, M. (2003). Updating the beers criteria for potentially inappropriate medication use in older adults. *Archives of Internal Medicine, 163*, 2716–2724.

Hirsch, C. H., Sommers, L., Olsen, A., Mullen, L., & Winograd, C. (1990). The natural history of functional morbidity in hospitalized older patients. *Journal of the American Geriatric Society, 38*(12), 1296–1303.

Inouye, S. K. (2006). Delirium in older persons. *The New England Journal of Medicine, 354*, 1159–1165.

Lipschitz, D. A. (2006). Nutrition. In K. C. Cassel, R. M. Leipzig, H. J. Cohen, E. B. Larson, & D. E. Meier (Eds.), *Geriatric medicine: An evidenced based approach* (4th ed., pp. 1009–1021). New York: Springer Science + Media, LCC.

Mentes, J. (2006). Oral hydration in older adults. *The American Journal of Nursing, 106*(6), 40–48.

O'Keeffe, S. T., & Lavan, J. N. (1999). Clinical significance of delirium subtypes in older people. *Age and Ageing, 28,* 115–119.

O'Mahony D. & Gallagher, P. F. (2008). Inappropriate prescribing in the older population: Need for new criteria (commentary article). *Age & Ageing, 37:* 138–141.

Perry, D. P. (1999). When medicine hurts instead of helps. *The Consultant Pharmacist, 14,* 1326–1330.

Plassman, B. L., Langa, K. M., Fisher, G. G., Heeringa, S. G., Weir, D. R., Ofstedal, M. B., Burke, J. R., Hurd, M. D., Potter, G. G., Rodgers, W. L., Steffens, D. C., Willis, R. J., & Wallace, R. B. (2007). Prevalence of dementia in the United States: The aging, demographics, and memory Study. *Neuroepidemiology, 29,* 125–132.

Reuben, D. B., Herr, K. A., Pacala, J. T., Pollock, B. G., Potter, J. F., & Semla, T. P. (2009). *Geriatrics at your fingertips* (11th ed.). New York: The American Geriatrics Society.

Sendelbach, S., & Guthrie, P. F. (2009). Acute confusion/delirium. In D. P. Schoenfelder (Series Ed.), *Series on evidence-based practice for older adults.* Iowa City: Hartford Center of Geriatric Nursing Excellence, The University of Iowa College. of Nursing.

Sendelbach, S., Guthrie, P. F., & Schoenfelder, D. (2009). Evidenced-based guideline acute confusion/delirium identification, assessment, treatment, and prevention. *Journal of Gerontological Nursing, 35*(11), 11–19.

Zwicker, D., Fulmer, T. Reducing Adverse Drug Events. (2008). In E. Capezuti, D. Zwicker, M. Mezey, & T. Fulmer (Eds.) *Evidence-based geriatric nursing protocols for best practice* (3rd ed.) (pp. 257–308). New York: Springer Publishing Company, Inc.

Case 5.2 What a Difference a Day Makes

By Cora D. Zembrzuski, PhD, APRN

Ms. L is an 82-year-old woman who resides at the skilled nursing facility for the past 3 years. She was referred to the gero-psychiatric clinician for "change in behavior". The staff states that she is "confused" and "very different from her usual self". They also state, "She was just fine yesterday."

She is generally in fairly good health with medical diagnoses of diabetes Type 2, hypertension, and peripheral vascular disease. She has a history of deep vein thrombosis (DVT). She has a surgical history of left total knee replacement (2003) and has experienced several episodes of symptomatic hypoglycemia over the past 2 months. She is widowed and has a daughter and son who visit periodically but who live out of state. According to the staff, she is negative for smoking and substance abuse. Ms. L's family history includes diabetes, heart disease, and hypothyroidism present in her two younger female siblings. Ms. L states, "The staff is putting kerosene in my juice," and "They sometimes poison my meals with alcohol." Ms. L's current medications include lisinopril, 20 mg by mouth daily; metformin, 500 mg by mouth 3 times daily; coumadin, 5 mg by mouth daily, accompanied by frequent blood work and dose adjustments; a baby aspirin daily; double strength acetaminophen, every 6 hours as needed for pain; lorazepam, 0.25 mg by mouth every 6 hours for distressful anxiety, which she uses 2–3 times weekly. She is allergic to penicillin as she breaks out in hives.

Case Studies in Gerontological Nursing for the Advanced Practice Nurse, First Edition.
Edited by Meredith Wallace Kazer, Leslie Neal-Boylan.
© 2012 John Wiley & Sons, Inc. Published 2012 by John Wiley & Sons, Inc.

OBJECTIVE

Ms. L presents as anxious, alert, and disoriented to place and time. She is dressed neatly and has her walker nearby for ambulation but forgets to use it. The review of systems revealed no shortness of breath. Respirations are 25 per minute and may be related to her anxiety; O_2 Sat is 95%. Her apical pulse is 90; blood pressure is 140/72; she has a negative Homan sign and no fever. Her weight is 110 lb; height is 5 ft; appetite is fair; no nausea and vomiting. She has a history of UTIs but is not experiencing frequency, burning upon urination, or hematuria. She is negative for constipation. She has a recent history of hypoglycemia with change in level of consciousness; blood glucose finger sticks range from 40–200, taken in the morning before meals. She is not hard of hearing (HOH) and has adequate eyesight with corrective glasses. There is no psychiatric history except for intermittent anxiety, for which she receives lorazepam.

Ms. L's thought processes are disorganized with undertones of paranoia. Rate and volume of speech is faster than her normal baseline. Her associations are loose and paranoid in nature. She talks about her childhood and sees her mother, who is deceased. Her flight of ideas take the form of "word salad" as Ms. L demonstrates difficulty with thought processes and language. She has difficulty with decreased attention and concentration, which make it challenging to elicit an accurate history. She presents with impaired short and long-term memory and is unable to recall discussions that occurred at the start of the assessment. Hand grasps are equal and strong. Her pupils are equal and reacting to light. She has a mild tremor in her hands that is exacerbated when she speaks. She is not on psychoactive medications and does not have an existing diagnosis of dementia or depression.

ASSESSMENT

Urinary tract or other infection: Infectious processes in older adults can manifest symptoms atypically, such as acute confusion, abrupt change in thought processes, and in logic and judgment, or presence of hallucinations or delusions (unfounded beliefs), as identified in Ms. L's case. Changes in thermoregulation in older adults predispose them to a reduction in sensitivity to metabolic and lymphatic changes, and thus a desensitized fever response (Beers & Berkow, 2000).

Hypoglycemia: The prevalence of diabetes, diagnosed and undiagnosed, doubles as individuals progress from the 40–59 year age group to the 60+ year age group (CDC, 2007) (Figure 5.2.1).

Estimated prevalence of diagnosed and undiagnosed diabetes in people aged 20 years or older, by age group, United States, 2007

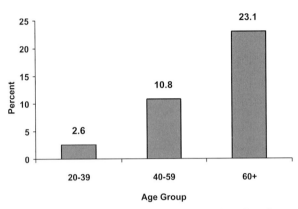

Figure 5.2.1. Estimated prevalence of diagnosed and undiagnosed diabetes in people aged 20 years or older, by age group, United States, 2007. Accessed from CDC. National Diabetes Fact Sheet, 2007. Source: 2003–2006 National Health and Nutrition Examination Survey estimates of total prevalence (both diagnosed and undiagnosed) were projected to year 2007.

As such, older adults are at high risk for diabetes. In Ms. L's case, her blood glucose levels were somewhat erratic suggesting that the efficacy of the current treatment with metformin was modest at best. Fasting blood glucose levels obtained in the morning before meals should range between 70 to 130, but are individualized given the person's symptomatic response to blood glucose fluctuations. In addition, Ms. L's variable blood glucose levels may have been a contributing factor to her difficulty with concentration and anxiety.

Cognitive impairment, but from what cause? As confirmed in her old medical records, Ms. L did not have a psychiatric history. Her change in thought processes, language skills, and notable change in behavior, with underlying paranoia and confusion, may suggest dementia. Alzheimer's and other dementias increase with age (Knopman et al., 2001). Alzheimer disease is the most prevalent of the dementias. The mortality rate from Alzheimer's has continued to increase by 46%, whereas mortality rate decreases for stroke, prostate cancer, breast cancer, and heart disease (Alzheimer's Association Fact Sheet, 2010). HTN and diabetes increase the risk of Alzheimer's and vascular dementia (Figure 5.2.2). Her PMH and family history suggest Ms. L may be at risk for dementia.

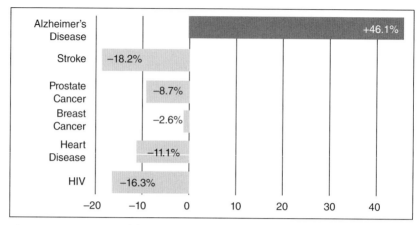

Figure 5.2.2.   Accessed from Alzheimer's Association *2010 Alzheimer's Disease Facts and Figures* at www.alz.org/statistics.

TABLE 5.2.1.   A summary of characteristics of delirium.

Acute versus chronic onset; intermittent symptoms with periods of lucidity.
Inattention, disorganized thinking, rambling, poor recall, and poor short-term memory.
Altered consciousness—hyper- or hypovigilance, slow responses to questions, stupor.
Hallucinations or delusions: stark misinterpretations of reality.
Sleep/wake cycle dysfunction—too much or too little sleep.
Mood changes: fear, anxiety, paranoia, depression, irritability, apathy, anger.
Polypharmacy and/or the new additions of medications.
Medical diseases associated with delirium: Infection, fracture/trauma, stroke, metabolic abnormalities, blood loss, decreased liver and/or kidney impairment, or diseases.

The incidence rate of delirium in the nursing home is estimated at 60% (Inouye, 2006). In Ms. L's case, cognitive impairment due to delirium is a strong possibility. Finding out the cause of the delirium, that is, UTI or metabolic abnormalities, is critical to treating and resolving the behavioral dysfunction (Waszynski, 2007). Clinical characteristics and variables to look for in the process of determining a delirium diagnosis versus other diagnoses are noted in the Table 5.2.1.

DIAGNOSTICS

- **UA, C&S:** The clinician should look for high leukocytes and specific bacterial growth in the results. The sensitivity will show whether the bacteria are sensitive or resistant to specific antibiotics (Kamel, 2004).

- **CBC with differential:** Older adults, in general, may not respond to infection with above-normal leukocytes. Comparisons should be made from previous CBCs.
- **Thyroid-stimulating hormone (TSH)** differentiates primary from secondary hypothyroidism. Commonly, hypothyroidism is treated with levothyroxine.
- **Vitamin B12 and folate:** Low levels of these nutrients can mimic depression and dementia. When levels are low, homocysteine increases and indirectly increases the individual's risk for cardiac events and nerve damage. Supplements have been shown to reduce homocysteine levels and neuronal breakdown (Mangoni & Jackson, 2002).
- **Electrolytes:** Abnormal electrolytes support a diagnosis of dehydration along with insufficient fluid intake. Older adults are very sensitive to electrolyte imbalance and are at risk for dehydration. The clinician should check oral fluid intake (OFI) and urinary output. Is the older adult dinking at least 1500 mL daily? Is the urine concentrated or clear? Is there an odor? Odor may indicate concentrated urine or suggest not enough fluid intake, or it may suggest a UTI. When urine is clear and lacking concentration, low sodium may be the culprit or may be a side effect of some medications, such as Depakote and antidepressants (Jacobson, Pies, & Katz, 2007). The syndrome of inappropriate antidiuretic hormone (SIADH) and the inability to concentrate urine are not uncommon in older adults and may present as possibilities.
- **Hg A1c and FBS:** Results will shed light on how well diabetes is being managed. For better regulation, insulin may be an option. Level of consciousness may change with very low or very high blood glucose levels.
- **CT and MRI:** These can determine whether the older person has sustained a stroke or other damage to the brain. They are expensive diagnostic options, to be used after ruling out other possible etiologies of the behavior.
- **CAM and MMSE:** These can inform the clinician of the cognitive specifics and presence of clinical characteristics associated with delirium.

CRITICAL THINKING

What is the most likely differential diagnosis and why? Are any referrals needed?

What is the plan of treatment? Are there any standardized guidelines that the clinician should use to assess or treat?

What is the plan for follow-up care?

Describe if and how the clinician might incorporate the family into a treatment plan.

What if this patient were male?

What if this patient lived in a rural, more-isolated setting?

RESOLUTION

What is the most likely differential diagnosis and why? Are any referrals needed?

Ruling out a UTI is an appropriate first step and the most likely diagnosis. First, Ms. L has a history of UTIs. We know that "history repeats itself" if disease prevention measures are not taken. A critical point of concern is that Ms. L did not present with a fever but presented with a change in mental status and thought processes consistent with a delirium diagnosis. In this case, Ms. L was positive for delirium based on assessment findings using the CAM. She was positive for a urinary tract infection and was treated with ABT. Ms. L's WBCs were elevated slightly above normal and were considerably higher when compared to previous values. Results from electrolytes indicated an increased BUN/Cr level consistent with insufficient OFI which was noted to be 800 mL/daily, below desirable values. Fasting blood glucose was below normal at 60, and the HgA1c results were 8—lower and higher, respectively, than what is typically desirable. In addition, the MMSE from 1 year ago was 21/30, but a dementia diagnosis was not fully confirmed. TSH findings were normal. Vitamin B12 and folate results were at low-normal. CT/MRI was not done at this time.

Important referrals at this point include referral to a geriatric assessment center for full workup for dementia by a geriatric team, which is comprised of a geriatric nurse practitioner, geriatrician, neurologist, social worker, psychologist, and nutritionist.

What is the plan of treatment? Are there any standardized guidelines that the clinician should use to assess or treat?

In Ms. L's case, UTI was positive and antibiotic treatment was started. Low OFI was treated by adding additional fluid with her medications. Better blood glucose management was achieved by starting an insulin regimen. Ms. L's behavioral symptoms resolved within 1 week. Standardized guidelines were used from the American Diabetes Association, the DSM-IV (for delirium) and the American Dietetic Association (for determining fluid requirements). The referral to a geriatric assessment center was critical to note whether there were symptoms related to short- and long-term memory loss and symptoms supporting a diagnosis of dementia. The MMSE could not be administered during Ms. L's symptoms of delirium but was administered in 1 month showing a decline in score from 21/30 to 19/30. It is likely that Ms. L may have early signs of dementia; but a follow-up MMSE in 3–4 months, plus a CT/MRI scan, are warranted.

What is the plan for follow-up care?

Findings and recommendations from the geriatric assessment center will guide follow-up care—for example, the addition of cholinesterase inhibitors if Ms. L is positive for dementia. Also, close monitoring of blood glucose levels and OFI is warranted to promote prevention of recurrent delirium.

The root cause of anxiety needs to be addressed since Ms. L had this symptom prior to the onset of delirium. There are more than 20 possible causes of secondary anxiety in older adults (Jacobson et al., 2007). A referral to a psychiatric clinician might elucidate the reason for her anxiety.

Describe if and how the clinician might incorporate the family into a treatment plan.

Part of diagnosing dementia is obtaining supportive data acquired from the family regarding histories of dementia, memory loss, impaired safety judgment, impairments in problem-solving abilities, substance abuse, and mood fluctuations including her response to stressors. Also, the family may be able to elucidate her past patterns of behavior, likes and dislikes, and previous occupation and hobbies—all critical pieces of information in designing an effective long-term care plan.

What if this patient were male?

The resident's gender is not as significant as the presence of acute illnesses. For example, the risk for delirium increases significantly with surgeries requiring anesthesia and where the older person experiences serious blood loss; falls including hip fractures; UTIs and sepsis; and end-of-life care situations. Likewise, the highest occurrences of delirium are in the hospital and sub-acute settings (Inouye, 2006). If Ms. L were male, we would be aware of the importance of a BPH or prostate cancer, as these might contribute to urinary tract infections. Also, the presence of cardiac diseases and renal impairment might be contributing factors in light of a diabetes diagnosis, but these are not necessarily gender related.

What if this patient lived in a rural, more-isolated setting?

In some instances, living in a rural setting may influence access to care (Agency for Healthcare Research and Quality [AHRQ], 2005). Given acute illnesses where a rapid response is necessary, such as in the case of delirium from various illnesses, the individual may not be able to get fast enough interventions needed for survival. If delirium is not treated, it may result in death.

REFERENCES

Agency for Healthcare Research and Quality (2005). Healthcare disparities in rural areas. Findings from the 2004 National Healthcare Disparities Report. AHRQ Publication No. 05-P022 retrieved on 7/1/2010 from http://www.ahrq.gov/research/ruraldisp/ruraldispar.htm

Alzheimer's Association Fact Sheet. (2010). Retrieved July 1, 2010, from http://www.alz.org/statistics

American Nurses Association and American Association of Diabetes Educators (2003). *Scope and standards of diabetes nursing practice*. Washington, DC: The Publishing Program of ANA.

Beers, M. H., & Berkow, R. (2000). *Merck manual of geriatrics*. Whitehouse Station, NJ: Merck Research Laboratories.

Centers for Disease Control. (2007). National Diabetes Fact Sheet 2007. Accessed June 9, 2011, at http://www.cdc.gov/diabetes/pubs/pdf/ndfs_2007.pdf

Inouye, S. K. (2006). Delirium in older persons. *New England Journal of Medicine*, *354*(11), 1157–1165.

Jacobson, S. A., Pies, R. W., & Katz, I. R. (2007). *Clinical manual of geriatric psychopharmacology*. Washington, DC: American Psychiatric Publishing Company.

Kamel, K. (2004). Managing urinary tract infections in the nursing home: Myths, mysteries and realities. *The Internet Journal of Geriatrics and Gerontology*, *1*(2), 1–12. Retrieved 6/24/10 from http://www.ispub.com/ostia/index.php?xmlFilePath=journals/ijgg/vol1n2/uri.xml

Knopman, D. S., DeKosky, S. T., Cummings, J. L., Chui, H., Corey-Bloom, J., Relkin, N., Small, G. W., Miller, B., & Stevens, J. C. (2001). Practice parameter: Diagnosis of dementia (an evidence-based review). Report of the Quality Standards Subcommittee of the American Academy of Neurology. *Neurology*, *56*, 1143–1153.

Mangoni, A. A., & Jackson, S. H. (2002). Homocysteine and cardiovascular disease: Current evidence and future prospects. *The American Journal of Medicine*, *112*, 556–565.

Waszynski, C. M. (2007). *From the Try This series: Best practices in nursing care to older adults*. Retrieved 6/26/10 from http://consultgerirn.org/uploads/File/trythis/try_this_13.pdf

Case 5.3 I Don't Feel Good

By Evanne Juratovac, PhD, RN (GCNS-BC)

Mr. P is an 81-year-old, divorced, Caucasian, first generation Scottish-American male, who presents to the primary care clinic upon referral from an emergency room (ER) visit 1 week ago. His chief concern is "I don't feel good. It got worse last week." Mr. P reports that he feels listless, apathetic, and unwell, with poor energy, appetite, and sleep, over the last 6 months. He is "pretty fretful and forgetful." "I lie awake worrying at night." On further inquiry, the clinician learns that Mr. P lies down during the day to catch up on his sleep. As of the last 3 months, he no longer drives, nor attends a local water exercise class and gatherings at the "VFW" lodge. He is a retired high school history teacher and lives alone on the second floor of an urban 2-story apartment building. He is disheveled and unshaven, but with no odor. He winces during ambulation.

Mr. P has a personal history of arthritis affecting his knees and borderline hypertension (HTN), with no surgical history and NKDA. Family/first-degree relatives' medical history is uncertain, as his parents, an older brother, and only son are deceased; and he seems reluctant to provide more family information. Tobacco use is remote (he quit 20 years ago), and EtOH use was probably moderate when he in the armed services and absent recently, due largely to a decrease in social gatherings. His only prescription medicine is atenolol, 25 mg daily; and he endorses no over-the-counter medications. He served as a U.S. Marine, with one combat tour in the Korean conflict circa 1950. He reports a similar experience of ill health upon his honorable discharge in the early 1950s. The "worse" feeling last week was characterized as intolerable insomnia.

Case Studies in Gerontological Nursing for the Advanced Practice Nurse, First Edition.
Edited by Meredith Wallace Kazer, Leslie Neal-Boylan.
© 2012 John Wiley & Sons, Inc. Published 2012 by John Wiley & Sons, Inc.

OBJECTIVE

Mr. P has equal pupils that react to light and accommodation (PERRLA). He wears no glasses and reveals mild presbycusis for high tones. His neck is supple. His BP (sitting): 142/82; HR: 78; R: 16; T: 36.7°. His abdomen is soft and nontender, consistent with an absence of self-reported GI/GU problems. Mr. P has nonpitting, bilateral, 1+ pretibial edema at 15:00.

ASSESSMENT

Sleep disorder: Approximately 50% of older adults report one or more sleep problems. Inability to fall asleep and sleep through the night are among the most frequent complaints of older adults. Sleep patterns are affected by both normal and pathological aging changes. Sleep assessment is the first key to successful sleep management.

Early dementia: Dementia is a general term used to describe over 60 pathological cognitive disorders that occur as a result of illness or brain injury. While normal aging results in some changes to brain vasculature and neurons, dementia is a pathological manifestation of aging that requires a full clinical evaluation.

Depression: It is estimated that by 2020 depression may be the second largest threat to older Americans' health and ability (Chapman & Perry, 2008) in a steadily growing aging population. Epidemiological studies suggest that prevalence rates for geriatric depression may be lower if the actual prevalence among older adults is not being captured; yet the trend is higher percentages for older adults receiving home care or long-term care (Hybels & Blazer, 2003; Jones, Marcantonio, Rabinowitz, 2003), as would be expected in the presence of chronic comorbid medical conditions. Unfortunately, the prognosis for geriatric depression may often involve relapse and suggests a chronic disease trajectory (Cole, Bellavance, & Mansour, 1999).

DIAGNOSTICS

Mr. P's blood chemistries reveal Chem 23, CBC, and TFTs (including TSH and thyroxine) that were drawn in the ER 1 week ago. These are available to review via a shared electronic medical record and are all within normal limits. His ADL score is 6, indicating relatively high functioning (http://consultgerirn.org/uploads/File/trythis/try_this_2.pdf). His IADL assessment suggests he needs considerable assistance with transportation, laundry, shopping, meal preparation, and housekeeping (http://consultgerirn.org/uploads/File/trythis/try_this_23.pdf). The clinician performs a mental status exam. His thought content is positive for intensified body concern, though negative for illusions, hallucinations, delusions, or suicide idea/risk for harm. His thought process is positive for distractibility. His MMSE score is 28 out of 30 points, with errors for the day and date. He denies sad mood and denies a history of exceptionally high mood or energy. Sleep is estimated at 3 hours at night, with late insomnia.

CRITICAL THINKING

What is most likely affecting Mr. P's health and functioning?

What if the clinician screened him but he did not meet enough criteria for a particular condition? That is, what does the clinician recommend in the case of subclinical symptoms?

What comorbid conditions may be affecting him? Why might he resist reporting or minimize symptoms?

Could his age and military service influence the depression?

What treatment considerations should the clinician keep in mind for geriatric depression?

RESOLUTION

What is most likely affecting Mr. P's health and functioning?
Mr. P doesn't feel good because depression is affecting his health and functioning. His symptoms suggest that he has a recurrent episode of major depression; however, his previous postdeployment experience suggests that he may have had depressive symptoms that did not meet the criteria for a diagnosis of depression at the time. Risks to his health and safety include self-neglect and the potential for suicide idea, a life-threatening depressive symptom. Mr. P's age, cohort influences, and life experiences may explain reluctance on his part to endorse depressive symptoms, which makes it important to acknowledge the stigmata associated with having depression.

Depression is classified as a mood disorder, yet depressive symptoms affect more than just the older person's mood. Depressed older people may not feel good because of prominent physical symptoms;

though depression also affects cognitive, affective, social, spiritual functioning, and, ultimately, the quality of life for older adults. Further, energetic and apathetic symptoms in Mr. P are likely causing intrapersonal and interpersonal distress, leading to interference with his social, ADL, and IADL functioning. The particularly distressing symptom for this man is "insomnia", so understanding a sleep–depression relationship will be important to his care. While sleep problems may be indicative of depression, sleep disorders may also be independent risk factors in and potential markers for recurrence of depression in an older adult (Cho et al., 2008).

For a detailed discussion of the specific criteria for a diagnosis of major depression, see the DSM-IV-TR (American Psychiatric Association [APA], 2000). According to this classification, in order to be considered to be depressed, the person has to have at least 5 of 9 symptoms, with at least 1 of the following 2 core symptoms—depressed mood and loss of interest/pleasure—persisting nearly daily for at least 2 weeks. In addition to 1 or both of these symptoms, the person must have at least 4 more of the 9 symptoms, again persisting nearly daily for 2 weeks, including weight and appetite changes; increased or decreased sleep; psychomotor agitation or retardation; fatigue; themes of worthless, helpless, hopeless, and guilt; difficulty with concentration and decision-making; and recurrent thoughts of death. Subjectively, these symptoms cause distress and impairment, and represent a departure from the person's typical functioning. A differential diagnosis for unipolar major depression includes ruling out bipolar disorder, where the person has documented episodes of both manic as well as depressed mood (APA, 2000), as in the colloquial name for this condition, manic depression. Further specifiers included in a depression diagnosis indicate whether a depression episode is chronic and whether the mood features are accompanied by a psychotic thought process (APA, 2000).

Screening for depression in primary care is necessary care and is facilitated by the brevity and age-appropriateness of instruments. Three instruments are highlighted here. Generally, items on scales that measure depressive symptoms detect somatic, thought, relationship, and safety problems, in addition to affective/mood features of depression. A 2-item instrument, part of a geriatric depression tool kit, assesses sad mood and low interest, indicating further screening if 1 or both symptoms are present (see instrument at http://www.gericareonline.net/tools/eng/depression/index.html), though this instrument will not capture other depressive symptoms. A 10-item Centers for Epidemiological Studies depression scale assesses somatic, mood, and interpersonal features and is quick and reliable for use in older adult populations (Andresen, Malmgren, Carter, Patrick, 1994), indicating further screening for a score of 4 or more. A 15-item Geriatric Depression Scale emphasizes nonsomatic features (http://consultgerirn.org/uploads/File/

trythis/try_this_4.pdf), indicating further screening for a score over 5. From the information the clinician has elicited, Mr. P would score at least 4 on the CES-D-10 and at least 6 on the GDS-15, indicating probable depression and warranting further workup. A geriatric depression workup should always include cognitive testing and may include an EKG and brain imaging to rule out comorbid problems involving cardio-vascular and cerebrovascular functioning (Blazer, 2003).

What if the clinician screened him but he did not meet enough criteria for a particular condition? That is, what does the clinician recommend in the case of subclinical symptoms?
In other words, why might depression not be the obvious answer for why Mr. P is not feeling good? Depressed older patients are at risk for misdiagnosis—or worse—a *missed* diagnosis. Two reasons in particular are notable: First, older adults may have atypical presentations of clini-cally significant depressive symptoms; and second, the DSM-IV-TR diagnostic criteria for depression actually require a persistence of depressive symptoms that older adults do not typically experience. More specifically, older adults tend to have intermittent symptoms; and the DSM-IV-TR specifies that the person experience the symptoms daily for 2 weeks (APA, 2000) for major depression. To illustrate via a counterintuitive twist, some older adults may not typically experience sad mood, yet have depression (Gallo & Rabins, 1999). Cognitive and somatic features often dominate; and thus, depression can be missed.

While it may sound more accurate to suggest that Mr. P has subsyn-dromal/subclinical depression (VanItallie, 2005), or minor depression (not a DSM-IV-TR diagnosis), this condition is by no means **minor** in its impact on his health and functioning. Thus, a misinformed clinician may not determine that Mr. P's impairment and distress are from treat-able depressive symptoms. Ultimately, both diagnostic criteria and clinician misinformation may contribute to missed depression and increased vulnerability for older adults. A fuller discussion of the barriers to depression detection and treatment in older adults can be found in the landmark U.S. Surgeon General's report http://www.surgeongeneral.gov/library/mentalhealth/chapter5/sec3.html (U.S. Department of Health and Human Services [USDHHS], 1999).

Depression can be deadly for older adults if undertreated, unmoni-tored, or missed; and a markedly higher suicide risk in older adults is well documented. The clinician should screen Mr. P using a "SAD PERSONS" mnemonic (Patterson, Dohn, Bird, Patterson, 1983), as he may have several risk factors for death from suicide, especially as an elderly, Caucasian, single man with chronic health problems and ques-tionable social supports. Adding to his vulnerability, depression may be an independent risk factor for mortality that is not due to suicide (Geerlings, Beekman, Deeg, Twisk, & Van Tilburg, 2002; Schulz, Drayer, Rollman 2002).

Continuity of care is essential, providing monitoring and support through his primary care setting. As suggested by the findings of two longitudinal clinical trials, depressed older adults with suicide idea responded favorably to formal intervention in primary care, with less suicide idea and no death due to suicide (Bruce et al., 2004; Unützer et al., 2006). Trends from one of the trials suggested that ideas of death were a risk for 5-year mortality among usual care patients, and the authors suggested that screening for ideas of death is important even without prominent depressive symptoms (Raue et al., 2010).

What if the clinician screened him but he did not meet enough criteria for a particular condition? That is, what does the clinician recommend in the case of subclinical symptoms?
Mr. P's health and functioning may be impacted by 2 comorbid conditions in particular—pain and anxiety. Comorbidity poses an additional challenge to clinicians in assessing older adults for depression. Since depression is known to co-occur with other chronic health conditions such as cardiac (McGann, 2000) and pain conditions (Leong, Farrell, Helme, & Gibson, 2007), then comorbidity is the rule rather than the exception with current cohorts of older adults. For the many older adults who have co-occurring anxiety and depression, disturbance in social functioning and future outlook pose additional burdens (Jeste, Hays, & Steffens, 2006). Indicating whether this is a first or subsequent episode will be important, as there are likely neuropsychological distinctions impacting the disease process and function in late-life depression (Rapp et al., 2005). Confounding the assessment further, symptoms common across several chronic health problems— fatigue, for example—could mask or mimic the depressive symptoms that interfere with Mr. P's function. Screen him for other chronic health conditions. If older adults have exacerbations of their other medical conditions, untreated depression may contribute to poorer outcomes (Gallegos-Carrillo et al., 2009; Lyness, Niculescu, Tu, Reynolds, & Caine, 2006).

Could his age and military service influence the depression?
A particular complexity in the care of older adult veterans is the "triple threat" of being old, veteran, and depressed. The clinician should assess for loss and grief, and consider whether Mr. P has a comorbid (i.e., distinct) anxiety condition or whether anxious features are part of his depression. Further, loss, grief, and trauma-related features in an older veteran may be contributory, in a complex interplay. His history of a similar experience post deployment suggests some posttraumatic stress disorder (PTSD) features. Explore whether his social isolation is related to recent functioning, compared with his history. PTSD may be prominent in older veterans who appear depressed (Kales, 2009), and possible past traumatic experiences may impact an older person's functioning in subsequent stressful circumstances (Izzo, 2010). Explore

social and practical supports for Mr. P informally, such as older veteran's social programs, or formally, such as psychotherapy or eligibility for veterans' services. Ultimately, the clinician should seek consultation with a mental health colleague if his presentation suggests he has more than one mental health disorder.

What treatment considerations should the clinician keep in mind for geriatric depression?

Geriatric depression is a brain disease. Imbalances in neurotransmitters such as serotonin and norepinephrine are implicated in the development and persistence of depressive symptoms. Medication and psychotherapy are considered very effective in older adults at treating depression and reducing excess disability (Reynolds et al., 2006). In particular, psychotherapy is known to be efficacious for older adults; but it may be hard to detect effects due to study designs (Pinquart, Duberstein, & Lyness, 2006). While a detailed listing of available medications with recommendations is beyond the scope of this discussion, clinicians should be familiar with classes of antidepressant medications commonly prescribed for older adults. Treatments may be selected in collaboration with a mental health colleague or geriatrician, and may include selective serotonergic reuptake inhibitors, abbreviated SSRI (such as escitalopram and sertraline), or combined action serotonin-norepinepherine reuptake inhibitors, abbreviated SNRIs (such as venlafaxine and duloxetine). (Note: exemplars provided by the author are illustrations and not endorsements). Some of these serotonergic acting medications may also be useful for Mr. P's comorbid pain, contributing to improved functional outcomes (DeVeaugh-Geiss et al., 2010).

A less obvious treatment consideration is examining other medications that the older adult patient is using. Note that some antihypertensive medications such as his beta-blockers have depressive effects (Fick et al., 2003), and consider whether a medication review would be helpful. Other somatic and social therapies may be helpful. Electroconvulsive therapy (ECT) is effective for severe depression and is conventional, safe care for older adults, many of whom have other chronic medical conditions (Kamat, Lefevre, Grossberg, 2003). Physical activity is an effective intervention, both as prevention and amelioration of depression in older adults (Phillips, Kiernan, King, 2003). Further, increasing this man's mobility has the potential to improve his overall health. The clinician should initiate a home care referral for physical and occupational therapy to rebuild his endurance. Home care colleagues will also be able to monitor his depressive symptoms and may help him with self-management strategies. Finally, local affiliates of the National Alliance for Mental Illness (http://www.nami.org) support recovery from depression in a community of peer support and psychoeducational groups.

REFERENCES

American Psychiatric Association (2000). *Diagnostic and statistical manual for mental disorders (4th ed.) (DSM-IV-TR)*. Washington, DC: American Psychiatric Press.

Andresen, E. M., Malmgren, J. A., Carter, W. B., & Patrick, D. L. (1994). Screening for depression in well older adults: Evaluation of a short form of the CES-D. *American Journal of Preventive Medicine, 10*(2), 77–84.

Blazer, D. G. (2003). Depression in late life: Review and commentary. *The Journals of Gerontology. Series A, Biological Sciences and Medical Sciences, 58A*(3), 249–265.

Bruce, M. L., Ten Have, T. R., Reynolds, C. F., III, Katz, I. I., Schulberg, H. C., Mulsant, B. H., Brown, G. K., McAvay, G. J., Pearson, J. L., & Alexopoulos, G. S. (2004). Reducing suicidal ideation and depressive symptoms in depressed older primary care patients: A randomized controlled trial. *Journal of the American Medical Association, 291*(9), 1081–1091.

Chapman, D. P., & Perry, G. S. (2008). Depression as a major component of public health for older adults. *Preventing Chronic Disease, 5*(1), 1–9. Accessed June 10, 2010, from http://www.cdc.gov/pcd/issues/2008/jan/07_0150.htm

Cho, H., Lavretsky, H., Olmstead, R., Levin, M., Oxman, M., & Irwin, M. (2008). Sleep disturbance and depression recurrence in community-dwelling older adults: A prospective study. *The American Journal of Psychiatry, 165*(12), 1543–1550.

Cole, M., Bellavance, F., & Mansour, A. (1999). Prognosis of depression in elderly community and primary care populations: A systematic review and meta-analysis. *The American Journal of Psychiatry, 156*(8), 1182–1189.

DeVeaugh-Geiss, A., West, S., Miller, W., Sleath, B., Gaynes, B., & Kroenke, K. (2010). The adverse effects of comorbid pain on depression outcomes in primary care patients: Results from the ARTIST trial. *Pain Medicine, 11*(5), 732–741.

Fick, D., Cooper, J., Wade, W., Waller, J., Maclean, J., & Beers, M. (2003). Updating the Beers criteria for potentially inappropriate medication use in older adults: Results of a U.S. consensus panel of experts. *Archives of Internal Medicine, 163*(22), 2716–2724.

Gallegos-Carrillo, K., García-Peña, C., Mudgal, J., Romero, X., Duran-Arenas, L., & Salmeron, J. (2009). Role of depressive symptoms and comorbid chronic disease on health-related quality of life among community-dwelling older adults. *Journal of Psychosomatic Research, 66*(2), 127–135.

Gallo, J. J., & Rabins, P. V. (1999). Depression without sadness: Alternative presentations of depression in late life. *American Family Physician, 60*, 820–826.

Geerlings, S., Beekman, A., Deeg, D., Twisk, J., & Van Tilburg, W. (2002). Duration and severity of depression predict mortality in older adults in the community. *Psychological Medicine, 32*(4), 609–618.

Hybels, C. F., & Blazer, D. G. (2003). Epidemiology of late-life mental disorders. *Clinics in Geriatric Medicine, 19*, 663–696.

Izzo, J. (2010). The experience of vulnerability in geriatric combat veterans with PTSD during times of disaster. In J. A. Toner, T. M. Mierswa, & J. L. Howe (Eds.), *Geriatric mental health disaster and emergency preparedness*. New York: Springer.

Jeste, N., Hays, J., & Steffens, D. (2006). Clinical correlates of anxious depression among elderly patients with depression. *Journal of Affective Disorders, 90*(1), 37–41.

Jones, R. N., Marcantonio, E. R., & Rabinowitz, T. (2003). Prevalence and correlates of recognized depression in U.S. nursing homes. *Journal of the American Geriatrics Society, 51*(10), 1404–1409.

Kales, H. C. (2009). High prevalence of PTSD among elderly depressed veterans (Abstract NR11). *American Association for Geriatric Psychiatry Annual Meeting. Honolulu, Hawai, March 6, 2009*. Retrieved June 10, 2010, from http://www.medscape.com/viewarticle/590037

Kamat, S., Lefevre, P., & Grossberg, G. (2003). Electroconvulsive therapy in the elderly. *Clinics in Geriatric Medicine, 19*(4), 825–839.

Leong, I., Farrell, M., Helme, R., & Gibson, S. (2007). The relationship between medical comorbidity and self-rated pain, mood disturbance, and function in older people with chronic pain. *The Journals of Gerontology. Series A, Biological Sciences and Medical Sciences, 62*(5), 550–555.

Lyness, J., Niculescu, A., Tu, X., Reynolds, C. F. 3rd, & Caine, E. (2006). The relationship of medical comorbidity and depression in older, primary care patients. *Psychosomatics, 47*(5), 435–439.

McGann, P. (2000). Comorbidity in heart failure in the elderly. *Clinics in Geriatric Medicine, 16*(3), 631–648.

Patterson, W. M., Dohn, H. H., Bird, J., & Patterson, G. A. (1983). Evaluation of suicidal patients: The SAD PERSONS scale. *Psychosomatics, 24*, 343–345.

Phillips, W. T., Kiernan, M., & King, A. C. (2003). Physical activity as a non-pharmacological treatment for depression: A review. *Complementary Health Practice Review, 8*(2), 139–152.

Pinquart, M., Duberstein, P., & Lyness, J. (2006). Treatments for later-life depressive conditions: A meta-analytic comparison of pharmacotherapy and psychotherapy. *The American Journal of Psychiatry, 163*(9), 1493–1501.

Rapp, M., Dahlman, K., Sano, M., Grossman, H., Haroutunian, V., & Gorman, J. (2005). Neuropsychological differences between late-onset and recurrent geriatric major depression. *The American Journal of Psychiatry, 162*(4), 691–698.

Raue, P., Morales, K., Post, E., Bogner, H., Have, T., & Bruce, M. (2010). The wish to die and 5-year mortality in elderly primary care patients. *The American Journal of Geriatric Psychiatry: Official Journal of the American Association for Geriatric Psychiatry, 18*(4), 341–350.

Reynolds, C. F., III, Dew, M. A., Pollock, B. G., Mulsant, B. H., Frank, E., Miller, M. D., & Kupfer, D. J. (2006). Maintenance treatment of major depression in old age. New England. *Journal of Medicine, 354*(11), 1130–1138.

Schulz, R., Drayer, R., & Rollman, B. (2002). Depression as a risk factor for non-suicide mortality in the elderly. *Biological Psychiatry, 52*(3), 205–225.

Unützer, J., Tang, L., Oishi, S., Katon, W., Williams, J. W. Jr., Hunkeler, E., Hendrie, H. . . . Langston, C. for the Impact Investigators. (2006). Reducing suicidal ideation in depressed older primary care patients. *Journal of the American Geriatrics Society, 54*(10), 1550–1556.

U.S. Department of Health and Human Services (USDHHS) (1999). *Mental health: A report of the surgeon general*. Rockville, MD: U.S. Department of Health and Human Services, Substance Abuse and Mental Health Services Administration, Center for Mental Health Services, National Institutes of Health, National Institute of Mental Health (Chapter 5: Older Adults) Retrieved from http://www.surgeongeneral.gov

VanItallie, T. (2005). Subsyndromal depression in the elderly: Underdiagnosed and undertreated. *Metabolism: Clinical and Experimental*, *54*(5, Suppl. 1), 39–44.

Case 5.4 Understanding Distress

By Eileen O'Connor Smith, BSN, RN-C, and
Kelly Smith Papa, MSN, RN

Mrs. A, an 80-year-old woman, presents to the Alzheimer's Resource Center for long-term care after being at a rehabilitation center. She is 3 weeks status post a right intertrochanteric hip fracture treated by open reduction internal fixation (ORIF). The rehabilitation center states that she is highly agitated. Mrs. A was diagnosed with Alzheimer disease at age 74. Over the past 10 years, she has experienced cognitive changes including word-finding difficulty, poor judgment, misplacement of meaningful objects, short-term memory loss, mood changes, irritability, and changes in her personality. Her past medical history also includes hypertension, hyperlipidemia, osteoarthritis, degenerative joint disease, and osteoporosis.

Mrs. A is a retired elementary school teacher, who loves cooking and sharing stories about growing up on a farm. Mrs. A is proud of her large Irish Catholic family. She has 3 sons and 10 grandchildren. Religion is very important to her. She has attended church regularly and prayed the rosary daily. Mrs. A's husband, George, passed away 15 years ago. Her son moved into her home to offer her support, as her memory loss was making living alone more difficult. Mrs. A's safety is a concern, as she is up most of the night. Nutrition and hydration are also concerns since she is no longer able to eat independently with her utensils. She has difficulty walking due to her knee pain and has had multiple falls without injury. Her communication is difficult as her vocabulary has decreased, and she no longer remembers her family's names. Mrs. A became irritable and frustrated when approached to

Case Studies in Gerontological Nursing for the Advanced Practice Nurse, First Edition.
Edited by Meredith Wallace Kazer, Leslie Neal-Boylan.
© 2012 John Wiley & Sons, Inc. Published 2012 by John Wiley & Sons, Inc.

bathe, use the bathroom, or eat. She has punched her son in the face when he has tried to help her bathe. Multiple times a day she asks for her husband George and gets very sad when they remind (inform) her that he is dead.

Three weeks ago, Mrs. A fell in the bathroom and fractured her right hip, was hospitalized for an ORIF, and then was transferred to the local rehabilitation center. The rehabilitation staff had difficulty providing care for Mrs. A because she would become resistive during ADL by yelling, hitting, biting, and grabbing. She was restless at night, crawling out of bed and yelling all night, which left her lethargic during the day. Mrs. A has been refusing meals and spitting out food and medications. She has been upsetting her roommate and other neighboring residents. Due to her behaviors, she has been placed on antipsychotic and anti-anxiety medications.

The care plan team feels they can no longer meet Mrs. A's care needs due to her behaviors and recommends that she be moved to a skilled nursing facility that specializes in person-centered dementia care. The following information arrived on the W-10 from the rehabilitation facility. Her medications include Risperdal, 0.5 mg by mouth at 9 a.m. and 5 p.m.; Risperdal, 1.0 mg by mouth at 9 p.m.; Ativan, 0.25 mg by mouth every 4 hours as needed; Diovan w/HCTZ, 80/12.5 mg by mouth daily; Lipitor, 10 mg by mouth daily; ASA, 81 mg by mouth daily; Tylenol, 650 mg by mouth every 4 hours as needed for pain; and an as needed bowel regime including Milk of Magnesia, Dulcolax suppository, and Fleet enema. She has no known allergies.

OBJECTIVE

Mrs. A is alert, confused, and disoriented to person, place, and time. Her blood pressure is 114/70; pulse: 68; respirations: 16; and O_2 Sat: 99%. She is afebrile. She is 5 ft 3 inches and weighs 110 lb. Her pupils are equal and react to light and accommodation (PERRLA). She has mild wax buildup in her bilateral ears. During the examination, she demonstrates difficulty in word finding, and speaks with word salad, repetitively yelling out "George". She is unable to be consoled or redirected. She wears glasses and hearing aids. Her lung sounds are clear. Mrs. A's abdomen is soft and nontender, with positive bowel sounds in all 4 quadrants. Her skin is pink and intact, with dry skin on her legs and arms. She has no edema. Her right hip incision is healed, clean, dry, intact, and open to air. She becomes resistant during range of motion (ROM) assessment, showing facial grimacing and pushing the clinician away. There is some rigidity of limbs and neck noted. Her oral mucosa is pink and moist. She intermittently licks her lips and gums.

ASSESSMENT

At the rehabilitation care facility, Mrs. A is described as agitated. Mrs. A exhibits signs of distress as evidenced by resistance to care, restlessness, biting, yelling, and grabbing. There are numerous causes of distress but only a few ways to show it, especially when dementia has impaired one's ability to verbally communicate feelings and needs. The advanced clinician's assessment should determine the cause(s) of her distress.

Physical cause: Individuals with dementia are at a high risk for unidentified or untreated pain (Miller, Nelson, Mezey, 2000) that would result in distress. Commonly used pain assessment tools rely on the person's ability to report their pain experience. The PainAD scale assesses pain in the person with advanced dementia by observing nonverbal objective observations and indications of pain—breathing patterns, vocalizations, facial expressions, body language, and consolability (Warden, Hurley, Volicer, 2003). Also, the clinician should assess for infections (urinary tract infections), gastrointestinal causes, and side effects of medications.

Cognitive cause: Depression is very common among people with dementia, yet it is frequently unrecognized and untreated. Other cognitive related causes of distress could include deficits such as delirium and hallucinations. Memory loss, forgetfulness, and impaired ability to communicate can result in unrecognized depression.

Caregiver approach and/or environmental cause: Due to cognitive, visual and auditory deficits, the person with dementia may misinterpret the approach of the caregivers or the chaos in their environment. Distress may be related to the speed of the caregiver's approach, not being able to see or hear their caregiver, or the feeling of loss of physical and/or emotional control. The noise level or stimulation of the environment (including intercoms, other residents, televisions, inappropriate music, rushing staff, clutter, and lack of light or personal connection) can also cause the person with dementia to have increased confusion and may result in personal distress.

DIAGNOSTICS

The following assessments were completed at the Alzheimer's Resource Center, and the results are as follows: Pain assessment for advanced dementia (PainAD): score of 6; Cornell scale for depression in dementia

(CSDD): score of 12; Mini-Mental State Examination (MMSE): score of 18; Functional assessment staging tool (FAST): score of 7a; and Abnormal Involuntary Movement Scale (AIMS): negative for movement disorder.

The following laboratory tests were ordered: urinalysis (UA) with microscopy; complete blood count (CBC); comprehensive metabolic panel (CMP); thyroid stimulation hormone (TSH); folic acid level; cholesterol, lipid panel; and 25-hydroxyvitamin D. The UA was negative for infection. The CBC, CMP, TSH, and folic acid levels were all within normal limits. Cholesterol levels were high. Mrs. A's vitamin D level was found to be insufficient at 27 ng/mL. Normal range is 20–80 ng/mL, <20 ng/mL is considered deficient, 20–30 ng/mL is insufficient, and >32 ng/mL is optimal. Vitamin D is necessary for bone health and calcium absorption and has an impact on many conditions including diabetes, falls, fractures, strengthening, balance, postural swaying, infections, and mood and cognitive impairments (Holick, 2007).

CRITICAL THINKING

What is the most likely cause of Mrs. A's distress?

What is the plan of treatment?

What steps can the clinician take as she approaches Mrs. A for care that will help Mrs. A feel more comfortable and prevent her from becoming distressed?

How does a person's psychosocial history impact their plan of care?

How are approaches to care different based on the type of dementia a person has?

What would the clinician see differently if Mrs. A had:
- Vascular dementia
- Frontotemporal dementia
- Early onset Alzheimer disease (EOAD)
- Alcohol-induced dementia
- Lewy body dementia

What can be done when Mrs. A does become combative or aggressive with care?

How can the care environment be modified to meet Mrs. A's needs as her Alzheimer disease progresses?

What would the clinician do if Mrs. A had a 10-lb weight loss in 2 months?

RESOLUTION

What is the most likely cause of Mrs. A's distress?

Mrs. A's diagnoses and assessment scores indicate that her distress is likely caused by a combination of pain, depression, and her perception of loss of control in her environment (Kovack, Logan, Simpson, Reynolds, 2010). As Mrs. A's distress is reduced, minimized, and alleviated, she will become more engaged and relaxed. She will eat better, have more restful sleep, and participate more in daily activities. Each potential cause of distress should be addressed as a plan of care is developed. Dementia caregivers should be educated to recognize and respond to signs and symptoms that the person is experiencing distress from pain, infection, comorbidities, depression, illness, environment, or approach (Kovack et al., 2010). The caregiver should monitor signs of distress and improvement when causes are treated and should look for improvements in mood, eating, sleeping, socialization, affect, and participation in personal care. As causes of distress are resolved, the plan of care must be adapted to meet new abilities.

What is the plan of treatment?

Mrs. A scored high on her PainAD; she was a 6 out of 10, indicating that she is experiencing moderately severe pain. Pain treatment includes PainAD assessments each shift, observations from the care team, and a combination of pharmacological and nonpharmacological interventions. Pain should be treated around the clock, with an oral analgesic or a transdermal patch for a more consistent level of relief. Consider pre-medicating for breakthrough pain 20–30 minutes prior to care or therapy with ibuprofen, NSAIDs, or other analgesics. Monitor for increased risk associated with the use of these medications, including constipation and bleeding due to increased risk of GI bleed with the use of NSAIDS. Mrs. A is also at a high risk of falling. Nonpharmacological interventions for pain relief should also be used. Consider consolidating personal care needs by having the nurse, nursing assistant, and/or therapists work together so that Mrs. A is not moved multiple times unnecessarily.

Mrs. A's CSDD was 12, indicating that an antidepressant should be added and monitored with consideration of the side-effect profile that would most appropriately fit Mrs. A's needs. A selective serotonin reuptake inhibitor (SSRI) such as Zoloft, Wellbutrin, Remeron, or Lexapro could be considered.

The high doses of Risperdal should be discontinued. The clinician may try a long-acting orally disintegrating medication that will rapidly dissolve. Zyprexa (Zydis), 5 mg each day, may be tried to eliminate the risk of her spitting it out or not swallowing it. The clinician should reassess in 30 days for the possibility of a gradual dose reduction (GDR) as other causes of distress are resolved. Upon assessment, she was licking her lips. Could this be a side effect of the antipsychotic medication? The AIMS (Guy, 1976a, 1976b) will help to monitor for signs of tardive dyskinesia, repetitive abnormal involuntary movements of the mouth, face, limbs, and neck, which are side effects of neuroleptic (antipsychotic) use. Follow facility policy for orthostatic blood pressure monitoring.

To treat her Alzheimer disease, the clinician may add titrating doses of Aricept, up to 10 mg by mouth daily, and Namenda, 10 mg by mouth twice daily, while monitoring for GI symptoms.

The clinician should follow up with the facility's earwax removal protocols. Be sure Mrs. A's hearing aids are working properly. Hearing loss can increase confusion and is frequently unrecognized in people with Alzheimer's.

The patient should be started on vitamin D3, 50,000 units by mouth twice a month, and Tums, 1 tab twice daily.

What steps can the clinician take as she approaches Mrs. A for care that will help Mrs. A feel more comfortable and prevent her from becoming distressed?

An **empathy-based**, person-centered approach is individualized and dignified and incorporates the person's life story to establish a connection that can help to prevent distress (Egan, 2007). An empathic caregiver is in tune with the feelings and emotions of a person with dementia. Ensure the environment is calm and use a slow approach that incorporates nonverbal communication. As dementia progresses, verbal communication decreases and people rely more heavily on nonverbal skills to communicate. Caregivers should be sure that Mrs. A can determine their presence and should offer her enough time to respond—sometimes 20–90 seconds. Caregivers should keep the sentences short with the most important word at the end of the sentence. The clinician may consider breaking down tasks into small steps. The caregiver must remain focused during conversations. The clinician should be sure not to rush or appear disinterested in what she is sharing. By mirroring her pace and feelings, the caregiver will help Mrs. A to feel safe and understood. Her feelings and emotions behind her words or actions should be validated. If Mrs. A is looking for George, whom we know passed away, ask her to describe him and how they met. Offer Mrs. A the time to share the feelings of love she has for him. As the disease progresses, caregivers may become the keeper of Mrs. A's stories and share them with her when she can no longer communicate.

How does a person's psychosocial history impact plan of care?

The more we know about a person's life story, the more we can develop personalized care that meets each individual's need. There are many clues in Mrs. A's story that offer us opportunities for relationship building prior to and after care. She loves her family; was a teacher; grew up on a farm; cooks; likes Irish culture, religion, and social conversation; and loves kids (Egan et al., 2007).

An empathic caregiver seeks to learn about events in world history and in personal lives that may be very real in a person's mind (war, abuse, a miscarriage, or the death of a loved one). As part of the care planning process, ask Mrs. A's family to share special stories from her life. Ask about her childhood and things she did as a mom, teacher, and friend.

How are approaches to care different based on the type of dementia a person has?

There are many causes and types of dementia. Alzheimer disease is the most frequent type of dementia. Alzheimer disease is a progressive neurological disorder that destroys brain cells. The first signs of Alzheimer disease are related to memory loss. Each type of related dementia has associated symptoms based on the effects the disease has on cognitive functioning. To treat the symptoms of dementia, there are a variety of pharmacologic treatments and nonpharmacologic approaches to care. Interventions need to be individualized and frequently assessed for effectiveness.

What would the clinician see differently if Mrs. A had:

- **Vascular dementia:** More inconsistent presentation of symptoms and course of disease; not as predictable as Alzheimer disease. Symptoms include confusion, memory loss, and progressive declines in cognition with a high risk of depression.
- **Frontotemporal dementia:** Symptoms include poor impulse control, restlessness, personality changes, and apathy.
- **Early onset Alzheimer disease:** With EOAD, the disease progresses quickly and has a devastating effect on families because of the young age of onset, between the ages of 30 and 60.
- **Alcohol-induced dementia:** Symptoms of alcohol-induced dementia include personality changes, depression, anxiety, confabulation, hostility, and irritability.
- **Lewy body dementia:** Symptoms include hallucinations and/or delusions with fluctuating cognitive impairments and high sensitivity to extrapyramidal side effects of neuroleptic medications.

What can be done when Mrs. A does become combative or aggressive with care?

As a person's ability to verbally communicate decreases, their communications may become physical, especially when they feel that they have lost physical and emotional control. Imagine lying sound asleep in bed at home, when all of the sudden a stranger enters the bedroom, turns on the light, and proceeds to lift off the covers. The role of a professional is to prevent the person from becoming distressed; but what if something happens that the individual perceives as threatening; and they grab, choke or bite? The first response is to remain safe and calm. Next focus on the hold, and determine if the use of a verbal or tactile cue would release the hold. If a maneuver to release the hold needs to be used, be sure that it is a move that protects both the person with dementia and the caregiver (Alzheimer's Resource Center, 2002). As a follow-up measure, the care team can determine if the use of Ativan as needed would lessen distress.

How can the care environment be modified to meet Mrs. A's needs as her Alzheimer disease progresses?
The atmosphere should be calm and free from chaos. It should offer meaningful music, natural lighting, with places to sit and rest. The use of televisions, overhead paging, and inappropriate music is distracting, confusing, and overwhelming to the person with dementia. The environment should offer support for the person to feel physically and emotionally safe.

What would the clinician do if Mrs. A had a 10-lb weight loss in 2 months?
As a person develops dysphagia, a speech therapist can be consulted to determine the appropriate food and liquid consistency. An occupational therapy consult will help to determine if adaptive equipment can be used to promote independence at mealtimes. The ED FED Nursing Assessment tool (Stockdell & Amella, 2008) can be used by the clinician to assess if weight loss is secondary to cognitive deficits, side effects of medication, poor appetite due to dislike of modified diet, environmental , or caregiver approach. Educate caregivers to use guiding-hand and caring-hand approaches during meals to keep the person with dementia engaged and social at mealtimes (Alzheimer's Resource Center, 2010). Mrs. A used to love to cook, so find ways to include her in meal preparation or in conversations about things she would cook for her family. To help supplement her calorie intake, offer to join her for a milkshake, yogurt, fruit smoothie, or protein shake.

REFERENCES

Alzheimer's Resource Center (2002). S.A.F.E. Response Techniques in Crisis Situations.

Alzheimer's Resource Center (2010). Dining with Friends: Innovative Approaches to Dining for the Person with Dementia.

Egan, M., Munroe, S., Hubert, C., Rossiter, T., Gauthier, A., Eisner, M., Fulford, N., Neilson, M., Daros, B., & Rodrigue, C. (2007). Caring for residents with dementia and impact of life history knowledge. *Journal of Gerontological Nursing*, *33*(2), 24–30.

Egan, G. (2007) *The Skilled Helper*, 8th ed. Belmont, CA: Thomson Brooks/Cole.

Guy, W. (1976a). *Abnormal involuntary movement scale. ECDEU: Assessment manual for psychopharmacology (revised)* (pp. 534–537). Washington, DC: US Department of Health, Education and Welfare.

Guy, W. (1976b). *ECDEU assessment manual for psychopharmacology*, revised ed. Washington, DC: US Department of Health, Education, and Welfare.

Holick, M. (2007). Vitamin D deficiency. *The New England Journal of Medicine, 357*(3), 266–281.

Kovack, C., Logan, B., Simpson, M., & Reynolds, S. (2010). Factors associated with time to identify physical problems of nursing home residents with dementia. *American Journal of Alzheimer's Disease and Other Dementias, 25*(4), 317–323.

Miller, L., Nelson, L., & Mezey, M. (2000). Comfort and pain relief in dementia. *Journal of Gerontological Nursing, 26*(9), 32–40.

Stockdell, R., & Amella, E. (2008). The Edinburgh feeding evaluation in dementia scale. *The American Journal of Nursing, 108*(3), 46–54.

Warden, V., Hurley, A. C., & Volicer, L. (2003). Development and psychometric evaluation of the pain assessment in advanced dementia (PAINAD) scale. *Journal of the American Medical Directors Association, 4*(1), 9–15.

Section 6

Issues of Aging and Independence

Case 6.1 Too Much of a Good Thing

By Susan C. Frazier, MS, NP-C, GNP-BC

Ms. M, an 86-year-old woman presents to the clinician's primary care practice with her daughter due a general decline in her condition over the last 3 months, including a fall for which she was evaluated in the emergency department (ED) over the weekend. Ms. M is transferring to the practice as she is moving into an in-law apartment at her daughter's home. Her last checkup was 6 months ago, and she brought her records with her. Ms. M has a past medical history that includes diagnoses of hypertension, hyperlipidemia, depression, osteoporosis, and osteoarthritis. She has had a remote cholecystectomy, a left total hip replacement, and 2 healthy pregnancies. She has a weekly social drink, but does not smoke. Her income comes primarily from social security and her deceased husband's pension. Her adult children are healthy. During this visit, her review of systems is notable for complaints of constipation, decreased appetite, and dry mouth; and her daughter reports new, intermittent confusion over the last 2 months. Ms. M denies shortness of breath, dyspnea on exertion, chest pain, palpitations, headaches, vertigo, vomiting, or diarrhea.

Ms. M's medications include lisinopril, 40 mg daily; atenolol, 25 mg daily; furosemide, 40 mg every day; potassium chloride (KCl), 20 mEq twice daily; fluoxetine, 20 mg daily; amitriptyline, 25 mg at bedtime; omeprazole, 20 mg daily; enteric-coated aspirin, 325 mg daily; simvastatin, 40 mg every evening; docusate sodium, 100 mg twice daily; Senna, 2 tabs at bedtime; alendronate, 70 mg once weekly; and calcium carbonate with vitamin D, twice daily. Her furosemide and KCl have been held since her ED visit due to concerns of dehydration. On further

Case Studies in Gerontological Nursing for the Advanced Practice Nurse, First Edition.
Edited by Meredith Wallace Kazer, Leslie Neal-Boylan.
© 2012 John Wiley & Sons, Inc. Published 2012 by John Wiley & Sons, Inc.

questioning, the clinician determines that she also takes ibuprofen, 400 mg 3 times daily as needed for arthritic pain, and Milk of Magnesia, 30 ml every other day as needed. She also admits to taking an acetaminophen with diphenhydramine tablet 3–4 times weekly to help with sleep. She has no known allergies (NKA).

OBJECTIVE

Ms. M is awake, alert, and appropriate. She has mild kyphosis. She appears clean and well kept. Her clothes are appropriate. She is 5 ft 2 inches and weighs 110 lb; BP: 160/90; P: 56; 02 sat: 97%. She is afebrile with a temperature of 97.6. Her lungs are clear. Cardiac exam reveals a regular heart rate, S1, S2, and no adventitious sounds. Her abdomen is slightly distended and tender. The clinician feels a distended bladder, and stool can be palpated in the right lower quadrant. Her bowel sounds are present but sluggish in all 4 quadrants. She has a scar from the open cholecystectomy on her abdomen, and her umbilicus is midline. Her skin is very dry but intact. She had no pedal edema and positive pedal pulses. Her eyes reveal clear normal sclerae with PERRLA. Her ears reveal normal tympanic membranes bilaterally. Her mouth indicates a dry oral mucosa and tongue. Neurological exam reveals 2+ deep tendon reflexes bilaterally and equal strength. Her gait is slightly ataxic, and she has some limited range of motion of her knees and hips. Due to her daughter's concern about her mental state, the clinician asks Ms. M to repeat and remember 3 words and to perform the Clock Drawing Test to determine her cognitive status. She has trouble figuring out where to put the numbers, but she puts them in the right order. However, she forgets to include the hands of the clock. She recalls 2 out of 3 of the words.

ASSESSMENT

Dementia, delirium, and/or depression: Ms. M's initial screen points to cognitive impairment and is the main concern of her daughter. She already carries a diagnosis of depression. It is possible for all 3 syndromes to coexist, making the diagnosis and treatment more challenging for the provider.

Dehydration: Ms. M's symptoms of dry mouth, constipation, and falls are consistent with this diagnosis. She was also recently treated in the emergency department for dehydration. However, her diuretic was discontinued 3 days ago; and her daughter reports that she has been encouraging her mother to drink liquids.

Polypharmacy: The clinician notices that Ms. M's medications could be contributing to her symptoms. She is on some medications that are considered inappropriate for older adults and others that may be contributing to her medical issues.

DIAGNOSTICS

Due to Ms. M's cognitive impairment and concern for continued dehydration, a workup should include a complete blood cell count, blood chemistries, liver function tests, a serologic test for syphilis, thyroid stimulating hormone, a vitamin B_{12} level, folate, urinalysis, and an electrocardiogram (Dick, 2008a, 2008b). A chest radiogram done in the ED was negative. The complete blood count, electrolytes, liver function tests, thyroid stimulating hormone, syphilis, vitamin B_{12}, folate, and urinalysis are within normal limits. Blood urea nitrogen (BUN) and creatinine (cr) are elevated at 28 (reference range 8–20 mg/dL) and 1.5 (reference range 0.44–1.03 mg/dL). Her blood urea nitrogen and creatinine were 40 and 2.0 upon admission to the ED and had normalized to her baseline of 20 and 1.0 by discharge after she had received intravenous fluids. Her electrocardiogram shows sinus bradycardia with a first-degree heart block, which is not new.

CRITICAL THINKING

What is the most likely differential diagnosis and why?

What is the plan of treatment?

What is the plan for follow-up care?

Does the patient's psychosocial history impact how the clinician might treat this patient?

How does the patient's kidney function impact treatment?

Are there any standardized instruments that the clinician should use to assess or treat this case?

RESOLUTION

What is the most likely differential diagnosis and why?
Ms. M has had a diagnosis of depression since the death of her husband 2 years prior. She was placed on an antidepressant (fluoxetine) at that

time by her primary care provider but did not seek counseling. When she complained at her last visit that she was still not sleeping well and had little appetite, a second antidepressant (amitriptyline) was added. Ms. M does exhibit the following signs of depression that are common in older adults: A focus on somatic concerns (her constipation and arthritic complaints), social withdrawal, a decreased appetite, and insomnia. Mild memory impairment is also possible in depression (Fournier, 2008), making the clinical picture more challenging.

Dementia affects approximately half of the population over 80 years of age. Memory loss, personality changes, difficulties with language, and problems with independent activities of daily living are common presenting symptoms of dementia. However, the changes are usually subtle and gradual (Dick, 2008a, 2008b). Ms. M's daughter states that her mother's mental status changes are new, within the past few months.

Delirium is characterized by fluctuations in mental status. There is an inability to focus, sustain, or shift attention, as well as a change in cognition (Dick, 2008a, 2008b). It may be caused by certain medications, systemic diseases, organic brain disease, metabolic disturbances, drug intoxication, and withdrawal from drugs or alcohol. Delirium, dementia, and depression have manifestations in common and can occur in the same patient at the same time. An episode of delirium may be the first sign of an unrecognized dementia in the setting of an acute illness (Dick, 2008a, 2008b).

Ms. M is taking 16 medications. Twenty-three percent of women and nineteen percent of men older than 65 take at least 5 prescription drugs. Fifty-seven percent of women take more than 5 medications when over-the-counter medications are included (Kaufman et al., 2002). Polypharmacy is the use of multiple medications, duplicative medications, medications prescribed at the wrong dose, and medications prescribed for the wrong duration (Planton & Edlund, 2010). Some consider it polypharmacy when there are simply too many medications to take (pill burden). Polypharmacy has a potential to cause more frequent adverse drug reactions and drug-drug interactions (Haque, 2009). Polypharmacy and biologic vulnerability for adverse effects also make the older person more prone to medication-induced delirium (Dick, 2008a, 2008b). Anticholinergic medications in particular have long been implicated as risk factors for delirium (Dick, 2008a, 2008b).

The development of any new signs and symptoms should be considered as a possible consequence of the patient's drug treatment. Ms. M appears to have been a victim of the "prescribing cascade". The prescribing cascade begins when an adverse drug reaction is misinterpreted as a new medical condition. A new drug is prescribed, and the patient is placed at risk of developing additional adverse effects relating to this potentially unnecessary treatment (Rochon & Gurwitz, 1997). In the case of Ms. M, this is evident by her prescription of fluoxetine for depression, followed by amitriptyline because of weight loss and continued insomnia. However, she continues to have insomnia and added over-the-counter acetaminophen with diphenhydramine, which she did not report to her physician. On followup, she began to complain of constipation and increasing joint aches from her arthritis. Ms. M began to use ever-increasing amounts of stool softeners and laxatives. She admits to using Milk of Magnesia almost daily, as well as enemas several times a week. Ms. M was told to take ibuprofen for her arthritic pains. Around this time, her blood pressure began to climb and her antihypertensives were titrated upward.

Fluoxetine likely contributed to Ms. M's insomnia and weight loss. The anticholinergics amitriptyline and diphenhydramine can cause dry mouth, constipation, confusion, and falls. Ibuprofen can increase blood pressure (Rochon & Gurwitz, 1997) and, especially with furosemide, can cause renal failure.

What is the plan of treatment?

All new patients should have a thorough review of all medications, including prescription and over-the-counter preparations; but it is especially important when delirium is suspected. Nonessential medications need to be tapered or discontinued (Dick, 2008a, 2008b). A priority would be to stop amitriptyline and diphenhydramine, which both have strong anticholinergic properties and are on the Beer's list of potentially inappropriate medications for the elderly (Fick, Cooper, Wade, Waller et al., 2003). Fluoxetine is also considered an inappropriate medication for the elderly due to its long half-life, and it is likely contributing to her insomnia and weight loss and should be discontinued. Mirtazapine is often used in the elderly as it has the beneficial side effect profile of weight gain and sleepiness. Ms. M was put on a proton pump inhibitor when she was hospitalized for her hip replacement several years ago, and it was never discontinued. As she denies ever having reflux, the omeprazole is discontinued. Ms. M and her daughter are educated about the hazards of nonsteroidal antiinflammatory drugs in the elderly. Ms. M is put on acetaminophen (less than 4 g daily) for her arthritic pain.

Ms. M's constipation is likely due to the anticholinergic medications, but it may also be worsened by the calcium supplements. This possibility is discussed with her and her daughter, and they decide to decrease her calcium carbonate tablets to once daily. This will hopefully reduce her need for the stool softeners and laxatives. As she has been on alendronate for 7 years, the option of taking a break from bisphosphonates is discussed. Also, there is no evidence to support the use of the daily aspirin on the development of cognitive impairment, so Ms. M and her daughter decide to discontinue it for now. Ms. M is now on 6 medications.

Due to her daughter's concern that her mother is not taking her medications correctly, the clinician orders home care to review the medication changes to make sure that she is taking them correctly and to monitor her blood pressure, pain management, and constipation. Ms. M is also referred to a grief support group when she is ready.

What is the plan for follow-up care?

Even removing the offending agents, delirium may take months to completely resolve (Dick, 2008a, 2008b). Ms. M should be followed closely for resolution of her confusion. In addition, her antihypertensives may need to be adjusted further as she stops the NSAIDS. Her other complaints of arthritis, depression, and constipation also need to monitored.

Does the patient's psychosocial history impact how the clinician might treat this patient?

Ms. M shows signs of intermittent confusion, and so it is important to include her daughter and health care proxy, Ms. D, in all discussions, while maintaining Ms. M's autonomy as much as possible.

How does the patient's kidney function impact treatment?

Prior to initiating any renal-eliminated medication in the elderly, the clinician must calculate the patient's kidney function (Planton & Edlund, 2010). Currently, the Cockcroft-Gault equation is recommended for drug dosage adjustments (Spruill & Wade, 2008; Planton & Edlund, 2010). Using this equation, Ms. M has a diminished creatinine clearance, even at baseline. The clinician will avoid prescribing any nephrotoxic drugs and will reduce renally eliminated medications as needed.

Are there any standardized instruments that the clinician should use to assess or treat this case?

Haque (2009) describes a functional tool that consolidates several recent recommended strategies. The ARMOR (Assess, Review, Minimize, Optimize, Reassess) tool approaches polypharmacy in a systematic and organized fashion. Although initially used in a long-term care facility, it is applicable in any setting. The restoration and maintenance of functional status and mobility are the primary outcome goals. The clinician assesses the individual for the total number of medications and for certain groups of medications that have potential for adverse outcomes. The medications are reviewed for possible drug-drug interactions, drug-disease interactions, drug-body interactions, impact on functional status, subclinical adverse drug reactions, and effects on primary body functions. The clinician then minimizes nonessential medications and those whose risks outweigh their benefits and optimizes the drug regimen by addressing duplication, adjusting renally cleared medications or medications that are metabolized in the liver, and adjusting certain medications such as oral hypoglycemics, antidepressants, beta-blockers, anticoagulants, and seizure medications. The last step is to reassess vital signs, functional status, cognitive status, clinical status, and medication compliance.

REFERENCES

Dick, K. (2008a). Delirium. In T. M. Buttaro, J. Trybulski, P. G. Bailey, & J. Sandberg-Cook (Eds.), *Primary care: A collaborative practice* (3rd ed., pp. 1037–1040). Philadelpha: Mosby.

Dick, K. (2008b). Dementia. In T. M. Buttaro, J. Trybulski, P. G. Bailey, & J. Sandberg-Cook (Eds.), *Primary care: A collaborative practice* (3rd ed., pp. 1040–1044). Philadelpha: Mosby.

Fick, D. M., Cooper, J. W., Wade, W. E., Waller, J. L., Maclean, J. R., & Beers, M. H. (2003). Updating the Beers criteria for potentially inappropriate medication use in older adults: Results of a US consensus panel of experts. *Archives of Internal Medicine, 163,* 2716–2724.

Fournier, D. (2008). Depressive disorders. In T. M. Buttaro, J. Trybulski, P. G. Bailey, & J. Sandberg-Cook (Eds.), *Primary care: A collaborative practice* (3rd ed., pp. 1388–1398). Philadelpha: Mosby.

Haque, R. (2009). Armor: A tool to evaluate polypharmacy in elderly persons. *Annals of Long-Term Care, 18*(6), 2–6.

Kaufman, D. W., Kelly, J. P., Rosenberg, L., Anderson, T. E., & Mitchell, A. A. (2002). Recent patterns of medication use in the ambulatory adult population of the United States: The Slone survey. *Journal of the American Medical Association, 287*(3), 337–344.

Planton, J., & Edlund, B. J. (2010). Strategies for reducing polypharmacy in older adults. *Journal of Gerontological Nursing, 36*(1), 8–12.

Rochon, P. A., & Gurwitz, J. A. (1997). Optimizing drug treatment for elderly people: The prescribing cascade. *British Medical Journal, 315,* 1096–1099.

Spruill, W. J., & Wade, W. E. (2008). Comparison of estimated glomerular filtration rate with estimated creatinine clearance in the dosing of drugs requiring adjustments in elderly patients with declining function. *American Journal of Geriatric Pharmacotherapeutics, 6*(3), 153–160.

ADDITIONAL RESOURCES

Try This, Issue 16.1—Beers' Criteria for Potentially Inappropriate Medication Use in the Elderly: Part I—2002 Criteria Independent of Diagnoses or Conditions: http://consultgerirn.org/

Try This Issue 16.2—Beers' Criteria for Potentially Inappropriate Medication Use in the Elderly: Part II—2002 Criteria Considering Diagnoses or Conditions: http://consultgerirn.org/

Case 6.2 Driving in My Car

By Valerie C. Sauda, RN-BC, MS

Mr. C is a 79-year-old man who presents to the primary care office for an unscheduled appointment with his oldest son due to his family's concern about his driving ability. He is a widowed American Indian man who lives alone. He has 2 children who live near his home and visit him daily. Mr. C receives income from social security and a retirement fund from his work as a teacher. He does not attend religious services, but he has shared on a previous visit that his inner peace comes from being out in nature. Mr. C sees the primary care provider annually and is up-to-date with all his vaccinations and preventive screenings. He has osteoarthritis in his hands and is able to perform his own activities of daily living. Mr. C has Type 2 diabetes mellitus, a history of 2 falls at home in the past year with no injuries noted, and a history of depression. He denies use of alcohol or tobacco. Upon review of systems, he wears glasses and is slightly hard of hearing. He denies shortness of breath, dizziness, chest pain, palpitations, nausea, vomiting, or diarrhea. He denies difficulty with urination or defecation and reports that he has regular daily bowel movements. He states that he is able to maintain his diet and takes his prescribed medications to manage his diabetes. He denies any complaints of pain. Mr. C's son shared that he is concerned that his father forgot the way home while driving recently and had an accident in which he was crossing a lane, turning left, and hit another vehicle. Mr. C denied any difficulty with driving.

Mr. C is taking the following medications: metformin 500 mg extended-release daily; ibuprofen, 400 mg 3 times daily; multivitamin

Case Studies in Gerontological Nursing for the Advanced Practice Nurse, First Edition.
Edited by Meredith Wallace Kazer, Leslie Neal-Boylan.
© 2012 John Wiley & Sons, Inc. Published 2012 by John Wiley & Sons, Inc.

1 tablet daily; and occasionally takes 1 tablet of over-the-counter Benadryl for sleep. He took 1 tablet of Benadryl 3 months ago for difficulty falling asleep. He has no known allergies (NKA).

OBJECTIVE

Mr. C is awake, alert, and oriented to person and place. He is unable to give the correct day of the week or the date. His speech is distinct, and he answers questions clearly. His posture is erect. His appearance is neat with pants pleated. Mr. C's height is 5 ft 8 inches, and his weight is 165 lb. His vital signs are as follows: BP: 130/72; pulse: 76 radial regular; respirations: 16 and even; temperature: 97.9° F oral. His skin is warm and dry to touch. His pupils are equal, round, and reactive to light and accommodation (PERRLA). His ears have no wax noted, but there is a diminished result noted on the whisper test. Mr. C's lungs are clear upon auscultation; his apical heart rate is regular. S1, S2 are present with no murmurs or extra heart sounds are noted. The abdomen has no surgical scars or lesions noted. His bowel sounds are present in all 4 quadrants. There is no tenderness, and no masses are palpable. There is no pedal or ankle edema; dorsalis pedis and posterior tibial pulses are palpable bilaterally. Deep tendon reflexes are 2+ bilaterally. His gait is steady, with full stride and full arm swings noted. There is reduced range of motion noted in both hands. His facial expressions are symmetrical, the Romberg test is negative, and finger-to-nose test and rapid alternating movements are performed slowly but accurately. In the Mini-Cog test, Mr. C recalled 2 listed items. In the Clock Drawing Test (CDT), he was able to draw the circle, but he did not place the numbers on the clock face in an organized manner or place the correct time as requested. Upon discussion about the driving incident, Mr. C stated, "That is just a one-time thing and is not serious."

ASSESSMENT

Memory loss with executive dysfunction: Mr. C's lack of remembering where he was going when driving, not identifying the seriousness of the driving issue, and indications that there is executive function impairment during the Mini-Cog screening may indicate that he has the beginning stages of memory loss or possibly dementia, which could potentially impair his driving.

Depression: Mr. C has a history of depression, lives alone, and has some memory loss. Functional impairments may indicate an exacerbation of depression.

Hypothyroidism: In older adults, hypothyroidism can contribute to lapses in memory.

Hypoglycemia: With Mr. C's history of Type 2 diabetes mellitus, which may be a contributing factor to memory loss, it is valuable to assess his diabetic status.

Nutrition impairment: Ruling out a nutritional issue is important as Mr. C has Type 2 diabetes mellitus, lives alone, and has some memory loss noted, putting him at risk for a nutrition deficit.

DIAGNOSTICS

A further neurological function consultation should be completed to ensure that there is not an organic problem associated with his cognitive function. A complete blood count (CBC) and metabolic panel with protein and albumin would be important to help rule out a nutritional deficit. TSH (thyroid stimulating hormone) and HgA1c are recommended to rule out hypoglycemia that could contribute to memory lapse. Vitamin B_{12}, folate, and urinalysis are recommended to rule out vitamin deficiency or urinary tract infection, which can also cause memory lapse. A geriatric depression screen is recommended to rule out depression contributing to his memory loss (AGS, 2009). Finally, it is recommended that he have an objective driving examination to determine whether he is having motor impairments that make him unsafe to drive (AMA, 2010).

Mr. C's complete blood count (CBC), metabolic panel, TSH, HgA1c, B_{12}, folate, and urinalysis are within accepted ranges. The geriatric depression screen score was negative. The driving examination revealed impairment in reaction time (the instructor hit the brakes 3 times during the examination) and an impaired ability to hear horns beeping, and Mr. C missed 1 stop sign at an intersection. It is noted that the instructor notified the Department of Motor Vehicles of the results of the driving examination, as required by state law.

CRITICAL THINKING

What are the most likely differential diagnoses and why?

What is the anticipated plan of treatment?

What will the clinician recommend for a follow-up plan?

What are the key factors in determining whether to recommend driver's license revocation?

What standard guidelines will the clinician use to determine whether to recommend revocation of his driver's license?

How will the clinician best manage an exacerbation of depression if the decision is made to revoke Mr. C's license?

What if the patient also had difficulty with his nutritional status?

How do culture and ethnicity affect the plan of treatment?

RESOLUTION

What are the most likely differential diagnoses and why?
Memory loss and mild executive dysfunction appear to be the differential diagnoses for Mr. C. The older adult with an onset of confusion from delirium, dementia, or depression is often able to function on a daily basis within normal daily activities and routines. As disease process progresses, the family may become more aware of the symptoms of confusion as the person starts to show impairments in judgment and activities of daily living like driving. The real challenge in this case is the role of the clinician in determining the older adult's fitness for driving. When looking at a patient's driving fitness, it is the best practice for the clinician to ensure that there is a complete medical review of all body systems, including current medication history, to identify factors that may be contributing to impaired driving fitness. In Mr. C's case, his nutritional risks, chronic illness management (such as his diabetes and mental health status for depression), as well as neurological function, are reasonable factors to consider before determining whether to recommend license alteration or revocation.

Nutritional impairments can impact an older adult's memory as well as their ability to respond to environmental stimuli, such as the reaction time required during driving. In addition, fluid and electrolyte imbalances can mimic symptoms of dementia; so it is important that the clinician assess these areas completely before determination of fitness to drive.

What is the anticipated plan of treatment?
The plan of treatment for Mr. C would be to recommend that he stop driving at this time in order to maintain personal safety related to the recent incident and his driving examination. Secondly, development of a person-centered plan of medical treatment for his underlying memory loss is recommended. Finally, encourage the family to offer transportation support to Mr. C for times when he needs to go out at night or to go longer distances. Development of a transportation plan is essential when recommending revocation of a license or stopping driving for an

older adult. This helps to ease the fear of isolation and potential loss issues associated with the loss of independence from loss of driving (ASA, 2006). The clinician would also need to ensure that findings are reported to the appropriate state agency such as the Department of Motor Vehicles, as required by state regulation. Documentation of a treatment plan is essential in order to ensure that any driving-specific recommendations that are made are clear and understood by the patient and his family (as permitted by patient).

What will the clinician recommend for a follow-up plan?

An additional office visit with the patient and a family member within 1 month for review of cognitive status, symptoms of depression, and transportation plan is needed. Encourage the family to contact a local area agency on aging or a local Alzheimer's association for support in developing a transportation plan for long-term community support for Mr. C.

What are the key factors in determining whether to recommend driver's license revocation?

The ability to drive is a significant issue for the older adult. There are many factors that need to be taken into consideration, including the person's medical status, psychological status, and functional status (AMA, 2010). Many times, the older adult has self-ability to recognize driving challenges, including decreased visual acuity, decreased ability to drive at night, or frequent near-miss accidents while driving (ASA, 2006). The older adult who exhibits cognitive impairment, however, may not have the executive ability to determine safety of self or others while driving. For the clinician, it becomes essential to conduct a complete review of the older adult's functional and physical factors that may lead to impaired driving ability. State driving regulations play a role in determining whether revocation is required, and the clinician should review state rules prior to revocation of a license. It is often recommended that a license be limited progressively over time as the functional status changes, so that the older adult maintains as much functional independence as possible (ASA, 2006). Safety of the person and the public are ultimately the primary determinants of permission to drive. The clinician plays a vital role in thoughtful driving outcomes for the older adult.

What standard guidelines will the clinician use to determine whether to recommend revocation of his driver's license?

The American Medical Association has developed an extensive tool kit for use by the primary care practitioner that helps to ensure a comprehensive review of an older adult's status related to driving. This is available at http://www.ama-assn.org/ama/pub/

physician-resources/public-health/promoting-healthy-lifestyles/geriatric-health/older-driver-safety/assessing-counseling-older-drivers.page. In addition, the American Society on Aging developed a tool kit for older adult drivers and their caregivers that can be very helpful in aiding in the determination of their next steps in driving. This is located at http://asaging.org/cdc/module4/home.cfm.

How will the clinician best manage an exacerbation of depression if the decision is made to revoke Mr. C's license?

As driving is an important factor in an older adult's ability to maintain independence, especially in rural settings, the revocation of a license needs to be viewed as a loss to the older adult. Careful monitoring for symptoms of depression is essential to ensure that the older adult's psychological health is maintained. In addition to depression screening, such as with the use of the geriatric depression scale, and treatment of depressive symptoms, the advanced practice nurse should frequently check in with the older adult and, with his permission, check in with family/friends to make certain that the established driving plan is working for the older adult and to offer additional community support services for transportation as needed.

What if the patient also had difficulty with his nutritional status?

If there is an indication of nutritional status deficiency, a referral for a home and nutritional assessment through a home health agency with occupational therapy and nursing may be helpful. Determination of whether the issue is a functional issue or an actual dietary or diabetes management issue would be helpful. Followup and action on recommendations would also be helpful to the older adult to aid in maintaining independence in the home for a longer period of time. Recommending temporary license adjustments would be appropriate since the older adult is still potentially unsafe in driving. The license can be returned back to its original status, if needed, upon resolution of dietary concerns and following another complete review of functional capacity for driving.

How do culture and ethnicity affect the plan of treatment?

Culture and ethnicity are key components in development of a transportation plan for an older adult. Older adults may not be familiar with public transportation options, may have cultural or ethnic beliefs about who is a caregiver or care provider, and may have strong values of independence and self-reliance. The clinician should ensure that there is a complete transportation plan that takes the patient's culture and ethnic beliefs and values into consideration to help maximize the potential for success of the transportation plan.

REFERENCES

American Geriatrics Society (2009). A Guide to Dementia Diagnosis and Treatment. Retrieved June 23, 2010, from http://dementia.americangeriatrics.org/

American Medical Association (2010). Physician's Guide to Assessing and Counseling Older Drivers. Retrieved June 4, 2010, from http://www.ama-assn.org/ama/pub/physician-resources/public-health/promoting-healthy-lifestyles/geriatric-health/older-driver-safety/assessing-counseling-older-drivers.shtml

American Society on Aging (2006). Road Map to Driving Safety. Retrieved June 4, 2010, from http://asaging.org/cdc/module4/home.cfm

ADDITIONAL RESOURCES

Burke, M., & Laramie, J. (2004). *Primary care of the older adult* (2nd ed.). St. Louis, MO: Mosby.

Duthie, E., Katz, P., & Malone, M. (2007). *Practice of geriatrics*. Philadelphia, PA: Elsevier.

National Highway Traffic Safety Association (2008). Resources for People around Older Drivers. Retrieved on June 7, 2010, from http://www.nhtsa.gov/Senior-Drivers

Reuben, D. (2009). *Geriatrics at your fingertips* (11th ed.). New York, NY: American Geriatrics Society.

Rosenthal, T., Williams, M., & Naughton, B. (2006). *Office care geriatrics*. Philadelphia, PA: Lippincott Williams and Wilkins.

The Hartford Financial Services Group, Inc. and MIT AgeLab (2007). Alzheimer's, Dementia, and Driving. Retrieved on June 4, 2010, from http://hartfordauto.thehartford.com/Safe-Driving/Car-Safety/Older-Driver-Safety/?KEY=AARP&PLCode=030313

Case 6.3 Sex Does Not Stop with Seniority

By Ashley Domingue, MSN, RN, ANP-BC, GNP-C

Mrs. B, a 73-year-old Caucasian female, presents to the primary care practice for her annual gynecological exam. Her gynecological history includes the onset of menses at age 15; 2 vaginal births (both daughters alive and well); the onset of menopause at age 52; no history of abnormal vaginal bleeding, spotting, discharge, pruritis, or dysmenorrhea; regular menstrual cycles approximately every 23 days; no current or previous use of birth control or hormone replacement therapy; and annual pap and pelvic exams until age 64. She reports that her last mammogram was 6 months ago and that her last colonoscopy was 2 years ago.

She performs monthly self–breast exams and has had 2 sexual partners during her lifetime. She denies any history of sexually transmitted infections (STIs) and no personal or family history of breast, gynecological, genitourinary, or colorectal cancer. She is currently sexually active with her husband of 51 years. She reports a recent increase in vaginal pain and discomfort, specifically itching and burning with urination and blood-tinged discharge after sexual intercourse over the last 3 weeks. Mrs. B notes an increase in frequency of urination and denies any changes in bowel patterns or stool consistency. Her last bowel movement was this morning.

Mrs. B has a history of hypertension (HTN). She has no surgical history and no hospitalizations other than 2 childbirths. She lives in a single-family home with her husband and feels safe at home. She is a retired elementary school teacher. Her 2 daughters live in the state; she sees them and her 4 grandchildren several times a month. Mrs. B goes

Case Studies in Gerontological Nursing for the Advanced Practice Nurse, First Edition.
Edited by Meredith Wallace Kazer, Leslie Neal-Boylan.
© 2012 John Wiley & Sons, Inc. Published 2012 by John Wiley & Sons, Inc.

for daily walks with her husband and sleeps approximately 8 hours each night. She denies any past or current use of tobacco or use of illicit drugs. She drinks a glass of red wine on most nights of the week with dinner and 2–3 cups of coffee daily. She denies any changes in mood, appetite, vision, or hearing. She denies any instances of dizziness, fatigue, fever, or headaches. Her medications include atenolol, 50 mg daily; Tylenol, as needed; calcium, 1000 mg daily; multivitamin; and vitamin D, 400 units daily. She denies other OTCs, herbals, vitamins, eye/ear drops, or inhalants. She is allergic to sulfa medications, which result in a rash. She denies allergies to food, latex, anesthesia, or seasonal.

OBJECTIVE

Mrs. B's vitals signs are as follows: height: 5 ft 4 inches; weight: 122 lb (9-lb loss since her last visit 6 months ago); BP: 150/70 (sitting), 154/66 (standing); P: 60; R: 18; T: 98.0. She is awake, alert, and oriented to person, place, and time. She appears well groomed, has an erect posture and clear and coherent speech, and maintains eye contact. Her head is normocephalic, with no lesions, lumps, or tenderness. Her face is symmetric, with no weakness or involuntary movements. Her visual fields are full; extraocular movements are intact; no nystagmus is noted. No ptosis, lid lag, discharge, or crusting are noted. Light reflex is symmetric and there is no strabismus. Her conjunctivae are clear, sclerae are white, and no lesions or redness are noted. Pupils are equal, round, and reactive to light and accommodation bilaterally (PERRLA). Her ears reveal no masses, lesions, scaling, discharge, or tenderness. The canals are clear, with minimal cerumen. Tympanic membranes (TMs) are pearly gray; landmarks are visible and intact, with no perforation. Nares are patent with pink mucosa and no lesions. The nasal septum is midline, with no perforation. There is no maxillary or frontal sinus tenderness with palpation. The oral mucosa and gingivae are pink, and no lesions or bleeding are noted. The neck is symmetric, with no masses, tenderness. Lymphadenopathy is noted. The trachea is midline, and the thyroid is nontender and nonpalpable.

Mrs. B's chest expansion is symmetric, and tactile fremitus is equal bilaterally. The lungs are clear to auscultation throughout. Normal S1 and S2 are auscultated with no murmurs, bruits or gallops. Her abdomen is rounded, soft, symmetric, and nondistended. Her skin is smooth, without lesions, scars, or striae. Bowel sounds are active in all 4 quadrants, no abnormal pulsations or bruits. Her breasts are symmetric, with no retractions or lesions. Her vulvae are without lesions. Vaginal walls are pale, pink, slightly rugated, with minimal discharge. Lubricant is required for insert of speculum; there is tenderness with insertion of a gloved finger. Watery, white, nonodorous discharge is seen near the cervix. The cervix is visible, clear, with no lesions, and positioned slightly to the left. The ovaries are nonpalpable and nontender.

ASSESSMENT

Atrophic vaginitis: Mrs. B's history of dyspareunia and vaginal dryness and the finding of pale, thin vaginal mucosa during her exam support this diagnosis. Atrophic vaginitis is a common cause of vaginal discharge and itching in postmenopausal females. The vaginal walls appear shiny and thin as a result of an inadequate amount of endogenous estrogen (Dains, Baumann & Scheibel, 2007).

Urinary tract infection (least concerning): Mrs. B's increase in frequency, itching, and burning with urination may be related to an infection of the genitourinary system. An elevated temperature is not always an indication of infection in older adults and still should be ruled out. Patients with UTIs can present asymptomatically (Dains, Baumann & Scheibel, 2007).

Endometrial cancer (most concerning): Mrs. B's vaginal bleeding, round abdomen (possibly due to an enlarged uterus), and 9-lb weight loss over the past 6 months can be considered red flags for cancer. Endometrial cancer is the most common female genital cancer in the United States and the average age of diagnosis is 61 years old. Possible risk factors include age greater than 40 years, weight greater than 200 lb, anovular cycles, nulliparity, infertility, tamoxifen use, and a family history of endometrial or colon cancer. Although Mrs. B's only potential risk factor is her age, cancer still should be included in the differential because she does present with possible symptoms (Telner & Jakubovicz, 2007). Earlier symptoms include painless vaginal bleeding and a rapidly enlarging endometrium, while weight loss and weakness are considered later symptoms (Dains, Baumann & Scheibel, 2007).

DIAGNOSTICS

Pelvic cultures, transvaginal ultrasound, complete blood count (CBC), urinalysis (dipstick and with microscopic examination), hemoglobin and hematocrit are ordered. Vaginal pH is 6.6. Wet mount reveals folded, clumped epithelial cells. Hematocrit and hemoglobin levels and CBC are within normal limits. Transvaginal ultrasound reveals an endometrial thickness less than 1.5 mm. A thickness of 5 mm is considered the cutoff point for a normal reading in postmenopausal women; anything greater is considered hyperplasia (Telner & Jakubovicz, 2007).

CRITICAL THINKING

What is the most likely differential diagnosis and why?

What is the plan of treatment?

What is the plan for follow-up care?

Does the patient's psychosocial history impact how the clinician might treat this patient?

Before giving this patient a diagnosis and treatment for vaginal atrophy, what other vaginal conditions should be ruled out?

Are there any best-practice guidelines that can be used to assess sexuality in older adults?

At what age should the clinician recommend that the female patient stop getting Pap smears?

RESOLUTION

What is the most likely differential diagnosis and why?

Atrophic vaginitis: Vaginal atrophy is a common, highly underdiagnosed condition in older women. An estimated 50% of postmenopausal women are affected, yet only 1%–5% seek treatment. It can have a negative impact on sexual health, urinary health, and overall well-being. Vaginal dryness is the number one complaint from sufferers (Moore, 2010).

What is the plan of treatment?
The goal of patient treatment will be symptom relief. Nonpharmacological options include regular sexual activity, lubricants for comfort, counseling regarding frequency of intercourse, and removal of genital irritants. Patient education should stress the importance of vaginal hygiene, which can be accomplished by avoiding heavily scented products, wearing loose fitting undergarments, cleansing with mild soap, and thoroughly drying the perineal area after swimming or showering. Nonhormonal vaginal lubricants and moisturizers are considered first-line for vaginal atrophy (Mehta & Bachmann, 2008).

What is the plan for follow-up care?

Symptoms should resolve within 30–60 days with first-line treatment. If symptoms do not subside, prescription therapy may be necessary. Although evidence is limited, low-dose local, prescription vaginal estrogen creams may be effective with minimal systemic absorption. In the United States, approved products are estradiol vaginal cream, estradiol vaginal ring, and estradiol hemihydrate vaginal tablet. If low-dose estrogen is being administered, progesten is seldom indicated. If symptoms still do not resolve, consider other causes, for instance, endometrial cancer, or refer the patient to a gynecological specialist (Mehta & Bachmann, 2008).

Does the patient's psychosocial history impact how the clinician might treat this patient?

This patient's experience with sexuality and her willingness to discuss her symptoms and their impact on her daily living need to be considered. The prevalence of sexual complaints among older men and women is high. However, few people seek assistance from a clinician and often attribute sexual troubles to normal aging or are embarrassed to discuss issues. Particularly for women, sexual function is often determined by the partner in the relationship. Exploring the patient's rapport with her husband and what she is looking for in terms of sexual satisfaction is very important in this case (Mehta & Bachmann, 2008).

Before giving this patient a diagnosis and treatment for vaginal atrophy, what other vaginal conditions should be ruled out?

Mrs. B's symptoms could be attributed to a variety of conditions. The possibility of infection, trauma, foreign body, inflammatory factors, and benign and malignant tumors should all be considered before initiating any nonpharmacological or pharmacological treatment (Mehta & Bachmann, 2008). In postmenopausal women, abnormal bleeding is considered to be any vaginal bleeding after 1 year of her last menstrual period, and it must be thoroughly evaluated (Telner & Jakubovicz, 2007).

Are there any best-practice guidelines that can be used to assess sexuality in older adults?

There are 5 recommendations that are available in geriatric nursing protocol for assessing sexuality in older adults. These include the following:

1. The PLISSIT model for talking about sexuality with patients recommends the following framework for addressing sexual issues(Annon, 1976): Seeking permission (P) to discuss sexuality with the older adult, sharing limited information (LI), providing specific suggestions (SS), and referring for intensive therapy (IT) when needed.

2. Ask open-ended questions. For example, "Can you tell me how your sexuality impacts your daily life?"
3. Explore normal physiological changes throughout the history, review of systems, and physical exam that may impact the patient's sexual function.
4. Review medications and specifically look for those that may impact sexual function such as antidepressants and antihypertensives.
5. Consider medical conditions that may be linked to poor sexual health and function. For instance, cardiac disease, stroke, Parkinson disease, diabetes, and BPH are all possible disorders that may have a negative influence on a patient's sexual well-being.

More details can be found at http://consultgerirn.org/topics/sexuality_issues_in_aging/want_to_know_more.

At what age should the clinician recommend that the female patient stop getting Pap smears?

Pap smears are used to routinely screen women for the presence of cervical cancer or abnormal cells that could progress to cancer. In the United States, cervical cancer screening guidelines are issued by 3 major groups: The U.S. Preventative Services Task Force (USPSTF), the American Cancer Society (ACS), and the American College of Obstetricians and Gynecologists (ACOG). It is mutually agreed that a woman should have her first Pap smear by age 21 or after her first sexual encounter. However, these 3 groups have differing recommendations for when Pap smears can safely be discontinued. The USPSTF advocates stopping Pap testing at age 65 and the ACS at age 70 if 3 consecutive tests within the past 10 years have been normal; and the ACOG encourages patients to discuss their individual "safe" age with their provider. It is important to realize that some women have a difficult time stopping because they consider having a normal Pap it to be a marker of good health. If the clinician decides that a patient no longer requires screening, pelvic exams can still be done to provide reassurance for the apprehensive patient and should be done to screen for vaginal cancers and ovarian masses (Robb-Nicholson, 2008).

REFERENCES

Annon, J. (1976). The PLISSIT model: A proposed conceptual scheme for behavioral treatment of sexual problems. *Journal of Sex Education Therapy*, 2(2), 1–15.

Dains, J. E., Baumann, L. C., & Scheibel, P. (2007). *Advanced health assessment and clinical diagnosis in primary care* (3rd ed.). Chicago: Mosby, Elsevier.

Mehta, A., & Bachmann, G. (2008). Vulvovaginal complaints. *Clinical Obstetrics & Gynecology, 51,* 549–555. Retrieved from Medline database.

Moore, A. A. (2010). Addressing Vaginal Atrophy With Your Patients: Modifying an Existing Therapeutic Approach—Part 1. MedScapeCME Ob/Gyn & Women's Health. Retrieved from http://cme.medscape.com/viewarticle/723563?src=cmemp&uac=133764SR

Robb-Nicholson, C. (2008). By the way, doctor. Is there an age when a woman no longer needs a Pap smear? *Harvard Women's Health Watch, 16,* 8. Retrieved from Medline database.

Telner, D. E., & Jakubovicz, D. (2007). Approach to diagnosis and management of abnormal uterine bleeding. *Canadian Family Physician, 53,* 58–64. Retrieved from Medline database.

ADDITIONAL RESOURCES

American Psychological Association. Aging and Human Sexuality Resource Guide. Retrieved from http://www.apa.org/pi/aging/resources/guides/sexuality.aspx

Hoffer, AP. Selected References on Sexuality and Aging. Retrieved from http://www.sexualityandaging.com/wp-content/uploads/2010/01/Hoffer_Selected-References-on-Sexuality-and-Aging-Rev-2010.pdf

Morley, J. E. Sexuality and Aging. Retrieved from http://media.wiley.com/product_data/excerpt/53/04700905/0470090553.pdf

The New England Journal of Medicine. A Study of Sexuality and Health among Older Adults in the United States. Retrieved from http://content.nejm.org/cgi/content/short/357/8/762

Case 6.4 Hidden Pathology

By Marie Boltz, PhD, APRN, BC

Ms. L, an 82-year-old female with Alzheimer disease (AD), presents to the emergency department (ED) with the chief complaint of change in mental status. The patient had been referred to the ED by a home care nurse who found the patient to be lethargic, with increased confusion, and incontinent of foul-smelling urine. These changes were reported to the nurse by the home care attendant who visits Ms. L 3 times a week to assist with showering. Ms. L resides with her son who is single and unemployed; her daughter lives out of state. Her son accompanies Ms. L to the ED and acts as respondent. He states that his mother has been more confused over the past 2 days and has not been eating well. He also reports that she has a history of hypertension, arthritis of the knees, and hypothyroidism, in addition to her Alzheimer disease. She sustained a fractured left hip 2 years ago, and her son states that she walks with a walker but has not left the house for the past 3 months. "She's deteriorating." According to the son, Ms. L has been receiving home care services for the past 2 months.

The primary care clinician was contacted by the ED physician, who confirmed the aforementioned diagnoses with the exception of dementia. The clinician reported that she had not seen evidence of cognitive impairment at the time of Ms. L's 2 prior examinations. She stated that Ms. L was alert and oriented when she last visited 3 weeks ago and was able to engage in her treatment decisions. The clinician further reported that she became involved with Ms. L's care upon referral from Ms. L's friend from church who was alarmed that Ms. L had become homebound. The friend had visited and then called the Area Agency

Case Studies in Gerontological Nursing for the Advanced Practice Nurse, First Edition.
Edited by Meredith Wallace Kazer, Leslie Neal-Boylan.
© 2012 John Wiley & Sons, Inc. Published 2012 by John Wiley & Sons, Inc.

on Aging to assist the son with help with caregiving. The clinician described some tension in the household at the time of her last visit. She described the son as "on edge", which she attributed to his unemployment status. Ms. L's medications include HCTZ, 25 mg daily, and Synthroid, 25 mcg daily. She has no known allergies (NKA).

OBJECTIVE

Ms. L is awake and oriented to person. She responds to questions with, "I don't know." She appears to drift off to sleep when undisturbed. She recoils when touched and avoids eye contact. She appears clean but is dressed in clothes not appropriate for the season. Ms. L's vital signs are height: 5 ft 3 inches; weight: 142 lb; BP: 164/92; P: 110; O_2 Sat: 98%; temp: 99.8. Her scalp has multiple raised, red, welt-like areas. She wears glasses; the frames are broken. Her oral mucosa is dry and pink; her lips are cracked; and her dentition is poor with several missing teeth. Her lungs are clear. Cardiac exam reveals a regular heart rate, S1, S2, and no adventitious sounds. She is tender to palpation over both sides of the anterior chest wall. Her abdomen is soft and nontender, with umbilicus midline; and bowel sounds are present in all 4 quadrants. Ecchymoses are visible on both deltopectoral triangles, both shoulders, her left pelvic rim, her right upper thigh, and the natal cleft. A well-healed scar is present over the left lateral thigh. No fractures are evident.

ASSESSMENT

Urinary Tract Infection (UTI): The presence of urinary symptoms (new incontinence and malodorous urine) and low-grade fever may indicate a urinary tract infection. The mental status changes also can represent atypical presentation of a UTI and may be related to insufficient oral intake.

Depression: Ms. L's mental status changes may be due to atypical presentation of depression. She has not been socially interactive (housebound for several months), and she avoids eye contact in the ED. This combined with the "I don't know" answers can indicate depression.

Delirium: Delirium or acute confusional state is a transient global disorder of cognition and may explain Ms. L's mental status changes. Delirium constitutes a medical emergency, as it is associated with increased morbidity and mortality rates. Prompt detection and treatment of the cause can reduce its risks (Inouye et al., 2008). A urinary tract infection is a common cause of delirium in older adults.

Suspected mistreatment: Elder mistreatment (abuse, neglect, exploitation, abandonment; Fulmer & O'Malley, 1987) is a commonly overlooked problem. Ms. L's risk factors for elder mistreatment include advanced age, social isolation, functional dependence, and a stressed caregiver who is financially dependent upon her (Laumann, Leitsch, Waite, 2008).

DIAGNOSTICS

If the older adult's responses indicate that there is potential for mistreatment, the older adult and caregiver should be questioned separately. Progressively focused questions should follow. An initial question might be, "Is there any difficult behavior in your family?" If the answer is yes, then the follow-up question might be, "Has anyone tried to hurt you?" Private interviews with the caregiver should focus on the needs of the older adult, as well as the caregiver's needs. The interviewer should be alert for signs of stress, isolation, or depression.

The Elder Assessment Instrument (EAI) is used to screen for elder mistreatment. This instrument is comprised of sections that review signs, symptoms, and subjective complaints of elder abuse (including bruising, lacerations, fractures, and evidence of sexual abuse); neglect (including pressure ulcers, depression, poor hygiene); exploitation; and abandonment. The tool is not scored. A patient should be referred to social services if one or more of the following exists:

1. there is evidence of mistreatment without sufficient clinical explanation,
2. there is a subjective complaint by the elder of elder mistreatment, or
3. the clinician believes there is a high risk for or probable abuse, neglect, exploitation, or abandonment.

Investigating and addressing emergent problems must be conducted while concomitantly evaluating for elder mistreatment. A urinalysis and urine culture and sensitivity (C&S) will determine the presence of a urinary tract infection. The Confusion Assessment Method (CAM; Inouye et al., 1990) will screen for and track the presence of delirium. A delirium workup, including a metabolic panel, complete blood count, nutritional parameters (serum albumin and prealbumin), B_{12} and folate level, and thyroid function are indicated. A referral to gero-psychiatry will help screen for depression.

In addition to the screening for mistreatment, Ms. L's urinalysis contains red blood cells, leukocytes, and many bacteria. The urine C&S is pending. The blood urea nitrogen (BUN) is high (48 mg/100 ml), and the TSH (thyroid stimulating hormone) level is high (5.5 mIU/L). Based on historical data provided by the clinician and the home care nurse, the CAM is remarkable for a delirium presentation (acute onset and fluctuating course of change in mental status, inattention, and altered level of consciousness). All other lab tests, including nutritional labs (serum albumin and prealbumin) are unremarkable.

There are several red flags that should raise suspicions of elder mistreatment of Ms. L, including:

1. Ms. L's social isolation, her physical withdrawal when touched, and her avoidance of eye contact can indicate exposure to mistreatment.
2. The appearance of welts on her scalp and multiple bruises are signs of potential physical abuse.
3. Other potential signs of mistreatment include broken eyeglasses, poor dentition, use of unseasonal clothing, and signs of insufficient oral intake.
4. Ms. L's son's behavior is suspicious. When she became homebound, (with no apparent indication), the son did not seek outside assistance. His characterization of her "dementia" (contradicted by the clinician) may be an attempt to exploit her and/or diminish her psychologically.

The EAI is remarkable for the following:

1. General appearance: Unseasonal clothing and poor dentition.
2. Evidence of signs of potential abuse: Bruising (ecchymoses and other various stages of healing bruises) as well as the statement by Ms. L, "I don't know why he hurts me."
3. Neglect indicators: Evidence of dehydration, potential depression, and evidence of failure to respond to the warning of obvious disease (homebound status).

CRITICAL THINKING

What is the most likely differential diagnosis and why?

What is the plan of treatment?

What is the plan for follow-up care?

Does the patient's psychosocial history impact how the clinician might treat this patient?

Are there any standardized guidelines that the clinician should use to assess or treat this case?

RESOLUTION

What is the most likely differential diagnosis and why?
Ms. L demonstrates evidence of elder mistreatment, specifically physical abuse and neglect. A UTI is an additional obvious differential diagnosis, given Ms. L's symptoms. The urinalysis confirms the diagnosis, and the culture and sensitivity testing of the urine sample will indicate the appropriate antibiotic to treat the UTI. There is evidence of delirium, likely secondary to the UTI, dehydration, undertreated hypothyroidism, and the injuries related to potential physical abuse. Given her clinical presentation and history, further evaluation of potential depression is warranted.

What is the plan of treatment?
Priorities of treatment include stabilizing Ms. L medically, promoting safety and comfort, and preventing further injury. Ms. L's daughter is contacted and apprised of her condition.

Treating the UTI with antibiotic therapy and hydrating her with intravenous therapy are immediate interventions. Additionally, Ms. L is assessed for sexual abuse and other physical mistreatment; that examination is negative. The social worker will contact Adult Protective Services (and/or another agency as mandated per state regulations), who will interview the son and conduct a full investigation related to the apparent mistreatment. Ms. L will also be interviewed when her mentation improves. The clinician should be careful to make sure this is done privately, without her son present. She will be checked frequently and provided with comfort, including emotional support and pain assessment and management. The CAM will be used to track her delirium status.

What is the plan for follow-up care?
Further evaluation and treatment of possible depression is indicated, through a consultation with gero-psychiatry. The primary care clinician will work with a psychiatric clinician to assess the decisional capacity of Ms. L. If she lacks decision-making capacity, issues of financial management, conservatorship, guardianship, and/or protective court orders will be discussed with Adult Protective Services. Ms. L will require new glasses and rehabilitation therapy to restore functional mobility and continence. The social worker will contact Ms. L's daughter and church to ascertain the possibility of additional social support. Discharge options will also be examined.

Does the patient's psychosocial history impact how the clinician might treat this patient?
The apparent mistreatment of the patient has implications for her ongoing care. Ms. L is at risk for depression, functional decline, and

related complications. Ongoing surveillance of risk factors and timely interventions to prevent and address complications are essential components of the plan of care.

Are there any standardized guidelines that the clinician should use to assess or treat this case?

To report suspected abuse in the community, contact the local adult protective services agency. For state reporting numbers, visit the NCEA Web site at www.ncea.aoa.gov or call the Eldercare Locator at 1-800-677-1116. Of course, if someone is in immediate danger, call 911 or the local police for immediate help.

The American Medical Association publishes "Guidelines for Doctors on Detecting Elder Abuse and Neglect" available at: http://findarticles.com/p/articles/mi_m1000/is_n367/ai_18200024/pg_2/?tag=content;col1

REFERENCES

Fulmer, T., & O'Malley, T. (1987). *Inadequate care of the elderly: A health care perspective on abuse and neglect.* New York: Springer Publishing Company.

Inouye, S., van Dyck, C., Alessi, C., Balkin, S., Siegal, A., & Horwitz, R. (1990). Clarifying confusion: The confusion assessment method. *Annals of Internal Medicine, 113*(12), 941–948.

Inouye, S. K., Zhang, Y., Jones, R. N., Shi, P., Cupples, L. A., Calderon, H. N., & Marcantonio, E. R. (2008). Risk factors for hospitalization among community-dwelling primary care older patients: Development and validation of a predictive model. *Medical Care, 46,* 726–731.

Laumann, E. O., Leitsch, S. A., & Waite, I. J. (2008). Elder mistreatment in the United States: Prevalence estimates from a nationally representative study. *Journal of Gerontology, B 63*(4), S248–S254.

ADDITIONAL RESOURCES

Baker, M. W., & Heitkemper, M. M. (2005). The roles of nurses on interprofessional teams to combat elder mistreatment. *Nursing Outlook, 53*(5), 253–259.

Donohue, W. A., Dibble, J. L., & Schiamberg, L. B. (2008). A social capital approach to the prevention of elder mistreatment. *Journal of Elder Abuse & Neglect, 20*(1), 1–23.

Elder Assessment Instrument. Retrieved at http://consultgerirn.org/uploads/File/trythis/try_this_15.pdf

Fulmer, T., Paveza, G., Abraham, I., & Fairchild, S. (2000). Elder neglect assessment in the emergency department. *Journal of Emergency Nursing, 26*(5), 436–443.

Fulmer, T., Paveza, G., VandeWeerd, C., Fairchild, S., Guadagno, L., Bolton-Blatt, M., … Norman, R. (2005). Dyadic vulnerability and risk profiling for elder neglect. *Gerontologist*, *45*(4), 525–534.

Heath, J. M., Kobylarz, F. A., Brown, M., & Castano, S. (2005). Interventions from home-based geriatric assessments of adult protective service clients suffering elder mistreatment. *Journal of the American Geriatrics Society*, *53*(9), 1538–1542.

Mosqueda, L., Burnight, K., Liao, S., & Kemp, B. (2004). Advancing the field of elder mistreatment: A new model for integration of social and medical services. *Gerontologist*, *44*(5), 703–708.

National Center on Elder Abuse Web site: http://www.ncea.aoa.gov/ncea-root/Main_Site/index.aspx

The National Criminal Justice Reference Service Web site: http://www.ncjrs.gov/App/Search/SearchResults.aspx?txtKeywordSearch=elder+abuse&fromSearch=1

Case 6.5 Taking Control of the Pain

By Alison Kris, PhD, RN

Mr. S is a 79-year-old man with Type 2 diabetes and chronic obstructive pulmonary disease (COPD). He has a history of a wound on his left heel that would not heal for more than 2 years. The wound began to worsen and became infected with methicillin-resistant *staphylococcus aureus* (MRSA). The decision was made to amputate below the knee of his left leg, and he is admitted to a long-term care unit because of this amputation. On day 3, Mr. S developed a pressure ulcer on his left buttock. It progressed from stage I through stage IV and is approximately 7 cm round. He has a history of obesity, hyperlipidemia, and hypertension. In addition to his aforementioned diagnosis, Mr. S has a long smoking history, beginning at age 16 and continuing until approximately 8 years ago. Prior to admission he lived at home with his wife, who is blind and therefore cannot drive. They have a daughter who lives 350 miles away, who has been visiting since admission. She will need to leave at the end of the week, when he is expected to be discharged back home. He has both Medicare and private insurance, which will pay for 7 days of subacute rehabilitation.

Mr. S is on oxygen, 2 L via nasal canula, to help manage his shortness of breath. He gets short of breath upon exertion and has been unable to participate in physical therapy. He denies any gastrointestinal or genitourinary difficulties. He has not been eating well since admission to the nursing home. Although the daughter states that she believes her father has lost weight, there has been some difficulty getting an accurate weight since admission. She explains that her father is in severe pain and she feels that the pain has caused him to

Case Studies in Gerontological Nursing for the Advanced Practice Nurse, First Edition.
Edited by Meredith Wallace Kazer, Leslie Neal-Boylan.
© 2012 John Wiley & Sons, Inc. Published 2012 by John Wiley & Sons, Inc.

withdraw, to eat less, and to resist participation in physical therapy. His medications include Combivent (ipratropium bromide, 18 mcg; albuterol 103 mcg) via nebulizer 3 times daily; simvastatin, 40 mg by mouth daily; metformin, 850 mg by mouth twice daily; regular insulin, per sliding scale; oxygen 2 L via nasal canula; captopril, 50 mg twice daily; acetaminophen, 650 mg, 2 tablets every 6 hours as needed; wet to moist dressing changes, daily. He has no known allergies (NKA).

OBJECTIVE

Mr. S is sleeping upright in bed. He is oriented to person, time, and place. Per his chart, he is 5 ft 10 inches and weighs 258 lb. This morning his blood pressure was 180/95 before medication. Following administration of his morning medications, his blood pressure has fallen to 135/80. Fasting blood sugar this morning is 212. His HEENT are unremarkable. He has poor peripheral circulation, and the pedal pulse in his right foot is not palpable. His right foot is cool to the touch with prolonged capillary refill. His lungs are clear with expiratory wheezes. He is slightly tachypneic with a respiratory rate of 28. His abdomen is soft, nontender and nondistended. He is learning to ambulate with a new prosthesis and walker following his amputation; however, he has not been able to participate in physical therapy since admission. He has a 7-cm, round stage IV pressure ulcer on his left buttock. The borders are clean, and there is no drainage. This pressure ulcer causes him extreme pain, 10/10. The surgical incision at the site of his amputation shows no swelling or erythema.

ASSESSMENT

Pressure ulcer: Mr. S has a large, stage IV pressure ulcer on his left buttock. In a patient with significant comorbidities (COPD, obesity) such an ulcer is a significant, serious diagnosis that can easily lead to **death** within 6 months.

Depression: Mr. S's daughter states that her father has lost weight, is withdrawn and has not been participating in physical therapy. Because there is a high concordance of depression with chronic pain, Mr. S should have his depression further evaluated.

Pain: Mr. S states that his pain is 10/10. A review of current pain management strategies and exacerbating factors (i.e., dressing changes) is a priority.

DIAGNOSTICS

Evaluation of the adequacy of the current pain management regimen would include a review of recent pain assessments by nursing staff, discussion of the adequacy of pain management strategies with the patient and/or the patient's family and a specific evaluation of the adequacy of pain management during dressing changes. If this patient was able to attend physical therapy, a consultation with the physical therapists about adequacy of pain management during therapy may be warranted. However, it should be noted that the best and most reliable indicator of the level of pain is the patient's own self-report. Mr. S states that his pressure ulcer causes him severe pain that he rates as a 10 on a 1–10 scale (10/10).

An evaluation of the current pain management regimen demonstrates that the patient currently is receiving acetaminophen , 650 mg, 2 tablets every 6 hours as needed. While it is clear that this level of pain management is inadequate, it is important to consider how much medication is necessary and how to approach pain in this situation. Figure 6.5.1 contains World Health Organization's guidelines to be considered.

CRITICAL THINKING

What factors contributed to the development of a pressure ulcer in this case?

What type of pain management protocol would the clinician recommend and why?

What is the plan for followup? What would lead the clinician to believe the protocol was adequate or inadequate?

What other factors might contribute to the adequacy of pain management? Is adjuvant medication necessary?

RESOLUTION

What factors contributed to the development of a pressure ulcer in this case?
There are several factors that contributed to the development of a pressure ulcer in this situation.

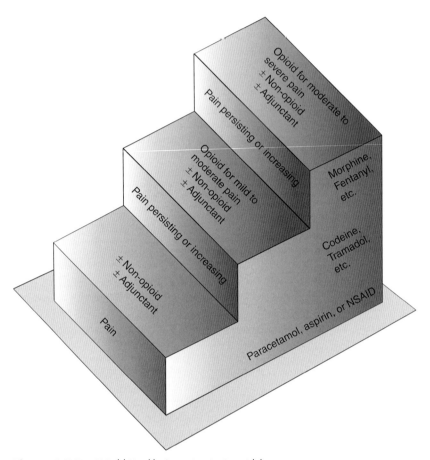

Figure 6.5.1. World Health Organization's guidelines.

1. **Cardiopulmonary factors.** This patient has poor circulation to his extremities and likely has poor perfusion throughout his integument, which will increase his risk for pressure ulcer. In addition to poor perfusion, the blood is poorly oxygenated secondary to the effects of COPD. The poor perfusion with poorly oxygenated blood again increases the risk of breakdown.

2. **Mobility factors.** In addition, there are factors that impair mobility—both the COPD, which creates dyspnea upon exertion (DOE), and the new below-the-knee amputation (BKA). Impairments in mobility increase pressure ulcer risk. Often patients with COPD prefer to sit upright for much of the day, creating increased risk of pressure ulcer development in the buttocks and sacrum. In addition, this patient is obese, creating increased pressure on the area.

3. **Nutritional status.** The patient's daughter comments that he has lost weight. While Mr. S is obese, nutritional balance is important to maintaining skin integrity. If the patient is losing weight at the expense of balanced nutrition, this could both contribute to skin breakdown and impair wound healing.

What type of pain management protocol would the clinician recommend and why?
In addition to the WHO guidelines, several other factors are important for consideration.

1. The maxim for older adults is to "start low and go slow".
2. It is important to consider any history that a patient may have had in using opiate analgesics in the past, as tolerance can develop.
3. Alterations in kidney and liver function can slow elimination of analgesics, so checking the most recent labs is important.
4. Consider the environment in which the pain management is being delivered. In situations where frequent assessments are not available, around-the-clock (ATC) medication may be more reliable than as-needed dosing. Research has demonstrated that less than 20% of as-needed pain medications prescribed are actually given to nursing home residents. Therefore, as-needed prescriptions written without followup may be of little value (Kayser-Jones, Kris, Miaskowski, Lyons, Paul, 2006).
5. Finally, any patient, particularly people over age 65, should be started on bowel regimens concurrent with the start of opiate regimens. Nutritional interventions, such as the addition of high fiber foods, together with fluids are important. Commonly, a stool softener such as docusate sodium (DSS), 100 mg by mouth daily or 250 mg by mouth daily, is added. The patient should be frequently assessed to determine the adequacy of the bowel management program.

A stage IV pressure ulcer requires both basal (ATC) pain medication as well as bolus pain medication for dressing changes. Extended release morphine can provide basal pain relief for 12 hours. Analgesic patch medication would be another option to provide stable opiate dosing over an extended period of time. Finally, additional medication (bolus dosage) should be provided at least 30 minutes prior to scheduled dressing changes. Nursing staff should be instructed about the importance of giving the pain medication prior to each dressing change.

What is the plan for followup? What would lead the clinician to believe the protocol was adequate or inadequate?
Followup should include review of the patient's chart to ensure that pain medications are being given as recommended. In addition, discussion with the patient should find that pain levels (currently 10/10) are significantly reduced. While 0/10 may not be realistic, pain should be manageable even during dressing changes. In addition, gastrointestinal

impact should be evaluated; and an abdominal assessment should be completed to check for distention and adequacy of bowel sounds.

What other factors might contribute to the adequacy of pain management? Is adjuvant medication necessary?

It is important to consider the close relationship between pain, anxiety, and shortness of breath (Kris & Dodd, 2004). The presence of these symptoms together can exacerbate distress from each symptom. Management of both shortness of breath and the anxiety that often results from shortness of breath will also be critical to ensuring adequate pain management. Better management of the patient's shortness of breath will impact the patient's ability to move comfortably, which is critical to wound healing. Adjuvant anxiety medication (e.g., lorazepam) may be considered if anxiety is associated with shortness of breath. In addition, the patient appears depressed as it was reported that he was sleeping during the day, not eating well, and not participating in physical therapy. Further evaluation of his psychological state may be warranted if his symptoms do not resolve with adequate treatment for his pain.

REFERENCES

Kayser-Jones, J., Kris, A., Miaskowski, C., Lyons, W., & Paul, S. (2006). Hospice care in nursing homes: Does it contribute to higher quality pain management? *The Gerontologist*, *46*(3), 325–333.

Kris, A., & Dodd, M. J. (2004). Symptom experience of adult hospitalized medical-surgical patients. *Journal of Pain and Symptom Management*, *28*(5), 451–459.

Case 6.6 The Road toward End-of-Life Decision Making: Who Has the Right of Way?

By Barbara L. Kramer, MSN, RN, CHPN, and
Christine M. Goldstein, LCSW-R, OCW-C

Ms. C is a 72-year-old African American and Native American woman who presents to the emergency department with complaints of fever, abdominal pain, bloating, and distention. She lives alone in a suburban 1-bedroom apartment. A college-educated professional, she is now retired due to her medical problems. Her medical history is significant for transient ischemic attack, anemia, gastroesophageal reflux disease, and metastatic vaginal cancer for which she received aggressive treatment for 5 years. This treatment included a course of pelvic radiation, multiple courses of chemotherapy, and surgical interventions, including total abdominal hysterectomy, bilateral salpingo-oophorectomy, and colon resection with colostomy.

Prior to seeking emergency attention for her current symptoms, Ms. C was receiving home hospice services. These services were terminated upon entry to the emergency department for evaluation and treatment. A complete medical workup was performed and included complete blood work, urinalysis with culture and sensitivity, abdominal and pelvic CT scans, and renal sonogram. The results revealed a massive distended urinary bladder, left hydroureter and nephrosis, a fungating mass in the rectum, and multiple pelvic masses. A supportive treatment plan was developed, and she was treated for a urinary tract infection and underwent insertion of a suprapubic tube (SPT) under fluoroscopic guidance. Additionally, Ms. C received physical therapy, nutritional counseling, and evaluation by the wound ostomy continence nurse (WOCN).

Case Studies in Gerontological Nursing for the Advanced Practice Nurse, First Edition.
Edited by Meredith Wallace Kazer, Leslie Neal-Boylan.
© 2012 John Wiley & Sons, Inc. Published 2012 by John Wiley & Sons, Inc.

The care manager worked with the patient throughout the hospital stay to formulate plans for her discharge needs. Ms. C was the eighth of 10 children, 9 of whom are living. She has 2 sisters who live within 75 miles of her home, and she has 1 daughter and grandchildren who reside in Georgia. In order to address her increasing care needs, her 2 sisters have arranged to stay with her in her apartment on a rotating basis, 1 week at a time. Her caregivers will require education in her care, including the care and management of her colostomy, suprapubic tube, and medication and symptom management. Ms. C was quite adamant that she no longer wishes to receive hospice services, and she has rescinded her do not resuscitate (DNR) order. Ms. C wishes to pursue aggressive cancer treatment. Receptive to home care services, she is referred for home care evaluation. The initial evaluation was completed and a plan of care developed to include the services of a registered nurse, home health aide, social worker, and physical therapist. Her care was guided by the palliative care (PC) team.

Ms. C's medications include fentanyl transdermal patch, 125 mcg/hour every 72 hours; oxycodone, 15–30 mg by mouth every 4 hours as needed for breakthrough pain; minocycline, 100 mg by mouth every 12 hours; docusate sodium, 100 mg by mouth twice daily; senna, 2 tabs by mouth at bedtime; ondansetron HCl, 4 mg by mouth every 4 hours as needed for nausea; omeprazole, 20 mg by mouth daily. She is allergic to morphine, penicillin, and latex.

OBJECTIVE

Ms. C presents to the primary care team at the weekly interdisciplinary case conference. Her clinician expressed that Ms. C was unrealistic about her prognosis, evidenced by her pursuit of continued cancer treatment and her decision to pursue aggressive resuscitative efforts. The clinician also shared that she was increasingly uncomfortable with the patient's wishes and was fearful that she may not be able to honor those wishes should she be called upon to initiate cardiopulmonary resuscitation (CPR). Following a discussion by the PC team, it is decided that the nursing team leader would make a visit. Upon evaluation, Ms. C presents lying flat in bed and appears pale, cachexic, and in no apparent distress. She is appropriately groomed and is wearing a nightgown. She is soft-spoken, articulate, and alert and oriented, although she admits to sleeping much of the day and "feeling down". She is 5 ft 8 inches and weighs 100 lb. Her vital signs are BP: 100/62; AP: 78, regular; RR:16; T: 98.2. Using the numeric rating scale, she rates her pain at 0/10 and appears comfortable at rest. However, when positioned for physical assessment and ambulated, she appears distressed and rates her pain at 8/10. Her pain is described as burning, sharp, and stabbing. She refuses the use of her breakthrough pain medication, stating that her current pain level is acceptable as long as she lies still and avoids the sitting position. Her colostomy is functioning every 2–3 days, and bowel movements are painful. Her stool is gray and hard. Her stoma is pale and irregular in shape, with peristomal protrusion attributed to tumor growth. Ms. C states that her colostomy appliance is causing her discomfort and is becoming more difficult to change. Her SPT is draining cloudy yellow urine; 500 cc is present in drainage bag. She requires biweekly irrigations to maintain patency. She has been advised that this tube will never be removed, as placement of a new catheter would be impossible due to her extensive tumor involvement. Her gait is slow and steady, and she uses a rolling walker to assist with ambulation. Upon physical examination of her perineum, she has a fungating tumor protruding from her rectum, tumor erosion in her vaginal area and bilateral groins, with open ulcerations, and a 10–15 cm deep cavity in her vaginal area. There is a large amount of foul-smelling drainage.

Following physical examination, a discussion was initiated to elicit her understanding of her disease, her goals of treatment, and her beliefs about end-of-life care. Ms. C demonstrates a clear understanding about her cancer, acknowledging that she is in the terminal phase of illness. However, she expresses that she never wants to eliminate the possibility of treatment that may help her to live longer or more comfortably. She understands that cure is not possible. She understands what resuscitation means but feels that "do not resuscitate" often means "do not treat" and cites that under hospice care she was discouraged from seeking emergency treatment for her abdominal discomfort. She feels that the placement of the SPT was necessary and has enabled her to live longer and more comfortably. She also verbalizes that she feels that treatment decisions are often made based on a person's worth—that an elderly, black female may not necessarily receive the same treatment options as "younger, white, male executive type who has more to contribute to society". Ms. C verifies that she plans to pursue continued aggressive cancer treatment, but she admits that 2 oncologists have discharged her from their services, expressing that further treatment would be futile. She reaffirms that she has rescinded her DNR order and has destroyed the prior directive. Additionally, she has revised her current health care proxy document and named an agent who would support her wishes.

ASSESSMENT

Pain and odor management: Ms C's abdominal pain is controlled to her satisfaction with the current analgesic regimen. However, her vaginal pain and buttocks pain increase with position changes and sitting, hindering her mobility and ability to participate in activities of daily living (ADL). Resistant to increasing her analgesic doses due to excessive sedation and constipation, she is agreeable to alternative nonopioid medications and local treatments if available.

Colostomy management: Due to tumor growth and a changing abdominal landscape and stoma dimensions, the current colostomy appliance is no longer effective, resulting in leakage and discomfort.

Conflicts in the patient's and the clinician's goals of care and ethical beliefs: Ms. C's expressed desire to pursue active treatment and aggressive resuscitation procedures is in conflict with the clinician's professional desire to provide compassionate care, relieve pain, minimize suffering, and maximize quality of life. The pursuit of futile treatment and aggressive life-sustaining procedures would likely result in increased pain and suffering and prolong death.

CRITICAL THINKING

What interventions might be applied to minimize pain and symptom burdens?

What is the plan of treatment?

Does the patient's psychosocial history impact how the clinician might treat this patient? What referrals are needed?

How can care be provided that will satisfy the ethical beliefs of both the patient and the professional staff?

A question of autonomy: Does Ms. C have the right to pursue aggressive futile treatments and refuse DNR status?

Is DNR a futile treatment in Ms. C's case?

How do we resolve the conflict between professional integrity and honoring a patient's wishes?

RESOLUTION

What interventions might be applied to minimize pain and symptom burdens?
Pain control and odor management are ongoing issues that adversely affect Ms. C physically, emotionally, and spiritually. Her persistent pain during position changes, ambulation, and sitting has resulted in the

need to remain lying flat in bed most of the day and night. This places her at risk for developing complications of immobility, including pressure ulcers, deep vein thrombosis, pneumonia, and constipation. Pain and persistent odor from tumor drainage have prevented Ms. C from participating in enjoyable social activities, making her essentially bedbound. Improved pain control and odor management would assist in maximizing quality of life.

Tumor growth has led to colostomy appliance failure and increased discomfort. This has caused leakage, placing Ms. C at risk for skin breakdown. Reevaluation of the abdominal landscape and stoma dimensions is necessary to obtain a colostomy appliance that will contain the leakage and maximize comfort.

What is the plan of treatment?
Due to the symptom burden of increased somnolence and constipation that would result from an increase in opioid therapy, alternative pain management options are explored. Pain described as sharp and stabbing suggests a neuropathic component. Use of adjuvant pain medications is explored, and gabapentin therapy is initiated at 100 mg twice daily and titrated upward to effect. An antidepressant is added to assist with the pain and mood disturbance (American Pain Society, 2008). Additionally, local treatment is initiated using a 1:1 mixture of lidocaine HCL external gel 2% and metronidazole external gel 0.75% is applied to the vaginal and rectal tumors twice daily, providing local analgesia and improved odor management.

A referral is made to the WOCN for evaluation and recommendations. A joint home care visit is performed with the palliative care team leader. A complete assessment is performed and includes full assessment of skin, abdominal characteristics, stoma, and colostomy appliance. Support surfaces and durable medical equipment in the home are also evaluated. Recommendations include a change in size and type of colostomy appliance to contain drainage and promote increased patient comfort and the addition of a support surface to the hospital bed for pressure relief and increased comfort. To promote improved comfort and reduced odor in the perineal area, a regimen is instituted using gentle warm-water irrigations and/or sitz baths as tolerated, along with the application of barrier cream to protect the skin from drainage. A topical antibiotic therapy was recommended to reduce the bioburden of fungating tumors and thus reduce drainage and odor.

Does the patient's psychosocial history impact how the clinician might treat this patient?
In exploring Ms. C's understanding of the extent of her disease, her prognosis, her desire for further treatment, and her wishes for full resuscitative efforts, she made some interesting comments that suggest that previous life experiences are influencing her current attitudes that are propelling her to seek aggressive treatments. References to racism,

ageism, social worth, and access to care are themes that emerged. Explorations of Ms. C's cultural background, history, and experiences would likely provide insight and understanding of her continued pursuit of futile treatment and aggressive resuscitative measures. Referral to social work and an agency chaplain are made to further explore these issues and provide emotional and spiritual support.

How can care be provided that will satisfy the ethical beliefs of both the patient and the professional staff?

In order to provide care that satisfies the goals and ethical beliefs of both the patient and the professional caregiver, there must be a full understanding of the motivation of all parties and the belief system that drives the decisions. It is easy to draw rapid conclusions, apply labels, and dismiss patient behavior that differs from that of the health care professional. Conversely, it is easy for the patient to assume that health care will be provided in the same way and with the same perceived inequities that she has experienced in the past.

In this case, the patient was quickly labeled as being in denial, not fully understanding the extent of her disease and her terminal prognosis. However, it became clear that this was not the case, that she was very knowledgeable, and that she understood the terminal nature of her illness. It has been well documented that inequities exist in access and delivery of health care to minority populations (Crawley, 2005; Freeman & Payne, 2000; Smedley, Stith, Nelson, 2003). Within this context, Ms. C's motivation became clearer to the professional staff. This, in turn, fostered an atmosphere of mutual understanding and trust. However, her goals and wishes continued to be at odds with those of some of the nursing staff. Ms. C's desire for aggressive resuscitation was incongruent with the clinician's vows to act in her best interest and do no harm. In order to resolve this conflict, a change in primary assignment was suggested and agreed to by all parties. In doing this, the patient's wishes were honored, and the clinician's beliefs about her professional obligations were respected.

A question of autonomy: Does Ms. C have the right to pursue aggressive futile treatments and refuse DNR status?

Over the last few decades, respect for autonomy has eclipsed other ethical principles (Tomlinson, Micholski, Pentz, Kuuppelomaki, 2001). Choices of individuals must be respected, and patients have well-established rights to determine the goals of their medical care and to accept or refuse any recommended medical intervention (Cantor, Braddock, Derse, et al, 2003). Due to the advanced nature of her illness, successful cardiopulmonary resuscitation would be unlikely and would more likely cause additional pain and suffering. Though the values of the patient and professional staff differ, the justification regarding resuscitation is not purely a matter of medical expertise and requires that the decision be made based on the values of the patient (Mappes

& Degrazia, 2006). Assessment of her quality of life requires a comprehensive examination of her views and values. Allowing patients to define goals, even when dying, is part of the process of improving quality of life (Bass, 2006). However, while patients have well-established rights to determine the goals of their medical care, it can be said that the rights of autonomy are negative rights. They include the right to refuse treatment or choose among treatment options. There is no right to demand whatever intervention a patient might choose, as this would make it impossible for health professionals to practice with integrity (Tomlinson et al., 2001). Offering ineffective treatments deviates from sound clinical judgment and professional standards. Forcing staff to inflict harmful procedures on patients makes them "agents of harm, not benefit" (Cantor et al, 2003). Ms. C may wrongly imagine that resuscitation would be beneficial, but this imagined benefit does not afford her a right to receive treatment.

Is DNR a futile treatment in Ms. C's case?

The basis of any futility dispute is a disagreement between the parties about what constitutes appropriate care. These disputes are fundamental disagreements about quality of life, its meaning, and decision-making authority and are often products of miscommunications (Fins, 2006). In Ms. C's case, the initial miscommunication occurred between her and the hospice staff. As Ms. C's disease advanced, she was provided with increased medication for pain control. However, she wanted to find the source of the pain and explore options for treating the cause of her pain and not just the symptom. In order to pursue her goal, she disenrolled in hospice care and sought care through the emergency department. Ms. C successfully found relief with the insertion of the SPT. This experience supported her belief that the medical community (i.e., hospice) did not necessarily have her best interests in mind, and this left her with a feeling of distrust. Establishing a therapeutic relationship with the patient within this atmosphere of distrust proved to be challenging.

How do we resolve the conflict between professional integrity and honoring a patient's wishes?

The principle of beneficence dictates that medical professionals caring for a patient are obliged to act in the best interest of that patient by evaluating the benefits and burdens of treatment (Bass, 2006). Basic to the conflict in this case is not only the question of whether CPR would provide a benefit to the patient, but whether CPR would be harmful. The principle of nonmaleficence dictates that medical professionals have a duty to redirect the efforts from lifesaving treatments that are no longer beneficial and will cause harm toward treatments that maximize the comfort and dignity of the patient (Schneiderman, 2008). The most clearly articulated description of this ethic of care can be found in the nursing literature where it is defined as a commitment to protecting and enhancing the patient's dignity (Schneiderman, 2008). Ms. C's unwillingness to pursue a DNR reflects a myriad of concerns that can be addressed through ongoing conversation. Her beliefs and values must be elicited using open-ended questions with the goal of learning her perspectives on illness, her expectations for care, and her wishes regarding end of life.

Building an environment of trust and cultural sensitivity with Ms. C can lead to mutual understanding and promote shared decision making. Professional integrity is maintained as there is a focus on the ethical duty to redirect efforts from the prolongation of life to comfort care (Schneiderman, 2008). Comfort care is not limited to physiological comfort, but also psychological comfort. Ms. C must be seen as a unique individual who will not be abandoned, but who will be treated with dignity, compassion, and respect.

REFERENCES

American Pain Society (2008). *Principles of analgesic use in the treatment of acute pain and cancer pain* (6th ed.). Glenview, IL: American Pain Society.

Bass, M. (2006). *Palliative care resuscitation*. Chichester: John Wiley.

Cantor, M. D., Braddock, C. H., Derse, A. R., Edwards, D. M., Logue, G. L., Nelson, W., Prudhomme, A. M., … Fox, E. for the Veterans Health Administration National Ethics Committee. (2003). Do-not-resuscitate orders and medical futility. *Arch Intern Med, 163*, 2689–2694.

Crawley, L. M. (2005). Racial, cultural, and ethnic factors influencing end-of-life care. *Journal of Palliative Medicine, 8*(Suppl. 1), S58–S69.

Fins, J. J. (2006). *A palliative ethic of care.* Sudbury, MA: Jones & Bartlett.

Freeman, H. P., & Payne, R. (2000). Racial injustice in health care. *New England Journal of Medicine, 342*(14), 1045–1047.

Mappes, T. A., & Degrazia, D. (2006). *Biomedical ethics* (6th ed.). New York: McGraw-Hill.

Schneiderman, L. J. (2008). *Embracing our mortality*. New York: Oxford.

Smedley, B. D., Stith, A. Y., & Nelson, A. R. (Eds.). (2003). Unequal Treatment: Understanding Racial and Ethnic Disparities in Health Care. Retrieved June 10, 2010, from http://www.nap.edu/catalog/10260.html

Tomlinson, T., Micholski, A. J., Pentz, R. D., & Kuuppelomaki, M. (2001). Futile care in oncology: When to stop trying. *The Lancet Oncology, 2*(12), 759–764.

Index

Case Studies in Gerontological Nursing for the Advanced Practice Nurse, First Edition. Edited by
Meredith Wallace Kazer, Leslie Neal-Boylan.
© 2012 John Wiley & Sons, Inc. Published 2012 by John Wiley & Sons, Inc.